Echo[...]
for th[...]
Neonatologist

For Churchill Livingstone

Commissioning Editors: Maria Khan/Deborah Russell
Project Managers: Carol Parr/Joanne Scott
Production Manager: Mark Sanderson

Echocardiography for the Neonatologist

EDITED BY

Jonathan Skinner
MBChB, DCH, MRCP(UK), FRCPCH, MD
Department of Paediatric Cardiology, Green Lane Hospital,
Auckland, New Zealand

Dale Alverson
MD
School of Medicine, University of New Mexico Health Sciences Center,
Albuquerque, New Mexico, USA

Stewart Hunter
MBChB, FRCP(Ed), FRCP(Glas), DCH
Department of Paediatric Cardiology, The Freeman Hospital,
Newcastle-upon-Tyne, UK

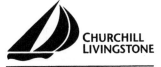

CHURCHILL
LIVINGSTONE

EDINBURGH • LONDON • NEW YORK • OXFORD • PHILADELPHIA • ST LOUIS • SYDNEY • TORONTO • 2000

CHURCHILL LIVINGSTONE
An imprint of Elsevier Limited

First published 2000
    Reprinted 2001, 2002, 2003, 2004, 2006, 2007 (twice), 2008

ISBN: 978 0 443 05480 8

British Library Cataloguing in Publication Data
A catalogue record for this book is available from the British Library

Library of Congress Cataloguing in Publication Data
A catalogue record for this book is available from the Library of
Congress

Note
Medical knowledge is constantly changing. Standard safety precautions
must be followed, but as new research and clinical experience broaden
our knowledge, changes in treatment and drug therapy may become
necessary r appropriate. Readers are advised to check the most current
product information provided by the manufacturer of each drug to be
administered to verify the recommended dose, the method and duration
of administration, and contraindications. It is the responsibility of the
practitioner, relying on experience and knowledge of the patient, to
determine dosages and the best treatment for each individual patient.
Neither the Publisher nor the editors assume any liability for any injury
and/or damage to persons or property arising from this publication.

The Publisher

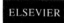

ELSEVIER your source for books,
journals and multimedia
in the health sciences

www.elsevierhealth.com

Working together to grow
libraries in developing countries

www.elsevier.com | www.bookaid.org | www.sabre.org

ELSEVIER   BOOK AID
International   Sabre Foundation

The
Publisher's
policy is to use
**paper manufactured
from sustainable forests**

Transferred to digital print 2009
Printed and bound in the United Kingdom

Contents

Contributors

Dale C Alverson MD
Professor of Pediatrics and OB/Gyn, School of Medicine, University of New Mexico Health Sciences Center, Albuquerque, New Mexico, USA

Carol Clericuzio MD
Associate Professor of Pediatrics, Department of Pediatrics, Chief, Division of Clinical Genetics/Dysmorphology, University of New Mexico School of Medicine, Albuquerque, New Mexico, USA

Andrew C Cook BSc
Cardiac Morphologist/Research Associate, Department of Fetal Cardiology, Guy's Hospital, London, UK

Mark R Crowley MD
Associate Professor of Pediatrics, University of New Mexico School of Medicine, Albuquerque, New Mexico, USA

Nick Evans DM
Senior Lecturer in Neonatal Medicine, Department of Neonatal Medicine, King George V Hospital, Camperdown, Sydney, Australia

S Yen Ho PhD, FRCPath
Senior Lecturer in Cardiac Morphology, Department of Paediatrics, Imperial College of Science, Technology and Medicine, National Heart and Lung Institute, London, UK

Gerard Holmes MD, PhD
Associate Professor of Pediatrics, Chief of Pediatric Cardiology, Director, Children's Hospital Heart Center, Children's Hospital of New Mexico, Albuquerque, New Mexico, USA

Stewart Hunter MBCHB, FRCP(Ed), FRCP(Glas), DCH
Consultant in Paediatric Cardiology, Department of Paediatric Cardiology, The Freeman Hospital, High Heaton, Newcastle-upon-Tyne, UK

John Madar BM, MRCP, FRCPCH
Consultant Neonatalogist, Department of Child Health, Derriford Hospital, Plymouth, UK

John Plowden MD
Associate Professor of Pediatrics, Department of Pediatrics, University of New Mexico Health Sciences Center, Albuquerque, New Mexico, USA

Jonathan Skinner MBChB, DCH, MRCP(UK), FRCPCH, MD
Consultant in Paediatric Cardiology, Department of Paediatric Cardiology, Green Lane Hospital, Auckland, New Zealand

J Deane Waldman MD, MBA
Professor of Pediatrics and Cardiology, Children's Hospital Heart Center, University of New Mexico, Albuquerque, New Mexico, USA

Tony A Whittingham PhD, F.Inst.P., FIPEM, C.Phys.
Head of Ultrasonics, Regional Medical Physics Department, General Hospital, Newcastle-upon-Tyne, UK

Jonathan Wyllie MBChB, MRCP, FRCPCH
Consultant Neonatologist, South Cleveland Hospital, Middlesbrough, UK

About the Editors

Jon Skinner trained first in paediatrics and neonatology to registrar level in the UK and Australia, gaining experience in three neonatal intensive care units. Becoming interested in neonatal haemodynamics, in 1990 he did a three year research project using echocardiography in the newborn leading to a doctorate. Recognising the importance of echocardiography in this regard, he began teaching echocardiography to neonatologists, and ran the first UK neonatal echocardiography course in 1991 with Stewart Hunter in Newcastle-upon-Tyne, and has run several courses elsewhere since. He then subspecialised in paediatric cardiology, and after training to a senior level in Birmingham (UK), Berlin (Germany), Bristol (UK) and Hamburg (Germany) he settled into a consultant paediatric cardiology position in 1998 at Green Lane Hospital, Auckland, New Zealand where he now resides.

Dale C Alverson, MD, is a practising neonatologist, teacher and researcher on faculty at the University of New Mexico Health Sciences Center, USA. He has had a long interest in determination of oxygen delivery and cardiac output in the newborn and its application to clinical practice and clinical or laboratory research. To that end, he was one of the early investigators studying and reporting on the use of Doppler ultrasound in the non-invasive estimation of cardiac output, other blood flow phenomena and hemodynamics in the human neonate. That initial work assisted in determining the accuracy and reproducibility of the Doppler method as applied to newborns and particularly their cardiac output measurements. Research with this technique has helped shed light on a variety of transitional or pathological states in newborns has assisted in diagnosis and provided a better understanding of the effects of medical management upon hemodynamics and oxygen delivery. He is enthusiastic in integrating echocardiography into the clinical practice of neonatology and hopes that the information and advice in this book will help to improve the care of our patients.

Stewart Hunter is a senior paediatric cardiologist at the Freeman Hospital, Newcastle-upon-Tyne, UK. He was involved with echocardiography at its inception and has personally trained a large number of eminent paediatric echocardiologists now dotted around the world. He established the first echocardiography courses in the UK during the 1980s, and these were extremely popular, attracting delegates worldwide. He has published and taught widely on paediatric, fetal and adult echocardiography and latterly has developed particular research interests in fetal and neonatal cardiology. He was the first president of the British Paediatric Cardiac Society and remains an important figure in British and European paediatric cardiology.

Preface

This book is aimed at neonatal paediatricians, including those in training, who wish to learn the essentials of echocardiography for use in neonatal intensive care. It will be valuable also to allied professionals who are skilled in echocardiography, but are occasionally called upon to provide opinions in the unwell newborn infant.

Neonatal echocardiography is an emerging subspecialty within echocardiography. We are not aware of any formal training program anywhere in the world, yet the training needs are different from those of paediatric cardiologists. For them the focus is the precise diagnosis of congenital, structural heart disease. The focus of this book, like that of the neonatologist, is the haemodynamic assessment of the newborn with a structurally normal heart, using echocardiography as part of the diagnostic armamentarium, and as such the book is unique. As with any clinical skill, echocardiography must be learnt within the clinical environment and the trainee needs to be supervised, and the echocardiograms reviewed and audited, by trainers. This book will be a complement to this process; it cannot replace it. Many trainees will find it useful to spend a period in a paediatric cardiology unit.

Each of the chapters, such as those on the assessment of pulmonary arterial pressure, cardiac output, atrial and ductal shunting are written by skilled neonatal echocardiographers with practical, clinical and research expertise in their area. They understand what neonatologists need to know, and what they can and cannot get from echocardiography. Some are paediatric cardiologists, others are neonatologists. The writers come from the UK, New Zealand, Australia and the USA.

The basic physics of ultrasound and Doppler echocardiography are explained straight forwardly by an ultrasound physicist, Tony Whittingham, with experience in teaching these concepts on many echocardiography courses in the UK. These chapters need not be read in detail to start with but will be useful for reference during training. From then on the apprentice should progress through the book from front to back, obtaining practical experience along the way.

This book is not intended for paediatric cardiologists in training - the sections on congenital heart disease focus on general principles but are far from all-inclusive. However, those paediatric cardiologists who do work with neonatologists frequently may find the haemodynamic assessment and ECMO sections useful for review.

JS, DA, SH, 1999

Terminology

Composing this book with writers from Europe, Australasia and the USA has inevitably highlighted the enormous differences between the different types of grammatical English and differences in medical terminology – particularly pertaining to cardiac anatomy. Neonatologists and paediatric cardiologists tend to use different jargon too. In Europe there has been an effort by cardiac morphologists to simplify nomenclature of complex cardiac lesions and to eschew Latin terms and eponyms in particular. This is of little relevance to the neonatologist, but there are some relevant conflicts in terminology. While most of us still use the term 'PDA', the new trend would be to call it the 'arterial duct' instead of the 'ductus arteriosus', and the 'oval foramen' instead of 'foramen ovale'. The respective abbreviations would be PAD instead of PDA and POF instead of PFO. Similarly, SVC becomes SCV as superior vena cava becomes superior caval vein!

These abbreviations are used interchangeably in this book in deference to the chapter author, being clarified as they arise, though we have tried to use as few pseudonyms and Latin terms as reasonably possible. You will of course use whichever you feel most comfortable with!

Abbreviations

A-A	arterioarterial		IMV	intermittent mandatory ventilation
ADC	analogue-to-digital converter		INN	innominate artery
AML	anterior mitral valve leaflet		IVC	inferior vena cava
A-mode	amplitude mode		IVCT	isovolumic contraction time
Ao or AO	aorta; aortic		IVRT	isovolumic relaxation time
AoCSA	aortic cross-sectional area		IVS	interventricular septum
AoSD	aortic stroke distance		IVSD	interventricular septum in diastole
ASD	atrial septal defect		IVSS	interventricular septum in systole
B-mode	brightness mode		L	left
BPD	bronchopulmonary dysplasia		LA	left atrium
BPs	systolic blood pressure		LAVV	left atrioventricular valve
CAT	computerized axial tomography		LCC	left common carotid artery
CAVSD	complete atrioventricular septal defect		LLE	low level enhancement
CCTGA	congenitally corrected transposition of the great arteries		LPA	left pulmonary artery
			LPEP	left ventricular pre-ejection period
CDH	congenital diaphragmatic hernia		LV	left ventricle
CFI	colour flow imaging		LVEDD	left ventricular end-diastolic diameter
CFM	colour flow mapping		LVESD	left ventricular end-systolic diameter
CHARGE	ocular coloboma, heart defects, atresia choanae, retarded growth and development, genital hypoplasia and ear anomalies		LVET	left ventricular ejection time
			LVETc	rate-corrected LVET
			LVIDd	left ventricular internal diameter in diastole
CHD	congenital heart disease		LVIDs	left ventricular internal diameter in systole
CS	coronary sinus			
CVP	central venous pressure		LVO	left ventricular output
CW	continuous wave		LVOT	left ventricular outflow tract
DAo	descending aorta		LVPW	left ventricular posterior wall
DGC	depth gain compensation		LVPWD	left ventricular posterior wall thickness in diastole
ECG	electrocardiograph			
ECMO	extracorporeal membrane oxygenation		LVPWESD	left ventricular posterior wall end-systolic dimension
EF	ejection fraction			
FiO_2	Inspired oxygen fraction		LVPWS	left ventricular peak systolic wall stress
FISH	fluorescence in situ hybridization		LVSV	left ventricular stroke volume
fps	frames per second		M-mode	movement mode
FS	fractional shortening		MPA	main pulmonary artery
FVI	flow velocity integral		MR	mitral regurgitation
HCM	hypertrophic cardiomyopathy		MV	mitral valve
HMD	hyaline membrane disease		NEC	necrotizing enterocolitis
IDM	infant of a diabetic mother		OF	oval fossa

PA	pulmonary artery
$PaCO_2$	arterial partial pressure of carbon dioxide
PAIVS	pulmonary atresia with intact ventricular septum
PAP	pulmonary arterial pressure
PASD	pulmonary stroke distance
MAP	mean airway pressure
PDA	patent ductus arteriosus
PEEP	positive end-expiratory pressure
PFC	persistent fetal circulation
PFO	patent oval foramen
PML	posterior mitral valve leaflet
PPAS	peripheral pulmonary artery stenosis
PPHN	persistent pulmonary hypertension of the newborn
prf	pulse repetition frequency
PTC	persistence of transitional circulation
PV	pulmonary valve
PWD	posterior wall dimensions
PWDD	posterior wall dimension in diastole
PWDS	posterior wall dimension in systole
PZT	synthetic ceramic used as piezoelectric material; name taken from constituent oxides of lead (P), zirconium (Z) and titanium (T)
Qp	pulmonary blood flow
Qpda	left-to-right ductal blood flow
Qs	systemic blood flow
R	right
RA	right atrium
RAM	random access memory
RAVV	right atrioventricular valve
RF	radiofrequency
RPA	right pulmonary artery
RPEP	right ventricular pre-ejection period
RV	right ventricle

RVET	right ventricular ejection time
RVSV	right ventricular stroke volume
RVO	right ventricular output
RVOT	right ventricular outflow tract
SaO_2	arterial oxygen saturation
SAM	systolic anterior motion
SV	stroke volume; single ventricle
SVC	superior vena cava
SVGA	super video graphics array
SVR	systemic vascular resistance
SVT	supraventricular tachycardia
TAPVC	total anomalous pulmonary venous connection
TGA	transposition of the great arteries
TGC	time gain compensation
ToF	tetralogy of Fallot
TPV	time to peak velocity
TR	tricuspid regurgitation
TS	tuberous sclerosis
TV	tricuspid valve
VACTERL	vertebral anomalies, anal atresia, cardiac defects, tracheo-esophageal fistula, renal/radial defects and other limb anomalies
V-A	venoarterial
VAo	temporal and spatial mean ascending aortic flow velocity
Vcf	velocity of circumferential fibre shortening
Vcfc	rate-corrected velocity of circumferential fibre shortening
VCF	velo-cardio-facial
VGA	video graphics array
VLBW	very low birth weight
VSD	ventricular septal defect
V-V	venovenous
ZCC	zero crossing counter

Physics of ultrasound and imaging the structurally normal heart

PART 1

Imaging

Physics, principles and safety of ultrasound scanning

TA Whittingham

BASIC PULSE-ECHO PRINCIPLES

During an ultrasonic scan, short pulses of high-frequency sound are transmitted into the patient and the echoes that are reflected or scattered back are recorded. Frequencies well above the limit of human hearing (ultrasound) are used because waves of such a high frequency can be made to propagate as a narrow beam, and thus can be directed in a well-defined course. In scanning systems, the interrogating beam is assumed to have negligible width, so that all echoes are treated as though they originate from structures lying precisely on the beam axis (the **scan line**).

It is also assumed that the echoes travel in tissue at a known constant speed: 1540 m/s. Assuming this speed, the time for a two-way trip to a target 100 mm deep is 130 µs, so the range of any echo-producing target can be inferred by allowing 1 mm range for every 1.3 µs that elapses between the pulse transmission and the return of its echo.

The transducer (Fig. 1.1.1) both transmits and receives. The transmit–receive process is repeated at a rate (known as the pulse repetition frequency, or prf) of several hundred or even thousand pulses per second, depending on the maximum depth. In order to avoid confusion over which transmission pulse generated which echo, a new pulse is not transmitted until sufficient time has elapsed for echoes to have returned from the deepest possible targets. Shallower target regions, such as occur in neonates, involve smaller 'go and return times', allowing higher prfs and the investigation of more rapidly moving structures.

The strength (intensity) of an echo from an interface is determined by the size and orientation of the interface and by the ratio of the characteristic acoustic impedances (Z) of the two media on either side of the interface. This quantity is a constant for any particular medium and its value depends on the density and compressibility of that medium (see p. 8).

Although it is common to refer to the reflection of echoes when describing ultrasonic scanning, in fact scattering is responsible for most of the echoes seen on most ultrasonic images. **Reflection** is a term normally associated with interfaces that are larger than the beam width, such as heart valve leaflets or chamber walls. If the surface is perpendicular to the beam, relatively large echoes may be reflected back to the transducer. **Scattering** occurs at smaller structures, such as the many tiny interfaces within each type of tissue (the walls of cells, collagen fibres, capillaries, etc.) and sends weak echoes in all directions. Reflections are important for investigating the size and movements of relatively large structures (such as valves), whereas scattering is important for differentiating between tissues (such as pericardium from myocardium).

THE VARIOUS MODES OF PULSE-ECHO SCANNING

A-mode scan

The simplest form of display, known as an A-mode scan (think of A for amplitude), is no longer used in cardiology. Here the transducer is held in a fixed position. The transmitted pulse and the resulting echoes are displayed as vertical spikes on a horizontal line (timebase) representing range (proportional to time after transmission), with the transmission spike at the start of the line; the height of each spike is proportional to the peak pressure amplitude of the corresponding echo (Fig. 1.1.2).

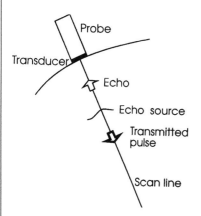

Fig. 1.1.1 Pulse-echo interrogation of a scan line.

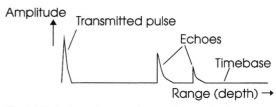

Fig. 1.1.2 An A-mode scan shows echo amplitude versus range (proportional to time taken for each echo to return).

M-mode scan

M-mode scans (think of M for motion) also interrogate a single straight line, but they are designed to reveal movements of interfaces along that line. However, amplitude is expressed as brightness rather than vertical deflections. The timebase is swept sideways (i.e. in a direction perpendicular to itself) across the display screen over a period of a few seconds, causing each echo of variable brightness to trace out a line (Fig. 1.1.3).

B-mode (cross-sectional or 2D) scan

The most common form of display is generally known as B-mode (think of B for brightness), but in cardiology the term 'cross-sectional' scan is preferred. This is a cross-sectional image of the body, built up by sweeping a beam sideways through a chosen scan plane in the body. At each position of the

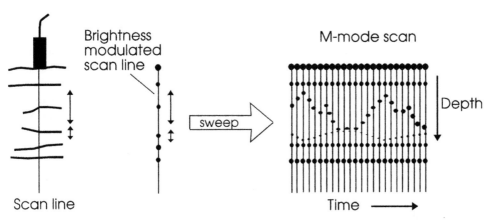

Fig. 1.1.3 An M-mode scan shows the ranges of targets along one scan line versus time. Grey levels (brightness) indicate echo strengths.

Echoes from stationary targets trace out straight lines perpendicular to the timebase, while echoes from moving targets trace out curves representing plots of range versus time. Thus the amplitude and velocity of movement of a heart valve leaflet can be measured directly from its frozen M-mode echo trace. M-mode scanning is particularly important as a non-invasive means of assessing the size and dynamic behaviour of the chambers and valves of the heart.

beam a pulse is transmitted down a new scan line and echoes from any targets in the beam are detected. These echoes are plotted as brightness modulations along a display scan line corresponding in position and angle to the ultrasound scan line (Fig. 1.1.4). As in an M-mode scan, the distance of each structure along the line is determined from the time of arrival of the echo, and its brightness or grey level is determined by the amplitude of the echo. The beam is automatically and repeatedly swept through

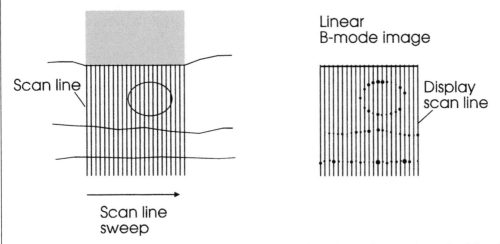

Fig. 1.1.4 A B-mode scan is formed by interrogating hundreds of scan lines in the same 'scan plane'. Grey levels indicate echo amplitudes.

all the scan line positions by mechanical or electronic means from a probe held still against the patient. The number of sweeps per second (frame rate) needs to be sufficiently high to follow the movements of the tissue, i.e. faster than the heart rate.

Various scan formats are used, according to the application (Fig. 1.1.5). In **linear** scanners the beam is stepped sideways by a fraction of a beam width between each transmission, all the beams staying parallel to each other. In **sector** scanners the beams fan out from a fixed point at or near the body surface. This format is useful in applications where gas or bone structures (such as ribs and lungs) near the body surface restrict the 'acoustic window' into the body.

Registration accuracy

This describes how well the displayed position of an echo matches the true position of the target.

Variations between the *speed of sound* in soft tissues, amounting to about ± 5% of the mean value, produce axial (range or depth) errors in the displayed positions of echoes of a few percent. Lateral errors can be produced by *refraction*.

Axial resolution

This is the ability to discriminate between targets that are closely spaced along a scan line (i.e. at different ranges).

If two such targets are very close together, their individual echoes may overlap and merge into one.

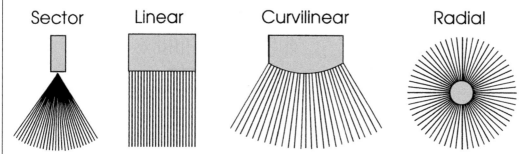

Fig. 1.1.5 Alternative formats of B-mode scans.

Linear scans give a wider field of view close to the surface, but have narrower fields of view at depth, and cannot be used if there are overlying gas or bone barriers to ultrasound. 'Curvilinear' scanners are a cross between linear and sector types and provide a wide field of view both close to the probe and at depth. 'Radial' or 360° scanning is an extension of sector scanning used with some 'endoprobes' designed for use inside the body, e.g. via the oesophagus or other accessible natural route, a blood vessel, or a surgical wound.

IMAGE QUALITY IN PRACTICE

In reality, the assumptions that the speed of sound is known and constant, that all echoes correspond to real targets situated precisely on the scan line, and that all targets will produce detectable echoes, are not entirely justified. The degree to which the scan is an accurate representation of the real distribution of targets may be described by a number of 'image quality' measures (terms in bold italic type are explained later in this chapter or in Chapter 1.2).

The crucial requirement for good axial resolution is a short *pulse length*. This is equivalent to a large *pulse bandwidth* since the latter is equal to the reciprocal of pulse length expressed as a time duration.

Lateral resolution

This is the ability to discriminate between targets that are closely spaced in a direction perpendicular to the scan lines.

Echoes from two or more targets at the same range but within the lateral limits of a single *beam* merge into a single echo. The crucial parameters for lateral resolution are therefore the width and transverse profile of the *pulse-echo beam*. The *beam width* can be up to several millimetres and varies with range.

Dynamic range

The dynamic range of a scanner is the ratio of the largest echo that can be displayed without saturation to the smallest echo that can be discriminated from *noise*.

Electrical noise can be reduced by careful

equipment design but it is always proportional to the *receiver bandwidth*. (Since the bandwidth of the receiver should match that of the pulse, there is a conflict between the need for a large bandwidth for good axial resolution and a small bandwidth for low noise.) In effect, dynamic range is a measure of the sensitivity of the scanner to very small echoes, i.e. from very weakly scattering or reflecting targets or from deep targets. Penetration, the maximum depth from which echoes can be detected, is limited by *attenuation* in overlying tissues, due to absorption and scattering within the tissues and reflection and refraction at the boundaries of organs and tissue masses. Both sensitivity and penetration also depend on the *power* and the *centre frequency* of the transmitted pulse and the size and shape of the pulse-echo beam.

Contrast resolution

This describes the ability of an M-mode or B-mode scan to show small differences in echo amplitude by perceivable differences in grey level. It is mainly determined by the electrical noise level, the precision with which the signal is digitized and stored and the settings of the *pre-processing* and *post-processing* controls (see Chapter 1.2). It may be degraded if the brightness and contrast settings of the display screen settings are not optimum or if the ambient lighting is too bright.

Temporal resolution

This describes how quickly the target can move or the probe position can be changed before the image fails to keep up. It is of crucial importance in cardiac scanning and is primarily determined by the *frame rate*, but the image persistence effect of using *frame averaging* to reduce noise can reduce it further. Frame rates are reduced if wide or deep fields of view are selected, or if *multiple transmission foci* are employed to improve lateral resolution (see Chapter 1.2).

Other artifacts also occur that can misrepresent the strengths and positions of echoes as well as generating spurious echoes. Some of these are discussed later throughout this chapter.

THE CHARACTERISTICS OF ULTRASONIC WAVES

The nature of ultrasonic waves

To consider the propagation of a pulse through a medium, it is helpful to imagine the undisturbed medium to be made up of many very thin (identical) elastic layers. The back and forth movements of the transducer face, acting like a piston, cause the layer of medium immediately in front to be alternately pushed forwards and compressed, pulled back and stretched, pushed forward and compressed, etc. Each layer pushes and pulls on the neighbouring layer in a similar way, resulting in the propagation of an alternating pressure disturbance away from the transducer (Fig. 1.1.6). Each peak and trough in the pressure wave travels at the same speed, i.e. the speed of sound (*c*). Note that each layer moves back and forth about its original position as it participates in the process of passing on the pressure disturbances.

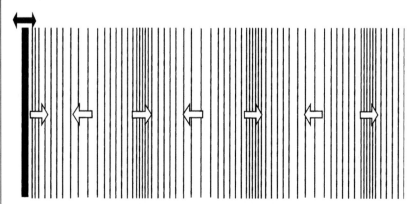

Fig. 1.1.6 A longitudinal wave in a medium, represented as a number of thin layers. High-pressure (compression) and low-pressure (stretching) disturbances travel away from the vibrating transducer face with the speed of sound. The 'particle velocities' (arrows) with which individual layers move back and forward are much lower, typically less than a few tens of cm/s for a diagnostic pulse.

This is a description of a longitudinal ultrasound wave; it is also a plane wave since it neither diverges nor converges.

The increase or decrease in pressure due to the sound wave is called the **excess pressure** or **acoustic pressure** and is given the symbol p. Being a pressure difference, it may be either positive or negative (Fig. 1.1.7).

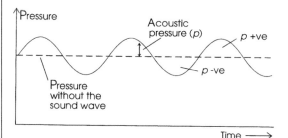

Fig. 1.1.7 Acoustic pressure is the difference between the actual pressure, and the pressure there would be without the sound wave.

The speed of sound (c)

The speed with which the wave propagates depends on the compressibility and density of the medium. An average value for c in soft tissues is 1540 m/s, but values vary by about ± 5%. Fat has the lowest speed and muscle one of the highest.

Wavelength (λ) and frequency (f) (Fig. 1.1.8)

Wavelength is the distance between two adjacent wave peaks, whereas the period (T) is the time between them. Frequency (f) is the number of cycles per second, thus $f=1/T$.

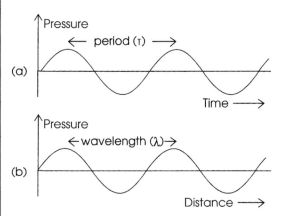

Fig. 1.1.8 (a) The time occupied by one cycle is the period. (b) The distance occupied by one cycle is the wavelength.

Wavelength and frequency are related by the equation:

$$\lambda = c/f$$

Frequencies used clinically are mostly between 3 and 15 MHz, corresponding to wavelengths between 0.5 mm and 0.1 mm, respectively.

Characteristic acoustic impedance (Z)

During ultrasonic wave propagation, a 'layer' is compressed (high positive p) when it moves forwards and stretched (high negative p) when it moves backwards. The acoustic pressure (p) and the induced **particle velocity** (v) therefore change sign in step with each other (they are 'in phase'; Fig. 1.1.9). Thus, for a plane wave in any medium, the quantities p and v are always in a fixed ratio. This constant ratio is known as the characteristic acoustic impedance (Z) of the medium.*

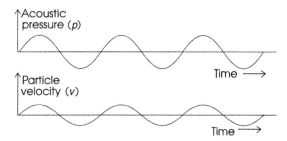

Fig. 1.1.9 For a plane wave, the acoustic pressure (p) and particle velocity (v) are in phase. The ratio p/v is a constant for each medium, called the characteristic acoustic impedance (Z).

Energy, power and intensity

The transducer does work when it pushes and pulls the medium. This is carried away as wave energy, eventually to become heat in the medium. The unit of energy is the joule (J). The energy leaving the probe every second is the acoustic power of the scanner; the unit is the watt (W), equivalent to one joule per second. The intensity of the wave is a measure of the 'local concentration' of power. It is defined as the energy per second

---

*It is sometimes erroneously stated that 'impedance' describes the degree of difficulty or resistance presented by a medium to the propagation of an ultrasound wave. This is not so; for example, ultrasound propagates well in both steel and water, but steel has a much higher impedance than water. The quantity that does describe the extent to which ultrasound is weakened as it propagates is the 'attenuation coefficient, p. 9'.

(i.e. the acoustic power) crossing unit area, with the unit of W/cm^2.

The peak intensity of a pulse determines how large an echo will be. The time-averaged intensity of a sequence of pulses has relevance to the safety of ultrasound since it determines the energy available for conversion into heat by the local tissue.

For continuous wave ultrasound, time-averaged intensity is half the peak intensity. The relatively long 'quiet' periods between transmissions in M-mode and pulsed Doppler means the time-averaged intensity is typically about one thousandth of the peak intensity of the pulse. In B-mode the scanning action means the ratio is smaller still.

The attenuation coefficient of a medium (α)

The rate at which the intensity of a plane wave decreases with distance in a particular medium is known as the **intensity attenuation coefficient** (α) of the medium. It is made up of contributions due to scattering and absorption, both of which increase with frequency. During absorption, part of the 'ordered' wave power is turned into the 'random' motion of heat.

The combined effect of scattering and absorption is to reduce the intensity of a wave by a particular fraction in every centimetre, resulting in an exponential decrease (Fig. 1.1.10), common to many forms of radiation (X-rays, γ-rays, light, etc.). Attenuation is highest in bone, followed by muscle, fat and other soft tissues, and is usually low in liquids, including blood.

PULSES

Pulse length and axial resolution

The **pulse length**, measured in the direction of travel, determines the axial (range or depth) resolution of the scanner.

Figure 1.1.11 shows a three-cycle ultrasonic pulse at one instant as it travels away from a transducer along the transmission beam. In this example the pulse length is 3 wavelengths.

The electrical signal produced by the transducer during echo reception lasts for as long as the echo lasts. The 'bright mark' produced on the displayed scan line therefore has a length proportional to the echo pulse length (Fig. 1.1.12). If targets are too close together, their representations on the displayed scan line can merge together to indicate just a single target.

Figure 1.1.12 illustrates three examples where a transmitted pulse is reflected from two interfaces (1 and 2) situated a small distance (d) apart, along the same scan line. In all cases the echo from interface 2 is a distance $2d$ behind that from interface 1, since an extra distance d has to be travelled by both the transmitted pulse and the resulting echo. In (a), the two echoes are clearly separate and the two interfaces will be resolved along the display scan line. In (b), the separation d is so small that the leading edge of the second echo is immediately behind the trailing edge of the first echo. This represents the limit of axial resolution and occurs when the distance between the echoes is equal to the pulse length, i.e. when the distance between the two interfaces is half the pulse length. In (c) the interface separation is substantially less than half the pulse length and the two echoes have merged into one.

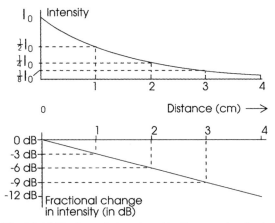

Fig. 1.1.10 The intensity is reduced by the same fraction in every 1 cm of travel. Here, a reduction by ½ per cm is shown, equivalent to –3 dB per cm.

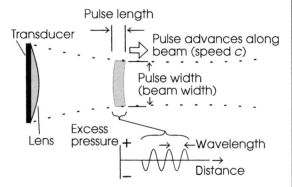

Fig. 1.1.11 Representation of a three-cycle pulse, at one instant in its travel along a beam.

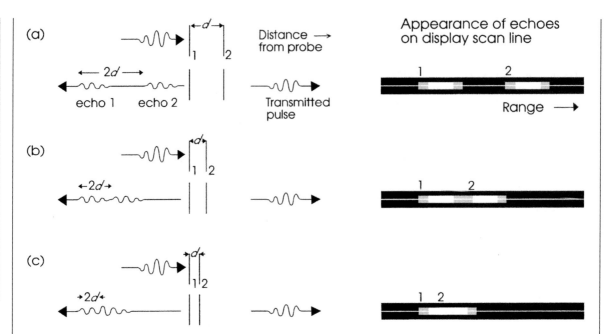

Fig. 1.1.12 Axial resolution. (a) Echoes from two reflecting interfaces separated by more than half the pulse length will be easily distinguished (resolved). In (b) the axial separation *d* is half the pulse length and the two echoes start to merge. For smaller separations (c), the two echoes merge into one. Note that scan lines are normally vertical on displays, not horizontal as here.

Pulse energy spectrum – bandwidth and centre frequency

Although it is common to refer to the 'frequency' of a pulse, this in fact refers to the **centre frequency** (f_c) of a spectrum of frequencies that make up the pulse. Only a continuous wave has a sufficiently simple or 'pure' form to be described by a single frequency. However, by adding together several sine waves of different amplitudes and frequencies, much more complex waveforms can be derived. In fact, a pulse of any shape can be considered as being equivalent to a range of sine waves of different amplitudes and frequencies (i.e. the spectrum of the pulse).

The **energy spectrum** of a pulse shows the range of frequencies making up the pulse and how its energy is distributed over that range (Fig. 1.1.13). Since most of the energy is contained in a central 'band' of frequencies, the term **pulse bandwidth** is used to describe this range of frequencies. It is defined as the width of the energy spectrum of the pulse, measured at half the maximum height of the spectrum. The shorter the pulse, the greater the bandwidth. In fact,

$$\text{bandwidth} = 1/\text{pulse length}$$

where bandwidth is expressed in MHz and pulse length is expressed in µs.

As they travel through tissue, the high-frequency components of each pulse are attenuated most, lowering the centre frequency and reducing the bandwidth (Fig. 1.1.14). Echoes from deep targets are therefore longer than those from shallower ones, and so axial resolution is poorer for deeper structures.

In high-performance scanners the bandwidth and centre frequency of the receiver are progressively reduced with time after transmission, to match the changes taking place in the spectra of

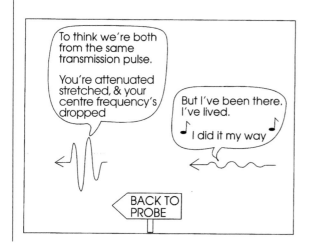

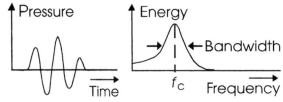

Fig. 1.1.13 A pulse is equivalent to a spectrum of continuous waves. A 6 MHz pulse really means a pulse with a 'centre frequency' (fc) of 6 MHz. The 'bandwidth' is the width of the spectrum at half height. Short pulses have large bandwidths.

the echoes as they return from greater depths. This is known as **dynamic filtering**.

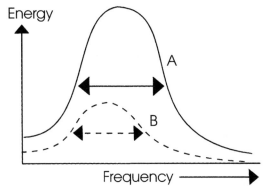

Fig. 1.1.14 Propagation through tissue changes the spectrum from A to B. The energies of all frequencies are reduced, but more so for higher frequencies. The centre frequency and bandwidth of B are lower than those of A.

The optimum pulse shape and frequency

Most pulses used for scanning consist of two to three cycles, irrespective of the frequency. Good axial resolution requires a short pulse, but high sensitivity requires a long pulse (i.e. a small bandwidth leading to lower receiver noise). A pulse length of about two or three cycles is about optimum.

The length of a pulse of a given number of cycles is inversely proportional to the frequency (Fig. 1.1.15), therefore higher frequencies give better axial resolution. However, attenuation will be worse, so sensitivity and penetration will be poorer. A compromise frequency is therefore necessary,

☞ *Practical Point*

● **Higher frequencies give better axial resolution but poorer tissue penetration.**

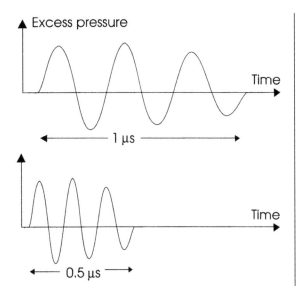

Fig. 1.1.15 For a fixed number of cycles (three shown here), the pulse length halves if the frequency doubles.

depending on the types of tissue involved and the maximum depth of the region to be scanned.

Frequencies as low as 2–3 MHz may be necessary for deep penetration, say in a large adult heart, whereas frequencies of 5 or 7 MHz may be used in infants. Frequencies of 30 MHz or higher may be used with intravascular probes (see Table 1.1.1). Axial resolution and maximum penetration both reduce inversely with frequency, so that whatever the application and frequency, the scale of the axial detail remains about the same fraction (about 1%) of the maximum depth of penetration.

Table 1.1.1 Applications of different ultrasound frequencies

Frequency (f)	Wavelength (λ)	Pulse length (say 2.5 λ)	Application examples
3 MHz	0.5 mm	1.3 mm	Adult abdomen, heart, late pregnancy
5 MHz	0.3 mm	0.8 mm	Child abdomen, heart, early pregnancy
7 MHz	0.2 mm	0.5 mm	Breast, thyroid, neonate heart and abdomen
10 MHz	0.15 mm	0.4 mm	Eye, peripheral blood vessels

BEAMS

Transmission, reception and pulse-echo beams

It is helpful to distinguish between three types of beam. The transmission beam is the region over which the transmitted wave has significant strength. The reception beam is the region in which an omnidirectional source of ultrasound might be located, such that waves (e.g. echoes) from it would be detected above background noise. The pulse-echo beam is the region from which echoes might be detected from scatterers, and depends on both the transmission and reception beam. For good lateral resolution, both transmission and reception beams must be as narrow as possible. This is achieved by using as high a frequency as possible, and by focusing.

Beam width and lateral resolution

Just as an ideal pulse would be very short, so the ideal pulse-echo beam would be very narrow. In reality, a pulse-echo beam may have a width of as much as a few millimetres, and therefore targets that are actually a few millimetres from the beam axis will be recorded as though they were precisely on the scan line. This has two important consequences for image quality.

First, it leads to the presentation of spurious echoes (acoustic noise echoes). For example, although a particular scan line may pass through the centre of a narrow liquid-filled structure (e.g. a blood vessel), and should therefore produce no echoes, the outer skirts of the beam may well be encompassing, and sending back echoes from, surrounding solid tissue (Fig. 1.1.16). The result is that what should be an echo-free region on the scan will contain some **noise** echoes.

Second, the wider the beam, the poorer the lateral resolution. A single small target at a particular range will lie within the beams associated with several adjacent scan lines. As the interrogating beam is swept across the scan plane (from left to right in Fig. 1.1.17a), the target will first be registered when it lies at the right-hand edge of the beam (scan line B). It will continue to be registered on all the following scan lines (Fig.

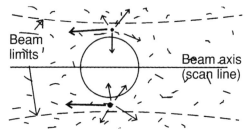

Fig. 1.1.16 Scatter from outside an echo-free region produces acoustic noise.

1.1.17b) until it lies at the left-hand edge of the beam (scan line F). In practice the scan lines are so closely spaced that the target is simply represented on the black background of the display (Fig. 1.1.17c) as a bright 'streak', perpendicular to the scan lines, having a length equal to the width of the beam.

Thus, the streaks produced by two targets at the same range that are closer than a beam width will overlap, and may merge into a single echo (Fig. 1.1.18).

Focusing beams – focal length, focal zone and strength of focusing

Focusing can be achieved by means of a lens, a bowl-shaped transducer or (rarely) by means of a concave mirror. A focused beam (Fig. 1.1.19) is characterized by a converging zone, a focal zone and a diverging zone. The narrowest part of the beam is the focal zone, usually defined as the region in which the beam width is within a factor of two of the minimum width. The intensity is greatest and the beam narrowest at the focus. The distance between the transducer and the focus is the focal length (F) of the transducer.

The width of the beam at the focus (w_F) is given by

$$w_F = F\lambda/a$$

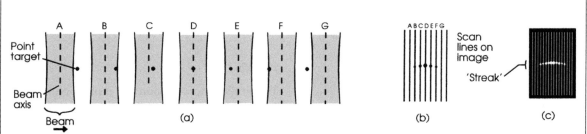

Fig. 1.1.17 (a) Seven consecutive positions of an interrogating beam in relation to a fixed point target. (b) An echo is registered on all the display scan lines corresponding to positions B, D, E and F. No echo is registered for positions A and G. (c) On the image these appear as a streak with the same width as the beam.

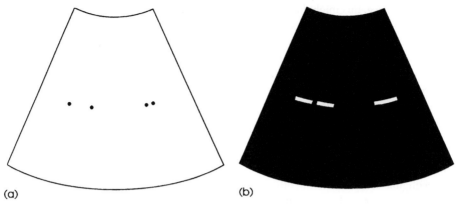

Fig. 1.1.18 (a) Point targets. (b) B-mode image. All targets produce a streak. The pair of targets on the left are resolved. Those on the right are closer together than the beam width and are not resolved.

where F is the focal length, a is the half-aperture (or radius) of the transducer and λ is the wavelength. Strength of focusing is defined as the ratio a/w_F. Strong focusing ($a/w_F > 2$) may be achieved by using a large aperture but this results in a short focal zone, so tissue at other depths is less well resolved. Consequently, if only a fixed focus is possible (as in some mechanical scanning), the beam should be weakly focused (Fig. 1.1.20).

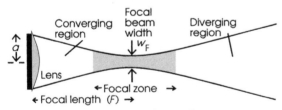

Fig. 1.1.19 Representation of a focused beam.

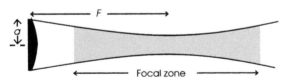

Fig. 1.1.20 A weakly focused beam has a moderate degree of narrowing but a long focal zone.

EFFECTS OF INTERFACES – REFLECTION, REFRACTION AND SCATTERING

Interfaces much larger than the wavelength: reflection and refraction

Reflection of a pulse or beam occurs at any large interface between media having different characteristic acoustic impedances (Fig. 1.1.21). If the surface is smooth (i.e. any roughness is much less than the wavelength) it is said to be a **specular**

reflector, behaving like a mirror. Examples include muscle fascia, healthy (i.e. smooth) heart valve leaflets and the diaphragm. Since

angle of incidence (θ_1) = angle of reflection (θ_1),

an echo from such a surface will only return to the transducer if the beam is incident perpendicular to the surface ($\theta_1 = 90°$).

☞ *Practical Point*

● **It is important to scan such surfaces with the probe oriented so that the scan lines are perpendicular to the surface, otherwise an echo of the surface may be missing from the image (specular reflection artifact).**

At most interfaces between soft tissues, the change in impedance is so small that only a small fraction of the incident power is reflected. At most,

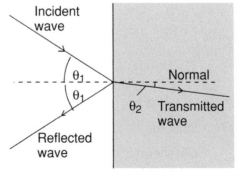

Fig. 1.1.21 Reflection and refraction at a smooth flat interface. The fraction of energy reflected depends on the ratio of the characteristic acoustic impedances on each side of the interface.

say at a fat–muscle interface, this might be 1%, but it could be 10 000 times less for, say, a blood–clot interface.

The change in impedance at a bone–tissue interface is very large, resulting in about half the incident power being reflected. This is one reason why tissues behind bone are difficult to examine with ultrasound; the other is the very high absorption and scattering that occurs in bone, particularly at higher frequencies.

If the impedances are so different that one of them is almost negligible compared to the other, there is nearly total reflection of the incident power. This is the case at a gas–tissue or a transducer–air interface, and is the reason why ultrasound cannot 'see' into air-filled lung or beyond the first surface of a pneumothorax or pocket of bowel gas. It is also the main reason why it is necessary to use coupling gel or some other liquid medium between the probe and the patient's skin (the other reason is that it acts as a lubricant).

☞ Practical Point
- **Large tissue impedance differences reflect a lot of incident power, such that tissues beyond bone or air cannot be resolved.**

If the surface is rough, as in the case of diseased valve leaflets or the irregular boundaries of many tumours, the surface is said to be a **diffuse** reflector. Diffusely reflecting surfaces send back echoes over a wide range of angles of incidence and, therefore, unlike specular reflectors, the beam does not need to be at right angles to them for them to be imaged.

Refraction is the deflection or 'bending' of a wave when it encounters an oblique interface at which there is a change in speed (Fig. 1.1.22). Refraction occurs if there is a change in speed at the interface and the incident wave meets the surface obliquely.

The most obvious imaging problem due to refraction is the lateral misregistration of the apparent position of a target when the beam has been deflected, for example at a fat–muscle interface. A target that is to the side of the scan line can return an echo that is presented as though it were actually on the scan line (Fig. 1.1.22a). A similar effect is known to spear fishermen who see their prey somewhat beyond its true position, owing to refraction of light at the water–air interface. By experience they learn to throw their spear a little short of the apparent position of the fish (Fig. 1.1.22b).

A particularly severe form of refraction is responsible for the type of acoustic shadow artifact that sometimes occurs when the beam is at very oblique incidence to a boundary where the speed of sound increases, such as a blood–muscle or fat–muscle boundary. The beam reflects rather than penetrates owing to a phenomenon called **total internal reflection**. Where this occurs there can be no echoes from targets directly beyond the interface (Fig. 1.1.23).

A less dramatic, but nevertheless troublesome, effect of refraction is the beam distortion produced when it passes through layers of

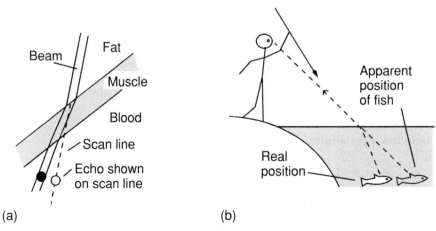

(a)　　　　　　　　　　　　　　(b)

Fig. 1.1.22 Refraction can produce a lateral shift in the apparent position of a target.

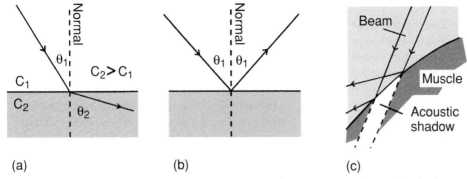

Fig. 1.1.23 Total internal reflection. If $c_2 > c_1$ and the angle of incidence θ_1 reaches a critical value, θ_2 reaches 90°. If θ_1 exceeds this critical angle, the beam is completely reflected. This is the cause of shadowing beyond obliquely insonated muscle interfaces.

subcutaneous tissue with an uneven nodular structure. Different parts of the beam experience different deflections on entering and leaving the various nodules, in the same way that light waves are distorted in passing through mottled bathroom glass (Fig. 1.1.24). This is one of the reasons why in some patients poor images always seem to be produced.

Interfaces smaller than the wavelength – scattering and speckle

Scattering

This occurs when the size of a structure is similar to or smaller than the wavelength. Occasionally, individual small structures (scatterers), such as calcifications or foreign bodies, may produce isolated echoes, but the commonest forms of

scatterers are the numerous tiny vessels, fibres, cells and other microstructures that make up the tissue itself.

As the beam travels through the tissue, the power of that part of the wave meeting the scatterer is redistributed as a new wave, radiating in all directions, although not necessarily with equal intensity in all directions (Fig. 1.1.25). If, like many microstructures in the body, the scatterer is much smaller than the wavelength, it is described as 'Rayleigh scattering'* (see p. 16) where the total power scattered is proportional to (scatterer size)[6] × (frequency)[4].

The sixth power dependence on scatterer size explains why echoes are seen (as speckle patterns, see below) in tissue, but not usually in blood. The fourth power dependence on frequency suggests that higher frequencies should be used when blood cells are the target, but in practice the weakness of the echoes from blood means that attenuation in the intervening tissue is a problem and that lower frequencies have to be used. The exception is intraluminal scanning, when frequencies up to 30 MHz may be used, producing visible speckle patterns from the echoes scattered by blood.

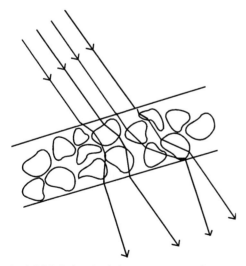

Fig. 1.1.24 Refraction in heterogeneous subcutaneous tissue can degrade image quality owing to beam distortion.

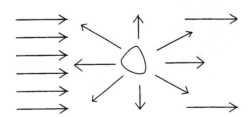

Fig. 1.1.25 Scattering of a wave by a small target redistributes power in all directions.

Speckle patterns

Most scatterers are too close together to be resolved separately in the image. Since the echoes arise from scatterers that have a fairly random distribution, there will be some instances when many of the echoes will be in phase or nearly so, and will produce a large sum (bright echo complex along the scan line); at other times they will all be at very different phases and will largely cancel each other out (dark region). The resulting 2D interference pattern of echo brightness is known as a speckle pattern. It may be tempting to interpret the detail within the speckle pattern as detailed structure within the tissue, *but this detail is random*. Tissue structure that is finer laterally than the beam width and finer axially than the pulse length cannot be resolved. In fact, although all the speckles are randomly different, their mean width is the beam width and their mean axial length is the pulse length.

The features of the speckle pattern that depend on the tissue are its mean brightness and its texture (speckle uniformity). Subtle differences in these parameters can be crucial in differentiating between tissues (contrast resolution).

THE SAFETY OF ULTRASOUND

The view of all authoritative professional bodies is that ultrasonic scanning is without hazard to the patient, *if used prudently*. However, some machines are capable of producing undesirable temperature rises and probably other biological effects. In the UK, machine output parameters are unregulated, but the Food and Drug Administration (FDA) in the USA does impose some limits. These are generally complied with by most manufacturers, although the limits do not guarantee absence of hazard in all circumstances. The responsibility for the safety of the patient in each individual investigation still lies with the doctor.

The most important mechanisms through which diagnostic ultrasound can create a biological hazard are heating and cavitation.

Heating

Heating is due to the absorption of ultrasound within the tissues. Unfortunately there is no single acoustic output parameter such as power or time-averaged intensity that can be used to predict the temperature rise in all 'target' regions of tissue. Many other factors are involved including the width of the beam (or scanned area), the attenuation introduced by the intervening tissue, the absorption coefficient of the target tissue, the frequency of the transmitted pulse, as well as the thermal conductivity and blood perfusion of the target and neighbouring tissues.

In general, heating is likely to be greatest whenever non-scanning modes are selected (particularly pulsed Doppler), whenever a high **power** setting selected, whenever a deep **focus** setting or a narrow deep **write zoom** box is selected, or whenever tissues with a high absorption coefficient (particularly bone) or poor perfusion (e.g. eye lens) are involved. (Continuous wave Doppler transmissions have low amplitude; their very low bandwidth means returning beams can usually be easily detected from noise, so high powers are not necessary.)

Calculations using the measured intensity distribution of commercial scanning equipment indicate that temperature rises of up to 6°C may be possible when directing pulsed Doppler beams onto

---

*It may be of interest to note that this frequency dependence explains why the sky is blue and sunsets are often red! The scattering of light by the molecules and other small particles in the atmosphere is another example of Rayleigh scattering. Blue light is at the high-frequency end of the visible light spectrum, while red is at the low-frequency end. Hence blue light is scattered more powerfully, and we see blue when we look at the sky. In the evening the sun is low in the sky and the sunlight travels through a greater length of atmosphere. Even more of the higher frequency colours are scattered to the side, leaving the sun itself looking red, and giving a red hue to any clouds illuminated by direct light.

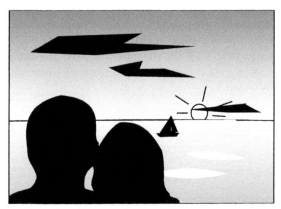

He: To think that this pleasing suppression of the high frequencies in the sun's light is governed by the same scattering laws that apply to ultrasound.
She: I love it when he talks physics.

---

a bone target, and about 2.5°C when the target is soft tissue.[1] In B-mode and colour flow modes, the temperature rises are between 1.5°C and 2°C in both soft tissue and bone. These calculations do not take into account the removal of heat by blood.

Cavitation

Bubbles can develop and collapse due to pressure variations in a liquid. Each negative half cycle of pressure of a sound wave encourages gas or water vapour to leave the liquid and increase the size of any pre-existing 'nuclei' bubbles. If the negative pressure excursion is great enough or lasts long enough, a bubble may grow so much within just one negative half cycle that it then collapses in the following high pressure half cycle in a violent implosion. The energy released by such 'collapse cavitation' appears as heat (local temperatures as high as that of the sun are theoretically predicted), light and shock waves, as well as leading to the production of free radicals such as OH⁻. This physical and chemical energy release is fatal to biological cells and is the basis of the mode of action of laboratory sterilization tanks.

A less violent form of cavitation, requiring lower pressure amplitudes, is 'stable cavitation'. This occurs when the natural resonant frequency of any bubbles matches the frequency of an applied sound wave. Bubbles or gas pockets of the appropriate size (around 1 μm for diagnostic frequencies) may already exist, or, if continuous waves or millisecond long pulses are used, smaller bubbles may grow under the influence of the sound wave until they reach resonant size. The resonating bubbles produce strong but localized swirling (microstreaming) in the surrounding liquid, which can damage nearby cells. A moderate form of this mechanism is thought to be responsible for the beneficial effect of physiotherapy ultrasound – the microstreaming stresses increase the permeability of the white cell membranes and thus accelerate the repair processes.

The likelihood of cavitation depends on many factors, but is greater for high peak negative pressure (high **output power**), low frequencies (choice of **probe**), long pulse length (large **gate widths** in pulse Doppler mode), high pulse repetition periods (small **gate depth** and high **frequency scale** settings in Doppler mode), free liquids, the presence of agitation to replenish nuclei

and gas supplies, and in tissues with pre-existing bubbles such as occurs in parents who have had lithotripsy in the previous 24 hr, or have received injections of ultrasound contrast agents.

In vivo tissue damage, consistent with cavitation, has been reported for exposure of animal lung tissue to diagnostic pulses.[2] This takes the form of superficial extravasation, and is associated with the presence of air pockets in the lung. It is not necessarily due to cavitation. Collapse cavitation due to diagnostic pulses has not yet been demonstrated in vivo in tissues devoid of pre-existing gas cavities, but it has been demonstrated in vitro and in gel, and it is known to occur during lithotripsy (which generates pulses in which the negative pressure lasts longer than in diagnostic pulses but which have similar negative pressures).

Thermal and cavitation hazards in cardiac scanning

The heart chambers are normally well cooled by blood flow, but heating may be a possible hazard within a thick mass of heart muscle or other soft tissue, or as a result of insonating the spine, ribs or other nearby bony structure. There is no report of cavitation being produced by diagnostic ultrasound within whole blood. However, the incidental insonation of neonatal lung tissue may produce local haemorrhage.

Thermal and Mechanical Indices

Until recently manufacturers seeking FDA approval had to ensure that certain acoustic output parameters were kept within specified application-dependent limits. An alternative means of gaining FDA approval now relaxes these limits in all applications to those of the application with the least stringent limits (peripheral vascular scanning), but requires that a constantly updated, application-specific, 'Thermal Index (TI)' and a 'Mechanical Index (MI)' be displayed on the screen.

These indices are intended to give some indication to the operator of the risk of thermal and cavitation hazard, but they should be used with caution since the calculations are simple and use many assumptions. Both TI and MI will underestimate the risk of hazard in a situation where the target tissue lies beyond a region of low attenuation, such as a liquid.

The FDA do not require either index to be

displayed if it cannot exceed 1, implying an assumption that values below this do not present a hazard. However, it should be noted that there can be as much as 100% error in calculating these indices and that the 'Statement on Non-human Mammalian in-vivo Biological Effects', issued by the American Institute of Ultrasound in Medicine, gives a TI value of 2 and an MI value of 0.3 as the lower limits for confirmed adverse biological effects in mammalian tissues.

REFERENCES

1. Whittingham TA, Henderson J, Jago JR. Temperature rise predictions using measured temporal average p^2 distributions from clinical scanners. IPEMB Ultrasound and Non-ionising Radiation Specialist Interest Group Meeting: *Estimating Thermal Effects of Ultrasound*. Bath Royal Literary and Scientific Institution, 1 November, 1995.
2. Dalecki D, O'Brian WD. Ultrasonically-induced lung haemorrhage in young swine. *Ultrasound in Med. and Biol.* 1997;23:771–781.

Basic features and controls of an ultrasound scanner

TA Whittingham

THE BEAM FORMER

The beam former is the part of the scanner that controls the shape and size of the pulse-echo beam and the way the beam is scanned.

Basics of transducer design

The transducer is the device that both transmits (launches) the outgoing pulse and receives the echoes, converting electrical signals to ultrasound pulses, and vice versa.

The design of a single-element transducer, which might be used for A-mode or M-mode scanning, or as the transducer in a single-element mechanical B-scanner probe, is shown in Figure 1.2.1. 'Array' transducers have the same basic features but are divided into a number of independent transducer elements to allow electronic beam forming (see later). A lens is usually incorporated to make the transducer transmit to or receive from one particular region on the transducer axis (the focal region) more effectively than others.

The transducer itself consists of a thin plate of a piezoelectric material. Piezoelectric materials change their size (their thickness in the case of a thin plate) when a voltage is applied across them, and a voltage is produced when their dimensions are changed, for example by compression. The piezoelectric used in medical scanners is usually a synthetic ceramic known as PZT (from the chemical symbols of its constituent components – the oxides of lead, zirconium and titanium). The PZT plate is coated with silver on the two flat faces, forming electrodes to which leads are connected.

In transmission, the flat faces of the plate can be made to behave as moving pistons by applying a varying voltage between the two electrodes. A sequence of voltage impulses is applied across the electrodes, with durations and timings designed to produce expansions and contractions in the PZT plate at its natural resonant frequency (Fig. 1.2.2). In reception, the pressure variations produced by the returning ultrasonic echoes produce thickness changes in the plate which generate proportional voltage changes between the electrodes, suitable for electronic amplification.

The impedance-matching layer is vital to the efficient transfer of energy between the transducer and the patient. PZT has a much greater characteristic acoustic impedance than tissue or lens material, so a large fraction (about 80%) of the energy of a pulse would be reflected from a PZT–lens or PZT–tissue interface. The matching layer helps the pulse to cross between transducer and lens (and thus into the patient) in easy stages. A backing layer absorbs the sound from the back face of the transducer, helping to keep the pulse short. It is made of a material with a high impedance, allowing good transmission from the PZT into the backing layer, and has the ability to absorb ultrasound strongly.

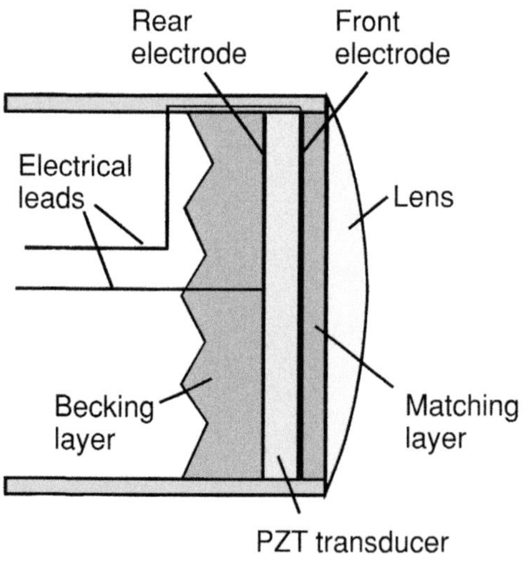

Fig. 1.2.1 Basic features of an ultrasonic transducer.

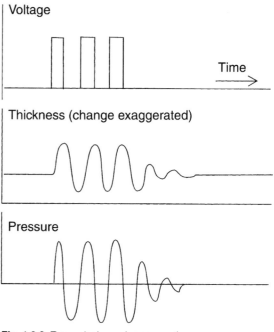

Fig. 1.2.2 Transmission pulse generation.

Single-element mechanical sector scanners

Beam forming in this type of scanner is achieved by simply swinging or rotating a single transducer in a hand-held probe.

The basic features of a mechanical B-scan probe consist of (Fig. 1.2.3):

- a probe case or housing. This usually carries a mark to indicate the scan plane;
- an electric motor;
- an angle-sensing device. This generates an electrical signal that uniquely identifies the angle of the transducer axis (scan line) relative to the probe axis;
- a mechanical linkage to produce the rocking (or in some makes a spinning) action with minimum vibration;
- the transducer assembly (PZT transducer, backing and matching layers, and a lens);
- an oil or water bath in which the transducer assembly moves;
- a flexible cable to the main console, containing leads to take power to the motor, carry the angle-sensing information, and a coaxial screened lead to the transducer itself.

Mechanically scanning probes can be made to have negligible vibration and can be inexpensive. They are often the best method of generating and scanning a high-frequency beam, but the involvement of moving parts and a water or oil bath mean that wear and tear can create maintenance problems.

Annular array mechanical sector scanners

Some mechanical scanners have a transducer assembly containing a set of several concentric ring-shaped transducer elements instead of a single disc (Fig. 1.2.4).

The operator can set the focus of the transmitted pulse at any point on the transducer axis by using the **transmission focus** control. This causes each element to be electrically excited, and thus transmit, at a slightly different time. The outer element transmits first, as it is furthest from any on-axis point, and the central disc transmits last. Thus, pulser from all the elements arrive simultaneously at the transmission focus, producing a large amplitude pulse.

The receive focus is also electronically (and automatically) controlled by the machine's computer. The echo signals from each element are electronically delayed (Fig. 1.2.5) by slightly different amounts to compensate for the slight differences in distance (pathlength) between each

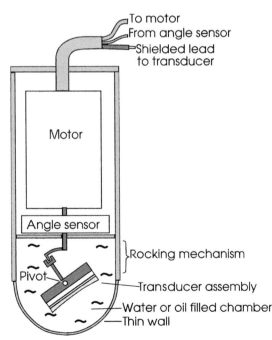

Fig. 1.2.3 Basic components of a mechanical sector scanning probe of the 'rocker' type. In practice the motor and angle sensor are often designed to be an integral part of the transducer assembly.

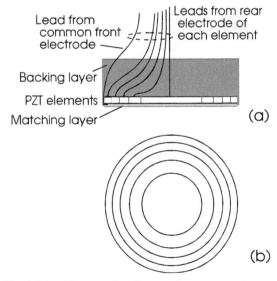

Fig. 1.2.4 (a) Construction of an annular array transducer assembly. This replaces the single-element assembly in Fig. 1.2.3. (b) Concentric arrangement of elements.

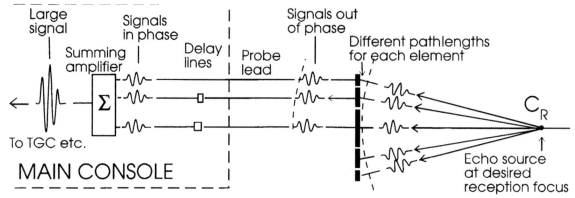

Fig. 1.2.5 A receive focus at a point C_R is produced by using delay lines to compensate for the differences in distance between C_R and the individual elements.

element and the receive focus. The delayed echoes are then added together in a summing amplifier to form a single echo. The signal generated by the summing amplifier is thereafter treated as if it had come from a single transducer.

Linear and curved arrays scanners

These scanners use probes containing a line of regularly and closely spaced rectangular elements in either a linear or curvilinear array (see Fig. 1.1.5, p 6). Beam forming is achieved by delaying the signals to and from each element, while beam scanning is achieved by using different combinations of elements.

Each transducer element is a rectangular PZT slab, sharing a common backing layer, matching layer and lens (Fig. 1.2.6). The elements are formed by cutting through a single slab of PZT. They share a common front electrode and lead, but each has its own rear electrode and lead.

Typically a linear array probe will have around a hundred elements, each about a wavelength wide.

The overall width of the probe is therefore inversely proportional to frequency, matching the reduction in penetration that comes with increasing frequency. As an example a typical 3.5 MHz probe, suitable for adult cardiac imaging, might have a probe width of 80 mm, and contain 128 elements. A 7 MHz array for the same scanner, suitable for the neonatal heart, would also have 128 elements, but in a probe of 40 mm width.

Only a limited group of adjacent elements (active group[1]) is used to form the transmitting and receiving apertures for each scan line, the other elements in the array being idle until they become part of the active group themselves. The interrogating beam is stepped from scan line to scan line across the array by dropping an element from one end of the active group and adding a new one to the other end (Fig. 1.2.7).

The number of elements in the active group can be changed to vary the active aperture, and delays can be introduced to the signals transmitted and

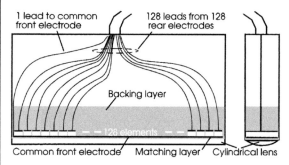

Fig. 1.2.6 Construction of a linear array probe. Each element is further 'sub-diced' (not shown) to reduce energy loss due to unwanted lateral vibrations.

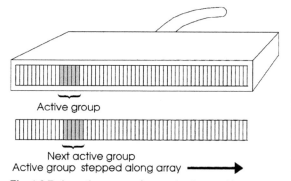

Fig. 1.2.7 An active group of several adjacent thin rectangular elements acts as a single larger rectangular or square transducer.

received by each element, in order to control the focal length in the same way as in an annular array probe.

Phased array scanners

'Phased array' scanners provide a sector scanning format by electronic beam steering (Fig. 1.2.8). They avoid the problems of wear and tear associated with mechanical sector scanners and offer useful mixed mode facilities (see next section). Modern phased array probes have similar numbers of elements as linear arrays, but are much narrower. A typical 3 MHz probe might have 128 elements in a radiating aperture 20 mm long.

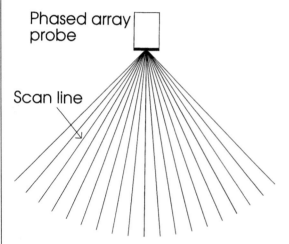

Fig. 1.2.8 Sector scan format of phased array.

Phased array scanners have one undesirable characteristic that is not shared by mechanical sector scanners – an increase in beam width and hence a decrease in lateral resolution towards the sides of the image. Unlike a mechanical sector scanner, the transducer of a phased array does not turn to face the target. Thus, for a focus on a scan line other than the probe's principal axis, the angle between rays from opposite sides of the transducer (φ in Fig. 1.2.9) is less than for targets on the principal axis. The formula $w_F = F\lambda/a$ (see Chapter 1.1) for the width of the beam in the focal region

---

> **☞ Practical Point**
> - **For best lateral resolution ensure that the target is near the centre line of an image produced by a phased array scanner.**

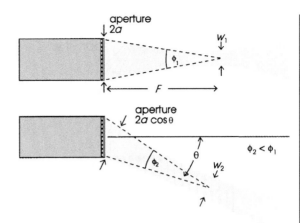

Fig. 1.2.9 Deflection of the beam to an angle θ causes the angular width of the aperture (φ) to decrease and hence the focal beam width to increase. Effectively the aperture reduces from $2a$ to $2a \cos \theta$.

may be expressed as $\lambda/\sin \varphi/2$, showing that the beam width increases as φ reduces. Thus the beam width increases, and lateral resolution degrades, as the angle of the scan line increases.

Mixed mode scanning

Both linear and phased array scanners are able to display a real-time M-mode scan of a specific scan line at the same time as displaying a real-time B-mode scan. This is particularly useful for phased arrays in cardiological applications. It is possible because, unlike mechanically scanned systems, there is no mechanical inertia associated with the beam sweep, and so the beam can jump instantly from one scan line to another in any order. Thus, after say two lines of B-mode echo acquisition (lines 1, 2 in Fig. 1.2.10), the beam can jump to a selected scan line and acquire one line of M-mode echoes (line 3), then jump back to continue the B-mode scan for the next two lines (lines 4, 5), then jump to the M-mode line (line 6), etc.

Another example of mixed mode scanning is 'duplex' scanning, where Doppler samples are recorded from a sample volume on a selected scan line of a simultaneous real-time B-mode image (see p.5). In duplex mode, the Doppler samples must be obtained at a high repetition frequency, so that even jumping to the Doppler line after every one or two B-mode lines is unlikely to be adequate. It is therefore more usual to allow the Doppler interrogation along the Doppler line to run for most of the time, with brief interruptions, typically only

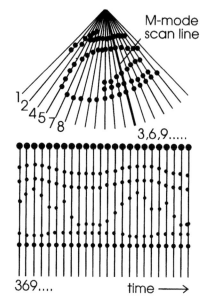

Fig. 1.2.10 Simultaneous real-time B-mode and M-mode scans. The numbers refer to the sequence in which the scan lines are interrogated. In this example, every third transmission is used to interrogate the selected line in M-mode.

20 ms every second or so, to perform one complete 'update' frame of the B-mode.

Defining the field of view

The **depth** control sets the maximum depth of the displayed scan lines, and inhibits the recording of echo information after the corresponding time. By itself, a reduced depth setting does not necessarily permit a higher pulse repetition frequency (prf) and hence a higher frame rate. Echoes will still be

returning from greater depths after the chosen echo acceptance period and, even though they are not being recorded, they would cause confusion if another pulse-echo reception sequence were to begin before they ceased. However, some machines increase the centre frequency of the transmitted pulses when a small depth is selected. This improves lateral resolution and allows a higher prf and frame rate, since penetration is reduced.

All phased array and many mechanical sector scanners have a **sector width** control. This normally produces an increase in frame rate, since fewer scan lines are interrogated when the angular width of the sector is reduced.

A more versatile way of reducing the field of view is **write zoom**. The operator first defines a 'region of interest' by means of a box superimposed on the image (Fig. 1.2.11a). On selecting write zoom, a magnified view of the selected region is displayed (Fig. 1.2.11b). No time is spent scanning outside the lateral limits of the box, and only echoes returning within the time limits corresponding to the near and far limits of the box are recorded. This allows the time saved by not scanning a large area to be traded for improvements in frame rate or lateral resolution.

☞ *Practical Point*

● **In general, narrowing the size of the field of view allows an increase in resolution. This is particularly important when accurate measurements are required from cross-sectional images.**

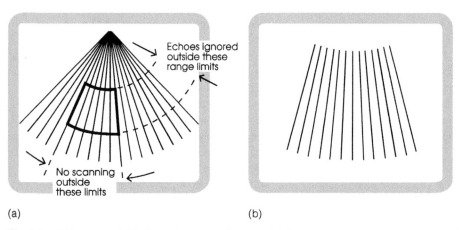

(a)   (b)

Fig. 1.2.11 Write zoom. (a) Defining the region of interest. (b) The write zoomed image has a higher line density and/or a higher frame rate.

SENSITIVITY CONTROLS

Transmission pulse generator

The peak voltages of the electrical excitation pulses to the transducer are set by the **output power** control. The larger the output power setting, the larger the amplitude of the transmitted ultrasound pulses and hence the echoes returned from all depths. This means greater sensitivity and greater penetration. However, some discretion should be exercised in increasing the output power, since this increases both peak negative acoustic pressure and time-averaged intensity. The former is relevant to the likelihood of cavitation occurrence, while the latter is relevant to tissue heating (see p. 16).

Radiofrequency amplifier

A radiofrequency (RF) amplifier is one specifically designed to amplify signals in which the voltage oscillates at frequencies of around a hundred kilohertz or higher, similar to those produced by radio circuits. The RF amplifier in the scanner is designed to amplify just the range of frequencies that lie within the pulse spectrum. The frequency response (a plot of amplification versus frequency) of the RF amplifier should have the same centre frequency and bandwidth as the echoes. The degree of amplification (gain) of the RF amplifier can be varied by the operator using the **overall gain** control.

☞ *Practical Point*
- **From a safety point of view, the most prudent way of varying sensitivity is to set the overall gain to a high level (but not so high that electrical noise is evident in the image), and then vary the output power to give the required sensitivity. This procedure ensures that the acoustic power delivered to the patient is never more than is necessary.**

SWEPT GAIN

The RF amplifier also uses a technique known as **swept gain**, time gain compensation (TGC) or depth gain compensation (DGC), that compensates for the fact that echoes from targets deep within the patient are extremely weak compared with those from targets near the probe (Fig. 1.2.12a). It does this by progressively increasing the amplification (gain) as echoes return from deeper

and deeper in the tissue, i.e. as time goes by after transmission (Fig. 1.2.12b). Provision is made for the operator to adjust how the gain varies with time (the TGC curve) according to the appearance of the image. The aim is to correct any general trends in echo brightness with depth (Fig. 1.2.12c). This does not mean that the operator should attempt to display all echoes with the same brightness (grey level), since there are diagnostically valuable differences in the reflecting and scattering ability of different interfaces.

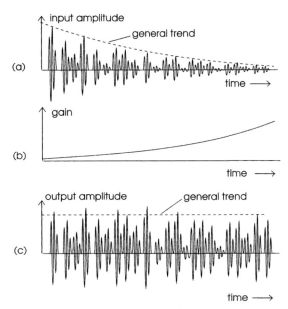

Fig. 1.2.12 (a) RF echo signals before swept gain. (b) Gain versus time curve needed to compensate for attenuation. (c) RF echo signals after swept gain.

In cardiac scanning, there may be layers of muscle, with a high attenuation coefficient, alternating with regions of blood, with a low attenuation coefficient. An appropriately complex TGC curve can be selected by having several slide controls, each dedicated to setting the gain independently over a specific narrow depth range (Fig. 1.2.13).

AMPLITUDE DEMODULATION

Up to this point in the receiver, the voltage versus time waveform of each electronic echo signal has been a replica of the pressure waveform of the ultrasonic echo. However, for display purposes, only the amplitude and the time of occurrence of each

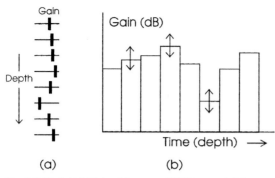

(a)   (b)

Fig. 1.2.13 (a) Multiple slider type of TGC control. (b) Example of the complex type of TGC curve that can be formed. Each slider sets the gain independently for a specific depth interval.

echo is needed. The RF pulse is therefore converted into a much simpler 'demodulated' pulse, but having the same overall shape and size (Fig. 1.2.14).

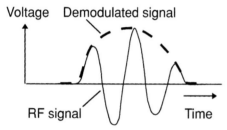

Fig. 1.2.14 Amplitude demodulation of an RF pulse produces a signal equal to the half-envelope.

ANALOGUE-TO-DIGITAL CONVERSION

An analogue signal is one that changes continuously in response to a change in another signal, no matter how small the change. For example, the RF echo signal produced by the transducer is an analogue of the pressure waveform of the ultrasonic echo signal returning to the transducer. While electronic amplification requires the echo signals to be in analogue voltage form, further processing and storage of the echoes after demodulation is better done by a digital computer. It is therefore necessary to convert the analogue voltage waveforms into digital form. A sequence of echoes is then represented by a series of binary numbers, which represent the amplitude of the echo sequence at closer intervals (for example 50 ns). This analogue-to-digital conversion is achieved using an analogue-to-digital converter (ADC). High performance scanners digitise the signal before the demodulator.

PRE-PROCESSING

The PRE-PROCESSING control defines the relationship between the number representing an echo amplitude stored in the image memory and the digital amplitude of that echo on leaving the ADC (i.e. following the TGC and demodulation stages). A plot of one against the other is called the pre-processing transfer characteristic, or pre-processing curve (Fig. 1.2.15). Selection of this curve, from the range provided by the manufacturer, or pre-defined by the operator, is one of the most important ways of determining contrast resolution. Although it might seem sensible to make this a straight line, i.e. to store values that are directly proportional to the incoming echo amplitudes, transfer curves of other shapes can often improve the diagnostic value of the scan. For example, when attempting to differentiate between, say, muscle and tumour tissue, it is more important to have good contrast resolution between the fairly low-amplitude echoes produced by these tissues than to be able to distinguish between the amplitudes of stronger echoes, say those reflected from tissue boundaries. In such cases the 'S' curve allocates most of the available storage levels to a limited range of moderately low level echoes. The 'low level enhancement curve' (LLE) would be more suitable for differentiating between very low-amplitude echoes, for example when searching for a blood clot in the heart.

Reject and **dynamic range** controls are also pre-processing controls. They both set a threshold for echo amplitude that echoes must exceed if they are to be displayed, and hence both reduce the dynamic range of the system. However, whereas the

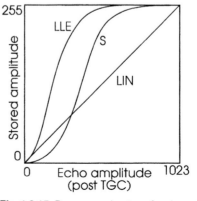

Fig. 1.2.15 Pre-processing transfer characteristics. L, linear; LLE, low level enhancement; S, 'S' curve.

reject control simply causes weak echoes or noise to disappear from the image, the dynamic range control adjusts the transfer curve so that the full range of the memory is used for the remaining echoes (Fig. 1.2.16). These controls are much used by some inexperienced operators because they 'clean up' the image and produce an apparent reduction in the complexity of the image. However,

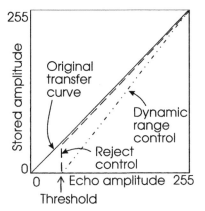

Fig. 1.2.16 Both reject and dynamic range controls set a lower threshold for echo amplitude.

☞ *Practical Point*

- **Don't overuse the REJECT and DYNAMIC RANGE controls when tidying up a 'noisy' image – some low-amplitude signals may be important, particularly in tissue differentiation.**

they should be used carefully since both involve the throwing away of low-amplitude echo information. Usually a reduction in overall gain or a change of transfer curve can achieve a similar result without losing the weaker echoes entirely.

IMAGE STORAGE AND PROCESSING

The image matrix

The scan plane is represented as a rectangular matrix of tiny rectangles called picture elements (pixels). Each pixel is uniformly filled with a single level of grey and has a horizontal (X) and a vertical (Y) 'address' (Fig. 1.2.17a). Typically X and Y addresses might range from 0 to 511 across the full width and height of the screen, respectively. For each pixel there is a corresponding location 'pigeon hole' in the image memory, having the same address coordinates as the pixel, in which a binary number defining the echo amplitude for that pixel is stored. The number of bits available for the stored number limits number of distinguishable amplitude values that can be stored, and hence the best contrast resolution the machine can achieve. Information is 'read' to the TV display by interrogating the memory, row by row, in synchronism with the TV scan lines.

Read zoom

The **read zoom** control allows part of the image, selected by the operator, to be viewed at a modest

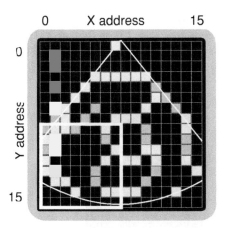

(a)

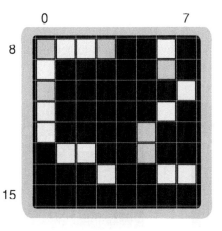

(b)

Fig. 1.2.17 (a) Each pixel in the image is identified by its X and Y address. This representation has addresses 0 to 15 only; addresses from 0 to (say) 511 are more typical in practice. The box (bottom left) defines an area to be magnified by 'read zoom'. (b) After read zooming, the defined area fills the screen. Note the magnified pixels.

magnification (Fig. 1.2.17b). It is achieved by restricting the read interrogation of the memory to a fraction of the full address range. The effect is similar to using a magnifying glass on newsprint – the ink dots simply look bigger with no real increase in image detail. If greater magnification is needed a reduced scan depth or write zoom should be considered (p. 24).

Frame freeze and cine loop

The **frame freeze** control inhibits the writing process, but allows the 'frozen' image data to be continually read to the TV display. A further development of the frame freeze principle is dynamic image review, often referred to as **cine loop** or **cine review**. This enables several seconds' worth of consecutive frozen frames to be reviewed at normal rates, in slow motion, or frame by frame. This is very useful when looking closely at detailed cardiac anatomy, particularly valve motion, at fast heart rates. A four-second sequence of around one hundred frames, 512 by 512 pixels and 256 possible grey levels (requiring 8 bits = 1 byte), acquired at a frame rate of 25 frames per second, requires approximately 25 megabytes of storage. This is well within the capability of the random access memory (RAM) used in the controlling computer.

☞ *Practical Point*
- **To review carefully valve or cardiac wall motion at fast heart rates, acquire a sequence on the cine loop and review it at your chosen speed.**

Frame averaging

This is a technique for improving the signal-to-noise ratio of a scan, at the expense of introducing a degree of persistence to the image, and hence degrading temporal resolution. In fact the persistence effect can be so pronounced that the **frame averaging** control is often referred to as the **persistence** control. Rather than simply replacing each stored frame of echo information with the following one, this control makes the new frame an average, pixel for pixel, of the old and the new. Noise signals come and go, and so are reduced by an averaging process, whereas genuine signals will be the same in consecutive frames (provided the frame rate is high enough for the target movement) and so will not be affected by averaging.

The weighting given to the old value can be varied by the **persistence** control: a low weighting produces only modest noise reduction but low persistence; a high weighting produces better noise reduction but greater persistence. In general, only modest levels of frame-to-frame persistence can be tolerated in cardiac imaging, except where the field of view is so small that very high frame rates can be employed.

If the frame rate is insufficient, frame averaging can produce **ghost artifacts** in frozen images, corresponding to partly faded images of rapidly moving structures (e.g. a heart valve leaflet) present in earlier frames, but either missing from, or in a different position in, the frozen frame (Fig. 1.2.18). If the weighting given to the old frame is high, it may take several frames for each image to fade away, and a frozen image may reveal several progressively weaker 'ghosts' in different positions.

Post-processing

The **post-processing** control allows the operator to select one of a number of post-processing transfer curves, defining the relationship between displayed

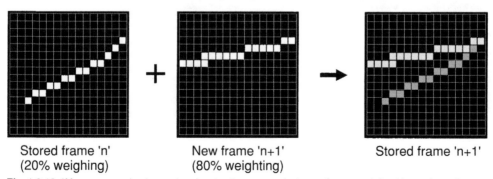

Stored frame 'n'
(20% weighing)

New frame 'n+1'
(80% weighting)

Stored frame 'n+1'

Fig. 1.2.18 If frame averaging is used and a structure moves between frames, a 'ghost image' may be seen on a frozen image.

grey level and stored amplitude (Fig. 1.2.19a). Together with the pre-processing transfer curve it defines the overall transfer curve, i.e. the relationship between the echo amplitude (post TGC) and the displayed grey level (Fig. 1.2.19b).

Post-processing has the advantage, compared with pre-processing, that the effect of different curves can be explored without needing to re-scan the patient. The disadvantage is that the dynamic range and contrast resolution are limited by the word length (number of bits) of the image memory.

DISPLAY

Some ultrasound systems now use special TV displays designed for digital interfacing to computers. They achieve greater spatial, contrast and temporal resolution than the PAL and NTSC broadcasting standard TVs which use 625 horizontal lines at a frame rate of 25 frames per second (fps) and 525 lines at a frame rate of 30 fps, respectively. The VGA (video graphics array) standard provides 640 by 480 pixels with 16 grey levels or colours, while the SVGA (super video graphics array) displays might have as many as 1024 by 768 pixels with 65 536 colours. Both can have frame rates of 72 fps.

☞ *Practical Point*
- **Whatever type of display is used it is important to ensure that the BRIGHTNESS and CONTRAST controls are set optimally. The background of the scan display area should be just brighter than the black background of the rest of the screen, and the grey-level calibration staircase should run from this level to a bright white, with clear differentiation of all the intermediate grey levels. Neglecting to check these control settings can reduce the image quality of a high-performance scanner to below that of a less expensive machine.**

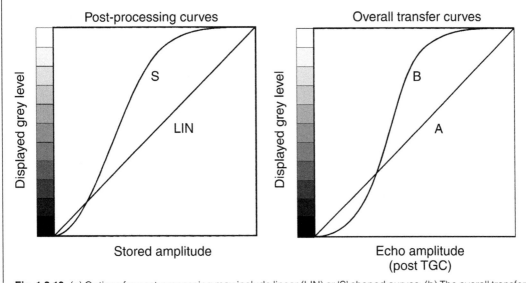

Fig. 1.2.19 (a) Options for post-processing may include linear (LIN) or 'S' shaped curves. (b) The overall transfer curve, defined by the post-processing and pre-processing curves acting together, may be linear (A) or more complex (B).

REFERENCE

1. Whittingham TA. A multiple transducer system for the heart, abdominal and obstetric scanning. *Ultrasound in Medicine*. Eds, Kazner et al. 1975. Excerpta Medica, Amsterdam.

Essential cardiac anatomy

Stewart Hunter
S Yen Ho
Andrew C Cook

INTRODUCTION

Cardiac anatomy is frequently badly taught in medical school and the majority of doctors practise with only the sketchiest idea of where the different parts of the heart lie. Knowledge of cardiac anatomy has not been helped in the past by the confusing nomenclature of many cardiac structures. Over the past 20 years a rationalization of the nomenclature of the heart has occurred in the UK and Holland and this has gradually percolated throughout the world.[1] The anatomical descriptions in this chapter eschew terms based on embryological structures and dead languages and concentrate on descriptive naming of the parts. When the nomenclature was revised there was a movement to remove the terms 'right' and 'left' when referring to the ventricles and atria. There is much sense in this in that the right-sided structures tend to be anterior and the left-sided structures posterior. It was, however, felt that the cardiological world was not ready for such radical change, and right and left have remained from the old nomenclature.

The heart develops and evolves continuously from conception throughout fetal life and continues to modify itself in the neonatal period. Obviously with the transition from fetal to neonatal circulation, shunts which were present in the fetus cease to exist. The right ventricular wall, previously similar in thickness to the left ventricular wall, gradually thins in the first month after birth. At this time also the left ventricular mass increases.[2] Nonetheless, the morphological features that distinguish morphologically right from morphologically left structures are the same in the fetal and the neonatal heart.

MORPHOLOGY OF THE NORMAL HEART

The arrangement of cardiac chambers in the normal heart is such that the right heart chambers are anterior relative to the left heart chambers. The left atrium is the most posterior cardiac chamber directly anterior to the oesophagus at the bifurcation of the trachea. The ventricles are inferior and leftward of their corresponding atria (Fig. 1.3.1). In the fetus and the small premature baby, more of the left ventricle is seen anteriorly than in the older infant. Indeed, because of the relatively large size of the abdominal contents, in particular the liver, the apex of the heart under these circumstances is tilted

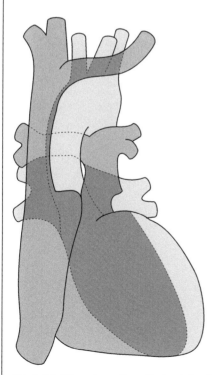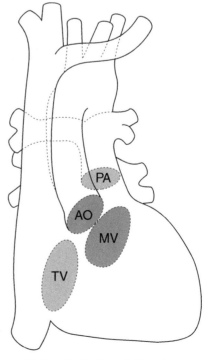

Fig. 1.3.1 When viewed from the front, the right heart structures (darker shading) over left heart structures (lighter shading). Ao, aorta; PA, pulmonary artery; MV, mitral valve; TV, tricuspid valve.

more towards the head and the long axis of the left ventricle lies more horizontally than in the older infant (Fig. 1.3.2).

The cardiac valves are arranged in a different plane, with the aortic valve normally in a central position. The pulmonary valve lies anterior and superior and the atrioventricular valves flank the inferior margins of the aortic valve. The most inferior valve is the tricuspid, which is in a nearly vertical plane and is attached to the septum closer to the cardiac apex than the mitral valve.

The atria both lie to the right of their respective ventricles, but are designated as morphologically left and right. Each has an appendage of distinct shape. In the fetus and infant, the appendages are relatively large compared with the rest of the heart. The broad triangular shape of the right appendage is easily distinguished from the crenellated and narrow outline of the left appendage. They have appropriately been described as appearing like Snoopy's nose and Snoopy's ear, respectively (Figs

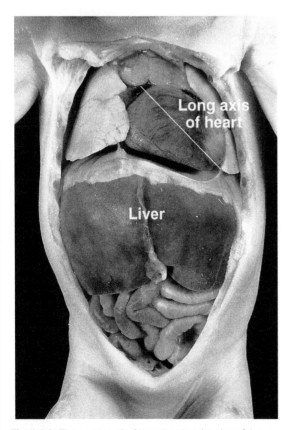

Fig. 1.3.2 The section of a fetus showing the size of the heart relative to the other thoracic structures and its orientation.

1.3.3a and 1.3.3b). The junctions between the appendages and the atria are different. The right appendage junction is broader than the left. A muscle band called the terminal crest gives rise to extensive pectinate muscles in the right atrium which extend all the way around the atrioventricular junction (Fig. 1.3.3c). This structure is not present in the left atrium and the pectinate muscles are only found within the atrial appendage (Fig. 1.3.3d). The pulmonary veins enter the posterior smooth-walled part of the left atrium and the systemic veins enter the venous component of the right atrium. In the neonate the superior and inferior caval veins enter at a sharper angle than in older children. The straightening of their insertions is an effect of growth on the chest. The Eustachian valve is a prominent structure in the newborn child as in fetal life it served to direct flow from the inferior caval vein towards the oval fossa. On the right atrial aspect of the septum, the muscular rim of the oval fossa is easily seen (Fig. 1.3.3c). On the left side, a flap-like valve apposes the rim (Fig. 1.3.3d). The valve starts off as a membrane in young fetuses, but gradually thickens and becomes more muscular towards term. Normally it has excessive fullness for the opening which it covers at the time of birth. This slackness disappears after birth when the valve starts to become adherent to the rim of the fossa. With the growth of the atrial chambers, the size of the oval fossa becomes relatively smaller. This is of importance to the paediatric cardiologist because it allows for gradual reduction in size of central atrial defects with the passage of time.

The ventricles have very distinctive shapes, with the right ventricle wrapping itself around the left ventricle. The cavity of the right ventricle is triangular in outline, whereas that of the left ventricle is ellipsoidal. The inflow and outflow tracts of the right ventricle are at an obtuse angle and those of the left ventricle at an acute angle. Because of this, the pulmonary outflow tract swings to the left and is superior relative to the aortic valve and root. The pulmonary valve is separated from the tricuspid valve by the supraventricular crest (Fig. 1.3.4). This crest is a fold of muscle with fatty tissue encasing the right coronary artery on its epicardial aspect. The crest is absent in the left ventricle where there is almost always fibrous continuity between the leaflets of the aortic and mitral valves (Fig. 1.3.5a). The mitral valve is tethered and supported by two groups of papillary

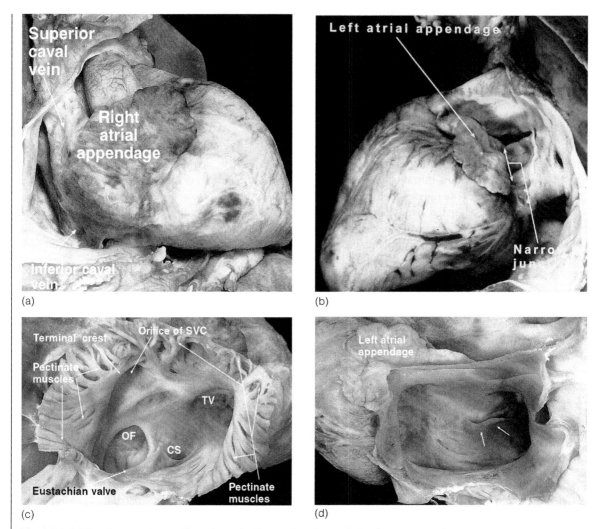

Fig. 1.3.3 (a) The right atrial appendage shown in this specimen has a distinctive triangular shape and a broad junction with the venous component of the atrium.
(b) The left atrial appendage is narrow, crenelated and shaped like a finger.
(c) A view into the right atrium showing extensive pectinate muscles and the terminal crest. A muscular rim surrounds the oval fossa and the Eustachian valve guards the entrance to the inferior caval vein. CS, coronary sinus; OF, oval fossa; SVC, superior vena cara (also called superior caval vein, SCV); TV, tricuspid valve.
(d) The inside of the left atrium is relatively featureless and lacks the terminal crest. The valve of the oval fossa (arrows) is seen in the centre.

muscles – the anterolateral and posteromedial groups. The aortic outflow tract is bordered on the medial side by the ventricular septum and laterally by the anterior leaflet of the mitral valve (Fig. 1.3.5a). In contrast, the tricuspid valve directly attaches its septal leaflet to the ventricular septum (Fig. 1.3.5b). A feature which distinguishes the right from the left ventricle is the trabecular pattern. Coarse trabeculations criss-cross the apical portion of the right ventricle. There is, in addition, a muscle band, called the moderator band, crossing the right

ventricular cavity. Trabeculations in the left ventricular cavity are fine and located in the apical portion, while the septal surface of the left ventricle is smooth (Fig. 1.3.5a).

The cardiac septa are largely muscular and comprise atrial, atrioventricular and ventricular components. The muscular atrioventricular septum exists because of the offsetting of the proximal attachments of the mitral and tricuspid valves. The atrial septum lies obliquely at 45° to the sagittal plane of the body. When viewed from the front, the

☞ *Practical Point*

- **Characteristic morphological features, identifiable on echocardiography, help to differentiate the right from the left ventricle in complex congenital heart disease. The tricuspid valve is always associated with the morphological right ventricle, is supported in part from the septum, is not in fibrous continuity with the outlet valve and arises from further down the septum than the mitral valve. The mitral valve is in fibrous continuity with the outlet valve, has no support from the septum and is always associated with the morphological left ventricle.**

right atrium overlies the left atrium.[3] The ventricular septum curves in a complex way from a plane which is nearly sagittal to one which is nearly coronal, separating respectively the inlet and outlet portions of the two ventricles. There is a tiny component of the septal wall which is not muscular, known as the membranous septum. It has atrioventricular and interventricular portions separated by the attachment of the septal leaflet of the tricuspid valve. In the neonate, the components of the membranous septum may not be particularly clearly seen.

☞ *Practical Point*

- **The ventricular septum curves in a complex way such that the exclusion of ventricular septal defects requires several different echocardiographic views.**

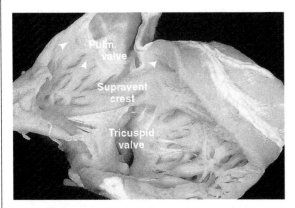

Fig. 1.3.4 The right ventricle is displayed to show the supraventricular crest which separates the pulmonary valve from the tricuspid valve. The pulmonary valve is supported by a sleeve or collar of muscle (arrowheads).

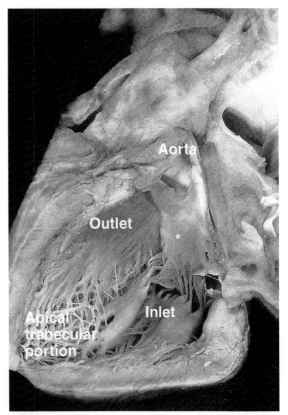

(a)

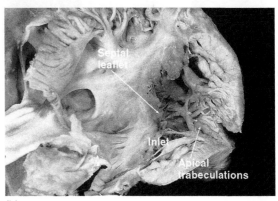

(b)

Fig. 1.3.5 (a) A dissection of the left ventricle to show the inlet, apical trabecular and outlet components. The aortic outflow tract is wedged between the ventricular septum and the aortic leaflet of the mitral valve (*).
(b) The right side of the heart is displayed in this dissection to show the inlet and apical trabecular components of the right ventricle. The septal leaflet of the tricuspid valve attaches directly to the septum.

The start of the aortic root rises to the right and posterior relative to the pulmonary tract. As it ascends, the aorta is related to the right atrial appendage, the right ventricular outflow tract and the pulmonary trunk (Fig. 1.3.6). On its right side is the medial wall of the right atrium, the superior caval vein and right-sided pleura. The transverse sinus of the pericardium lies behind the aorta, separating it from the left atrium and the right pulmonary artery. The ascending aorta passes superiorly, obliquely to the right and slightly forwards towards the sternum. In this position the thymus lies outside the pericardium interposed between the ascending aorta and the sternum. The arch of the artery begins just above the pericardial reflection, proximal to the origin of the brachiocephalic or innominate artery. It runs superiorly for a short distance before passing backwards and to the left. The arch finishes on the lateral aspect of the vertebral column after origin has been given to the arteries supplying the neck and arms.

The pulmonary trunk comes from the anterior aspect of the heart, just behind the left lateral edge of the sternum from a position just in front of the

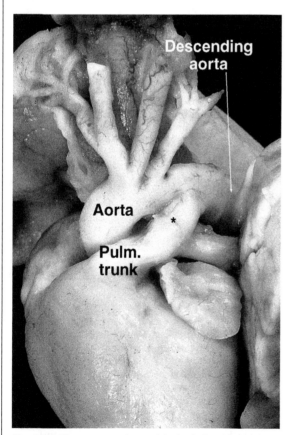

Fig. 1.3.6 The great arteries and their relationships are shown in this fetal specimen which demonstrates the pulmonary trunk, the arterial duct (*) and the aortic arch.

☞ *Practical Point*
- **The aortic valve is in a central position within the heart.**

aorta and the left coronary artery. It swings to the left side of the ascending aorta. Immediately after this it bifurcates into the left and right pulmonary arteries. The arterial duct extends onwards to the anterolateral aspect of the aorta, which it joins as the arch merges into the descending aorta (Fig. 1.3.6). There are changes particular to this area of the heart and great arteries as the individual moves from fetal to neonatal life. In the fetus the pulmonary end of the duct is related to the left margin of the sternum at the upper border of the second rib. Sometime after birth this point descends to the second intercostal space. The duct is patent throughout fetal life and loses its patency typically by the fourth day in term infants (and healthy preterm infants over 28 weeks' gestation). In most instances it is a ligament by 3 months of age.

☞ *Practical Point*
- **The most anterior part of the heart is the right ventricular outflow tract and the pulmonary valve, and the most posterior part is the left atrium and pulmonary veins.**

The pulmonary artery branches traverse the central part of the thorax with some important relationships. The left pulmonary artery passes in front of the descending aorta and superior to the left main bronchus. The right pulmonary artery is longer and traverses the mediastinum under the arch before passing behind the superior caval vein anterior to the main bronchus to reach the hilum of the right lung.

RELATING ECHOCARDIOGRAPHIC VIEWS TO CARDIAC ANATOMY

Echocardiographic access to the heart is much greater than it is later in infancy and childhood. From each of the echocardiographic windows, two main series of planes are available for scanning at right angles to one another, but a multiplicity of intermediate views can be obtained. The parasternal and apical windows produce planes along the orthogonal axes of the heart, while views through the subcostal and suprasternal approaches show the cardiac structures in planes that are nearer to the orthogonal planes of the body rather than of the heart.

The heart can be viewed parasternally through the second left, third left and fourth left intercostal spaces, producing a series of short or long-axis views. The short-axis sections towards the apex show the cross-sections of the ventricles and the curvature of the ventricular septum. Scanning upwards towards the base of the heart, the aortic root is visualized, and with slight angulations of the transducer both right and left coronary artery origins can be imaged. Sections at right angles to the short axis lie within the cardiac long-axis planes. Sections to the right and left of the main long-axis view show only right heart or left heart structures, respectively. In the standard long-axis view of the left ventricle the aortic leaflets usually visualized are the right coronary and non-coronary cusps (Fig. 1.3.7). From the fifth intercostal space (the 'apical' approach) the heart can be viewed along its two orthogonal long axes. One series of sections profiles the cardiac septum, producing the four-chamber

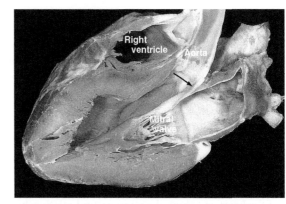

Fig. 1.3.7 This dissection shows the left side of the heart in a parasternal long-axis approach focusing particularly on the area of aorto-mitral valvar continuity (arrow). A small part of the right ventricular outflow tract is seen superiorly. An equivalent echocardiogram is shown in Figure 1.4.5a.

views inferiorly and the four-chamber plus aortic route anteriorly (Figs 1.3.8a,b). There are a series of sections at right angles to the four-chambered view showing two chambers of the heart which are similar to the parasternal long-axis planes.

The subcostal approach is very easy to obtain in

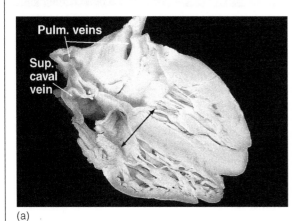

(a)

Fig. 1.3.8 (a) This is a four-chambered section showing the atrial septum, the position of the oval fossa (*), the ventricular septum and the muscular part of the atrioventricular septum (double-headed arrow).
(b) This section is superior to the four-chambered view and shows the aortic valve, ascending aorta and left ventricular outflow tract (*).

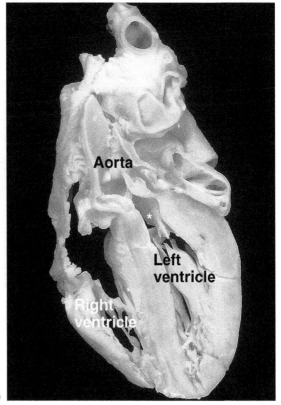

(b)

the infant as the transducer can be manipulated more readily under the diaphragm. Two series of planes are viewed from this aspect. One approximates to the coronal plane of the body while the other is almost in the sagittal plane of the body. The coronal series demonstrates right heart chambers in the anterior sections and approximates to a four-chambered view in the sections towards the diaphragm (Fig. 1.3.9). The atrial septum is particularly well seen in this series of views. At right angles to this series are sections in the parasagittal plane; these are nearly in the short axis of the heart and show the wrap-around relationship of the right ventricle to the left ventricle. Near the base of the heart, these sections demonstrate a more cranial position of the pulmonary valve relative to the aortic valve and the sweep of the right ventricle (Figs 1.3.10a and 1.3.10b). The aortic valve is seen in this view in cross-section.

Through the suprasternal notch the ascending aorta, aortic arch and its branches and the proximal portion of the descending thoracic aorta can be visualized. Scan planes at 50° to the coronal plane pass through the ascending aorta, aortic arch and descending aorta (Fig. 1.3.6). Beneath the lower aspect of the aortic arch, the right pulmonary artery is seen in cross-section passing into the right hilum. Rotation of the scan plane through 90° cuts the aortic arch into cross-section and shows the longitudinal section of the right pulmonary artery, perpendicular to the superior caval vein.

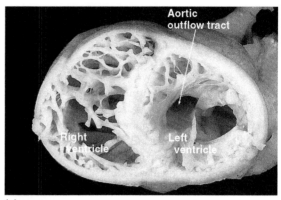

(a)

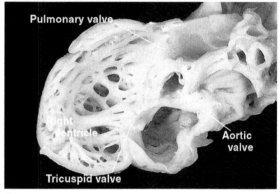

(b)

Fig. 1.3.10 (a) This is a short-axis, subcostal view from the heart of a neonate with the mitral valve seen in cross-section. The heavily trabeculated right ventricle lies to the left of the picture.
(b) This cut is more superior than the preceding short-axis subcostal view and shows the sweep of the right ventricle from its inlet portion, right to the outlet under the pulmonary valve. Part of the aortic valve is seen in cross-section in the centre. An equivalent echocardiograph section is shown in Figure 1.4.6.

REFERENCES

1. Anderson RH, Ho SY. Sequential segmental analysis – description and categorisation for the millennium. *Cardiology in the Young* 1997;7:98–116.
2. St John Sutton MG, Gewitz MH, Shah B *et al.* Quantitative assessment of growth and function of the cardiac chambers in the normal human fetus: a prospective longitudinal study. *Circulation* 1984;69:645–654.
3. Walmsley T. The heart. In: Sharpey-Schafer E, Symington J, Bryce TH (eds), *Quain's Elements of Anatomy*, vol 4. London: Longman's Green & Co., 1929.

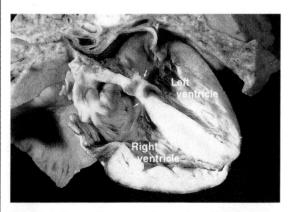

Fig. 1.3.9 The cardiac septum is seen in profile in the four-chambered view and the offset arrangement (arrows) of the mitral and tricuspid valves is particularly evident. A sample echocardiograph is shown in Figure 1.4.7.

Obtaining the standard echocardiographic views

John Madar
Stewart Hunter
Jon Skinner

INTRODUCTION

This chapter concentrates on how to obtain good cross-sectional ultrasound pictures of the heart. It covers:

- positioning of the infant
- appropriate imaging equipment
- positioning of the probe for specific views.

Echocardiographic 'windows' are better in babies than at any other age because the lungs (impenetrable to ultrasound) do not get in the way as much, and the heart and great vessels are nearer the probe.

POSITIONING THE INFANT

It is important to undertake examinations in an environment that keeps the baby comfortable. Cold babies may cry and struggle, with the result that the opportunity to get good pictures is lost and any haemodynamic information is less meaningful. Note that in an incubator the temperature may fall once the ports are open. There are often monitoring leads applied to the chest and abdomen which need to be moved before gel can be applied. In the critically ill and premature infant handling should be minimized and the gel should be warmed before use.

The infant must be exposed in the supine position with the chest and abdomen exposed (Fig. 1.4.1). Rolling onto the left side brings the heart closer to the chest wall and may improve image quality for precordial views. Extending the neck by placing a roll under the shoulders is helpful in obtaining good suprasternal images. Limitations on

movement may be imposed by the presence of other devices such as ventilators or vascular catheters.

APPROPRIATE IMAGING EQUIPMENT

The ultrasound machine needs to be configured appropriately for the neonate. It should be able to provide not just cross-sectional images, but also M-mode as well as pulsed and continuous wave Doppler. Colour flow imaging is becoming extremely valuable for the diagnosis of complex congenital heart disease in the neonate, and makes detection of ductal shunting much easier. High-frequency imaging probes of 5 MHz and 7 MHz provide the best images with adequate penetration. The transducer may be either a mechanical sector scanner or an electronic phased array. The 'footprint' (the part of the probe which touches the chest wall) varies in size. The larger the footprint and the bigger the probe, the harder it is to manoeuvre and obtain optimal views, particularly when dealing with preterm infants in incubators. Ultrasound gel is needed for the connection with the skin (acoustic coupling) and, as mentioned earlier, it should be warmed!

MANIPULATING PROBES

The probes used in conventional echocardiography are sector probes (as opposed to linear or curvilinear arrays), which provide a fan-shaped image with the point of the cone next to the transducer. The manoeuvres required to obtain

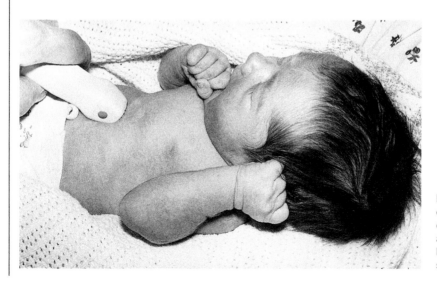

Fig. 1.4.1 Infant undergoing echocardiographic examination. Chest and abdomen exposed with infant lying supine. Probe is in the subcostal position.

appropriate images make use of three possible types of movement (Fig. 1.4.2).

- *Rotation* – the probe is rotated about the central longitudinal axis of the transducer.
- *Tilt* – the probe is moved in an axis at right angles to the image plane, bringing a new slice of the heart into view.
- *Angulation* – the probe is moved in an axis described by the image plane, extending the view at one or other of the ends of the image.

POSITIONING THE PROBE FOR SPECIFIC VIEWS

There are, by convention, a number of 'standard views' obtained from a variety of sites on the chest and upper abdomen. These will be covered in turn, highlighting variations that can be obtained where appropriate.

Once the **orientation of the heart** (see below) has been determined there are three axes which are conventionally used in describing cross-sectional images. These cut the heart in **long-axis, short-axis** and **four-chamber** planes. These three planes are at *right angles* to each other and, generally speaking, it is possible to view most of the structures of the heart through images obtained in these planes.

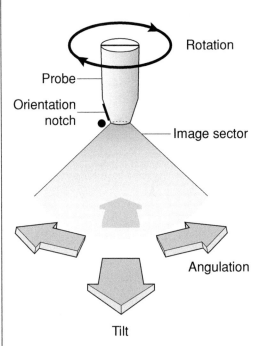

Fig. 1.4.2 Manipulation of ultrasound transducer using rotation, tilt and angulation.

It is the ability of a structure to reflect the ultrasound signal back – i.e. the echogenicity – that determines its visibility. Structures perpendicular to the oncoming ultrasound beam will be more effective reflectors. This is important with thinner elements such as the interatrial septum where 'drop-out' in certain views may appear as defects. It is important to use the most appropriate positions for the structures examined; in the case of the atrial septum, the best views (where the ultrasound beams are perpendicular to the atrial septum) are from the subcostal position, whereas apical views (with the beams in line) may give artificial drop-out.

ORIENTATION OF THE HEART

The apex of the heart is usually in the left chest, although in the neonate the bulk of the heart is often more midline. It is important to define not just the position but also the orientation of the heart, as this has implications for other structures both within and without the heart. The orientation can be defined in terms of the direction of the apex and the position of the great vessels. Only once the position and orientation are known can the transducer be manipulated to obtain the standard echocardiographic views. For the purposes of the rest of this discussion the heart will be assumed to be in the left side of the chest and normally oriented with the apex to the left (see Fig. 1.3.2). The orientation of the great vessels and abdominal viscera can be helpful in determining the orientation of the heart. Further details are given later, in Chapter 8. Normally the descending aorta is to the left of the spine and the inferior caval vein somewhat anterior and to the right within a right-sided liver (Fig. 1.4.3).

ECHOCARDIOGRAPHIC WINDOWS

Since ultrasound cannot pass through the air within the lungs the ultrasonic approach to the heart is through echocardiographic 'windows' where there is little or no air between the transducer and heart. In the newborn there are large echo windows, making imaging easier than in older children and adults. Poor quality ultrasound pictures are frequently the result of failure to place the transducer appropriately over a good echo window, or where the window is obscured by hyperexpanded lungs as in chronic lung disease, or by a pneumothorax.

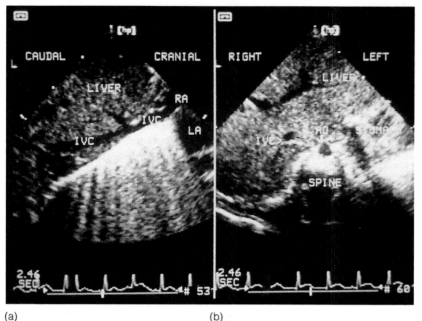

Fig. 1.4.3 (a) Subcostal saggital abdominal view showing drainage of the inferior caval vein (or inferior vena cava, IVC) into the right atrium (RA). LA, left atrium. (b) Subcostal transverse abdominal view demonstrating normal orientation with the IVC visible within the liver on the right, and the descending aorta (Ao) posteriorly to this and to the left of the midline.

There are a number of points from which good images can be obtained and it may be necessary to try all of these in order to obtain optimal images. The echocardiographic windows used most frequently (Fig. 1.4.4) are the:

- subcostal
- apical
- left parasternal
- suprasternal.

The 'standard' views can often be obtained from more than one place. Although the orientation on screen changes depending on the direction of the scanning head and screen configuration, the images are similar.

THE THREE AXES

The heart lies at an angle within the chest. Thus the 'standard' anatomical cuts (coronal, saggital, etc.) are not used. The scanning planes are related to the axis of the heart.

There are three axes which form the majority of standard views. They correspond to the mathematical x, y and z axes and are at right angles to each other. They create the long-axis, short-axis and four-chamber views. You will find it helpful to have a three-dimensional model of a normal heart beside you while going through this next, very important, section.

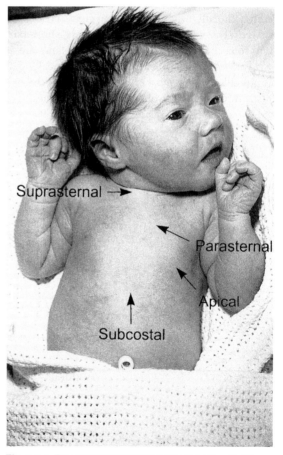

Fig. 1.4.4 The ultrasound 'windows' commonly used in cross-sectional echocardiography.

Long-axis plane

The scanning plane transects the heart along its longitudinal axis from the base and root of the aorta towards the apex (akin to slicing a green pepper longitudinally, leaving the stalk protruding from the slice). This provides an image of the left heart structures from the left atrium to the aorta with the interventricular septum and a small part of the right ventricle anteriorly. It does not show the right atrium or right ventricular outflow tract (RVOT). This image, when obtained from the left parasternal position, is the standard view from which M-mode echocardiography can assess left atrial and left ventricular dimensions and function (see Chapters 1.5 and 4). By convention parasternal long-axis images have the apex of the heart to the left and the outflow tract to the right of the picture (Fig. 1.4.5). The long axis can also be imaged from the apex of the heart.

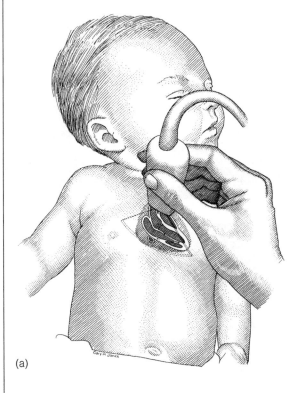

(a)

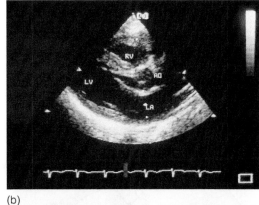

(b)

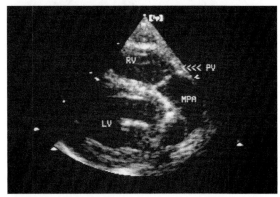

(c)

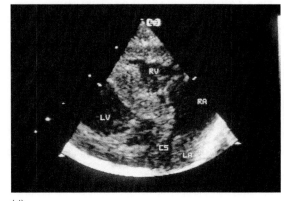

(d)

Fig. 1.4.5 (a) Diagram showing the position of the transducer and orientation of scanning plane to provide a parasternal long-axis image of the heart (see also Figure 1.3.7).
(b) Echocardiogram showing a standard parasternal long-axis image of the heart, ideal for demonstrating the left heart. The mitral valve is widely open in this diastolic frame. Ao, aorta; LV, left ventricle; RV, right ventricle.
(c) Tilting towards the left shoulder reveals a long-axis view of the main pulmonary artery (MPA) and pulmonary valve (PV).
(d) Tilting to the right, away from the left shoulder, reveals the tricuspid valve between the right atrium (RA) and right ventricle (RV). The coronary sinus (CS) is seen draining into the right atrium. LA, left atrium.

Short-axis plane

The short axis is at 90° to the long axis and cuts the heart transversely (rather like slicing rings from the green pepper). Short-axis views are obtained from the parasternal position by rotating through 90° from a long axis. Tilting of the probe allows different structures to be visualized. The standard 'midlevel' cut provides an image of the right heart as it wraps round the left ventricle and outflow tract. The right atrium, tricuspid valve, right ventricle, RVOT and main pulmonary artery can be seen around the central aortic valve and coronary arteries. By tilting up towards the sternal notch a higher cut demonstrates the right ventricular outflow, pulmonary arteries and, if present, the arterial duct (Fig 1.4.10). Tilting down towards the apex brings the left ventricle into view in a cross-section with the mitral valve structures gaping like

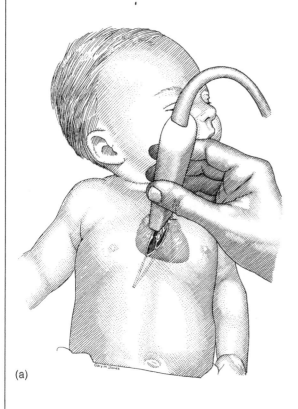

(a)

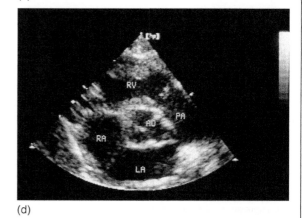

(b)

(c)

(d)

Fig. 1.4.6 (a) Diagram showing the position of the transducer and orientation of the scanning plane to provide a parasternal short-axis image of the heart at the aortic valve level.
(b) Parasternal short-axis echocardiograph at the level of the papillary muscles (towards the apex of the left ventricle).
(c) Tilting away from the apex (towards the right shoulder) brings this view of the mitral valve. AML, anterior mitral valve leaflet; PML, posterior mitral valve leaflet.
(d) Further tilt shows this cut at the aortic valve (as in part (a)). The anatomical section is shown in Figure 1.3.10. Note here how three aortic valve leaflets are seen, and how the right heart wraps around the aorta. Tilting the probe further still away from the apex demonstrates the pulmonary artery bifurcation – see Figure 2.2.9.

a 'fish mouth' as the leaflets open and close. Further manipulation of the probe in this position allows better views of RVOT, pulmonary arteries, duct and descending aorta. Short-axis images are often obtained from the parasternal position (Fig. 1.4.6) but can also be obtained subcostally.

Four-chamber plane
This third plane is at 90° to the other two and provides further images along the long axis of the

heart, cutting through the four chambers of the heart. Four-chamber views are possible from the apex (Fig. 1.4.7) and subcostal positions (Fig. 1.4.8), but not from the parasternum. The probe is placed at the apex in a near coronal plane (at 90° to the orientation that allows a 'longitudinal axis' view and parallel to the bed the infant is lying on). Tilting up towards the front of the chest brings the left ventricular outflow tract (LVOT) into view, providing the so-called 'five-chamber' view (the fifth

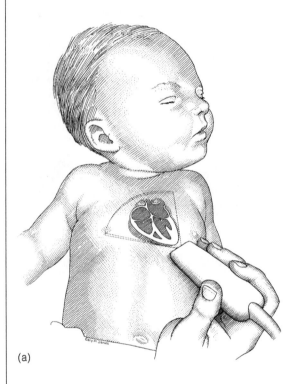

(a)

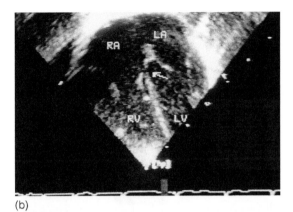

(b)

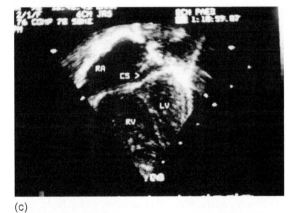

(c)

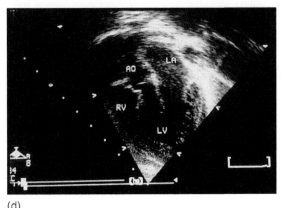

(d)

Fig. 1.4.7 (a) Diagram showing the position of the transducer and orientation of scanning plane to provide an apical four-chamber view of the heart.
(b) Apical four-chamber echocardiogram. Note that the screen has been inverted. The arrow indicates the lower position of the tricuspid valve as it arises from the septum. This region between the two atrioventricular valves is known as the atrioventricular septum, dividing the left ventricle from the right atrium. This is also shown in the anatomical section, Figure 1.3.9.
(c) Apical view of the heart with the probe angled posteriorly to bring the coronary sinus into view (not to be confused with a low atrial septal defect!).
(d) Apical view of the heart with the probe angled anteriorly bringing the left ventricular outflow tract and aortic valve into view – the so-called 'five-chamber view'.

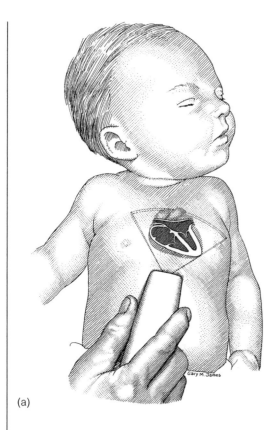

(a)

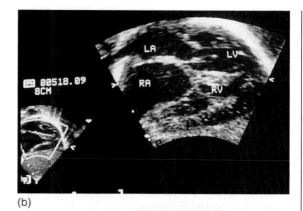

(b)

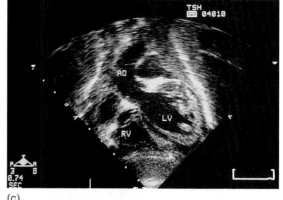

(c)

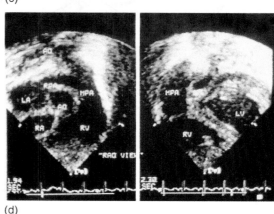

(d)

Fig. 1.4.8 (a) Diagram showing the position of the transducer and orientation of the scanning plane to provide a subcostal four-chamber image of the heart.
(b) Subcostal four-chamber image demonstrating the structures which can be seen. Note again that the screen has been inverted.
(c) Tilting the probe anteriorly brings the ascending aorta into view.
(d) *Left*: rotating anticlockwise brings the right ventricular outflow tract and pulmonary arteries into view (subcostal short-axis or 'RAO' (right anterior oblique) view). MPA, main pulmonary artery; RPA, right pulmonary artery. *Right*: rotating clockwise shows the interventricular septum and another view of the right ventricular outflow tract.

'chamber' being the aorta). Tilting back may bring the coronary sinus into view behind the left atrium.

The subcostal position allows these views to be developed and is a good position for examining the interatrial septum and much of the interventricular septum as they lie at 90° to the ultrasound waves and thus are maximally echogenic. By tilting the probe anteriorly and posteriorly much of the atrial and ventricular septums can be seen. With posterior tilt the floor of the atria, the entry of the pulmonary

veins into the left atrium can be seen, as can the coronary sinus running in the atrioventricular groove behind the left atrium and opening into the right atrium.

Rotating the probe anticlockwise in the subcostal position brings the RVOT into view anteriorly, with the right atrium posteriorly and aorta centrally. This is then a subcostal short-axis view and is analogous to the 'right anterior oblique' view in cardiac catheterization. Tilting the probe in this orientation allows other short-axis views to be obtained from the base to the apex of the heart.

GREAT VESSELS

The origin of both pulmonary arteries can usually be seen in the standard short-axis views.

The LVOT and some of the descending aorta can be seen in some of the views described above, but the ascending aorta, arch and descending aorta can only be seen in their entirety from the suprasternal window (Fig. 1.4.9). It is often useful to extend the infant's neck by placing a small roll under the shoulders so that the scanning head can be placed in the suprasternal notch. (Take care not to extubate your patient in the process!) The probe is angled so that the scan plane follows the line of the aorta. This is tilted and rotated slightly from a sagittal cut (towards the left shoulder) since the ascending arch passes to the right of the midline and the descending aorta lies to the left of the midline. By tilting the probe in this plane the aortic valve, ascending aorta, arch and descending aorta can be seen along with the distal end of the arterial duct. The right pulmonary artery is seen in cross-section as it passes underneath the ascending aorta.

A transverse cut in the suprasternal position, angled slightly posteriorly, demonstrates the innominate vein as it comes across anteriorly from the left subclavian vein to join the superior caval vein (SCV – also known as superior vena cava). (This cut, and modifications of it, is useful in assessing central lines placed from the neck or shoulder.)

The inferior caval vein (ICV – also known as inferior vena cava), in its course through the liver,

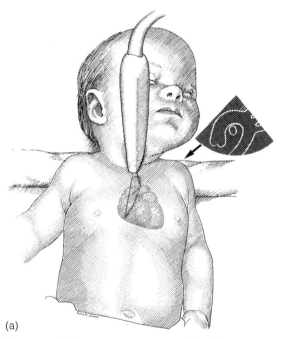

(a)

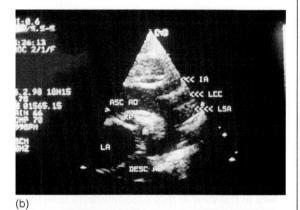

(b)

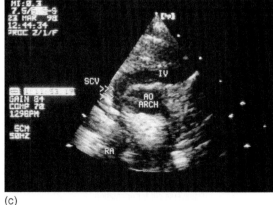

(c)

Fig. 1.4.9 (a) Diagram showing the position of the transducer and orientation of the scanning plane required to obtain views of the aortic arch with a conventional left-sided aorta. Note that a roll has been placed behind the shoulders to extend the neck.
(b) Image of the aortic arch and branches obtained from the suprasternal window. IA, innominate artery (or right brachiocephalic artery); LCC, left common carotid artery; LSA, left subclavian artery.
(c) With a transverse scanning plane, the innominate vein (IV) drains to the superior caval vein (SCV; or superior vena cava).

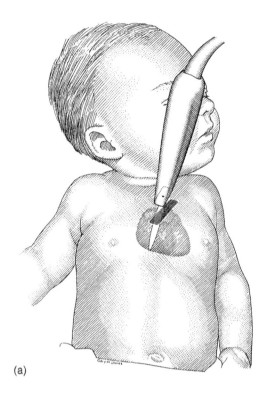

(a)

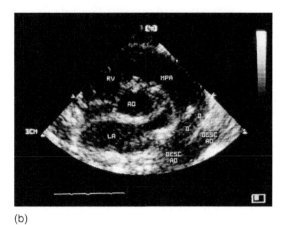

(b)

Fig. 1.4.10 (a) Drawing showing the movement of the foot of the probe required to bring the ductal view, roughly half-way between a parasternal short-axis view at the aortic valve level and a suprasternal view of the aortic arch. (b) The so-called 'ductal view'. D, the arterial duct, connects the main pulmonary artery (MPA) to the descending aorta (desc Ao). See Chapter 7.

can be seen well from the subcostal position by scanning in a sagittal orientation, vertically through the liver (Figure 1.4.3a). Angulation allows the vessel to be followed into the right atrium. The ICV is a right-sided structure and by tilting the probe slightly to the left, the descending aorta can be brought into view in a more posterior position. The mesenteric and coeliac axis arteries can often be seen in this view as they arise anteriorly from the descending aorta (Figure 7.7b).

The pulmonary veins can usually be seen entering into the back of the left atrium. However, it is often not possible to identify all four veins in a

single image, and a number of cuts from different positions may be necessary (Figure 2.23).

Table 1.4.1 summarizes the echocardiographic windows and the views often obtained from these with the heart in the usual orientation. Figure 1.4.10 shows the movement of the probe from the short axis view to obtain a view of the arterial duct; figures 1.4.11–1.4.14 summarise all the standard views described thus far.

CONCLUSION

During the first scan of an infant, it is important to follow a logical, sequential process, identifying venous return, orientation of the heart, and whether the connections between the inflow, ventricles and great arteries are normal or not. Normal anatomy must never be assumed – it should be proven. This important process is covered in more detail in Section III, Putting it into Practice, later in the book (Chapter 8). However, for now, we will continue to assume that the heart is normal in structure and orientation. The next chapter introduces M-mode echocardiography, before going on to Doppler echocardiography in part 2.

Table 1.4.1 Obtaining the standard echocardiographic views

Position	Views commonly obtained
Parasternal	Long-axis Short-axis Ductal view
Subcostal	Four-chamber Short-axis Outlet views Sagittal (descending aorta and ICV) Transverse cut for orientation
Apical	Four/Five-chamber Long-axis

Summary diagrams of standard echocardiographic views

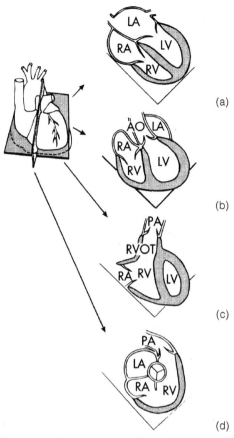

(a)

(b)

(c)

(d)

Fig. 1.4.11 Subcostal views. Figures (a), (b) and (c) are in the transverse or four chamber plane. (a) shows the four chambers. (b) is obtained with a slight anterior tilt to show the aortic outlet ('five chamber view') and (c) is further anterior showing the right ventricular outlet. To obtain the view in (d), the transducer is rotated anticlockwise through ninety degrees and shows a subcostal short axis view. (Reproduced with permission from Park Mk. *Pediatric Cardiology for Practitioners*, ed 3. St. Louis, Mosby, 1995.)

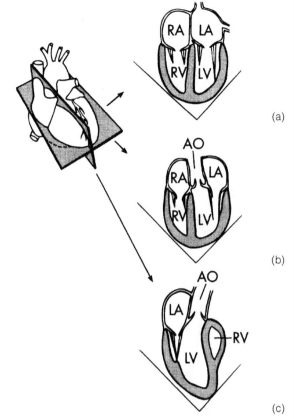

(a)

(b)

(c)

Fig. 1.4.12 Apical views. (a) is the four chamber view, and (b) the apical five chamber view including the aorta, from an anterior tilt. (c) is ninety degrees to (a) and (b) and is an apical long axis view. (Reproduced with permission from Park Mk. *Pediatric Cardiology for Practitioners*, ed 3. St. Louis, Mosby, 1995.)

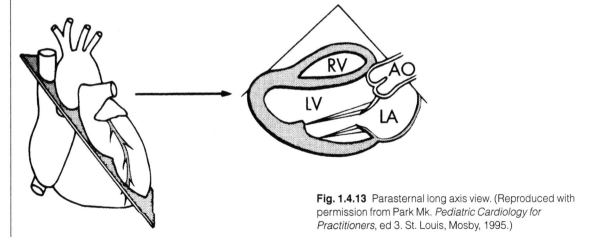

Fig. 1.4.13 Parasternal long axis view. (Reproduced with permission from Park Mk. *Pediatric Cardiology for Practitioners*, ed 3. St. Louis, Mosby, 1995.)

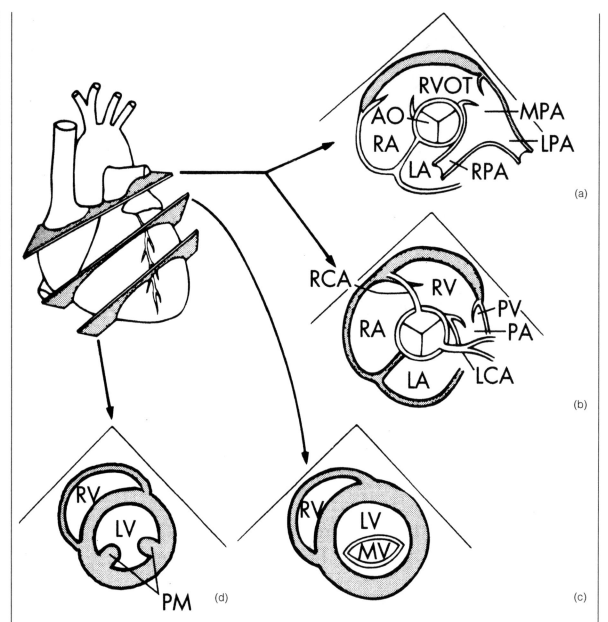

Fig. 1.4.14 Family of parasternal short axis views sweeping from the base of the heart (a) which shows the bifurcation of the pulmonary arteries, (b) shows the right and left coronary artery origins (RCA and LCA), (c) cuts through the mitral valve, and (d) cuts through the two papillary muscles near the apex of the left ventricle. (Reproduced with permission from Park Mk. *Pediatric Cardiology for Practitioners*, ed 3. St. Louis, Mosby, 1995.)

M-mode echocardiography

John Madar

INTRODUCTION

This chapter discusses the principles underlying M-mode (movement-mode) echocardiography. Examples are given of images achieved in this modality and its main indications are described.

WHAT IS M-MODE?

Cross-sectional images of the heart are generated from multiple single line scans from different parts of the heart. M-mode pictures display consecutive single lines through part of the heart, each line representing the same structure but at a different time. The lines are placed next to each other in sequence and build up a detailed picture of movement with time. This is explained more fully in Chapter 1.1 (and shown there in Fig. 1.1.3).

M-mode thus views the same structures over time during the cardiac cycle. Comparison of structure, chamber size and motion can take place with much higher frequency sampling than with cross-sectional scanning. Thus, the main value of M-mode is its ability to allow more detailed analysis of the change in cardiac structures over time and related to the cardiac cycle. Since measurement of left atrial and left ventricular dimensions are very repeatable, M-mode is the modality of choice for quantitation of dynamic indices of left atrial and ventricular function.

☞ *Practical Point*
- **M-mode is particularly good at timing cardiac events (such as the opening and closing of cardiac valves) because of the very high frequency of sampling.**

OBTAINING M-MODE IMAGES AND GENERAL PRINCIPLES

Although M-mode was available before cross-sectional echocardiography, the ability to generate a cross-sectional image of the heart before laying down the cursor defining the M-mode beam allows greater accuracy in positioning. Most machines not only allow the cursor defining the M-mode image to be overlaid on the cross-sectional image, but also display a miniaturized version of the cross-sectional image on screen simultaneously. This ensures that the operator

knows precisely where the cursor lies. If the cursor is not placed accurately, then foreshortened or otherwise inadequate and misleading images are generated.

Detection of structures is best if they lie perpendicular to the ultrasound beam, maximizing the signal, and it is important to remember that M-mode only detects movement of these structures towards and away from the probe. Parasternal views are most useful for assessing the left heart because the interventricular septum, left ventricular posterior wall, aorta and left atrial posterior wall lie perpendicular to the interrogating beam.

A simultaneous electrocardiograph (ECG) trace (which can usually be taken from the back of a standard monitor as an analogue signal and connected to the ultrasound machine) helps relate the movements of the various structures to the cardiac cycle. The 'sweep rate' of the display is analogous to the speed of an ECG trace and can usually be varied between 25 and 100 mm/s. It is usually set at 50 mm/s for most analyses.

RULES IN MAKING MEASUREMENTS ON M-MODE

1. Measurements are by convention made from 'leading edge to leading edge'.[1] The leading edge is the surface of a structure first reflecting the ultrasound signal, in practical terms that closest to the transducer, and is usually the most sharply defined.
2. Be certain the M-mode line is perpendicular to the structures being interrogated.
3. Have clear definitions of when *exactly* during the cardiac cycle measurements are to be made.

CURRENT CLINICAL USES FOR M-MODE ECHOCARDIOGRAPHY

The two main uses are outlined below.

1. To assess left ventricular function objectively by measurement of left ventricular fractional shortening, using a parasternal cut through the tips of the mitral valve.
2. To assess left atrial size as an indirect measurement of left-to-right ductal shunting, using a parasternal cut through the aortic root and left atrium.

THE NORMAL M-MODE APPEARANCES FROM THE LEFT PARASTERNUM

It is usually possible to record the movement of all four cardiac valves and gain an impression of both ventricular chambers, the left atrium and the left ventricular outflow tract. However, accurate assessment of the dimensions of right heart structures with M-mode is difficult and unreliable due to the complex way that they 'wrap around' the aorta and the nature of right ventricular contraction. The movements of the **tricuspid valve** are similar to those of the mitral valve, though more difficult to profile. The **pulmonary valve** movement is essentially the same as that of the aortic valve, but is also difficult to see well on M-mode. Timing of opening and closure of these two valves can be measured accurately with practice, and can be used to derive right ventricular systolic time intervals (discussed in more detail in Chapter 6). In M-mode echocardiography both static and dynamic measurements of both ventricular wall thickness and left atrial and left ventricular chamber size are useful. Myocardial wall thickness changes during the cardiac cycle, as do the chamber dimensions, so it is important that measurements are made at a standard time during the cardiac cycle. The usual timing for static measurements is at the end of diastole.

M-mode images can be obtained anywhere in the heart. However, in general there are two particular M-mode images which are found to be useful in analysis:

1. at the level of the mitral valve
2. through the aortic valve.

Both are obtained from the parasternal position.

M-MODE AT THE LEVEL OF THE MITRAL VALVE

The cursor is dropped through the parasternal long-axis image at the level of the mitral valve tips (see Figs 1.5.1 and 1.5.3). At this point the cursor lies across the left ventricular cavity at its widest diameter and passes through the anterior wall of the right ventricle, the right ventricular cavity, interventricular septum, left ventricular cavity and posterior wall of the left ventricle. The mitral valve leaflets should be visible throughout the cycle, opening in diastole and closing in systole. The M-

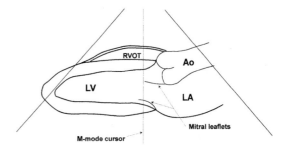

Fig. 1.5.1 Diagram to show positioning of M-mode cursor on the long-axis parasternal view.

mode derived from this view is illustrated (Fig. 1.5.4). A similar view can be obtained from an appropriate short-axis image at the same level (Fig. 1.5.2).

The **right ventricle** lies anteriorly. The shape of the ventricular cavity is such that it is not possible to place a cursor confidently across the point of maximum diameter. However, right ventricular end diastolic dimension is usually much less than that of the left ventricle (except in the first hours of life), so it can be useful to compare the two. If RV dimension (at end diastole) is similar or greater to LV dimension (at end diastole) it is likely that it is dilated – as seen in subjects in the first few hours of life or during persistent pulmonary hypertension of the newborn (PPHN), and in subjects with atrial septal defect in later life.

The **interventricular septum** is beneath the right ventricle in this section. It tends to be slightly thicker than the left ventricular posterior wall in the newborn (unlike in the adult or older child). Ratios of less than 1.3:1 (septal thickness: LV posterior wall thickness) are usual although higher ratios may be seen, particularly in PPHN. A ratio much higher than this is a classical feature of

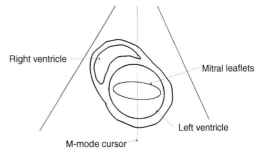

Fig. 1.5.2 Diagram to show positioning of M-mode cursor on the short-axis parasternal view; the cursor passes through the centre of the mitral valve tips.

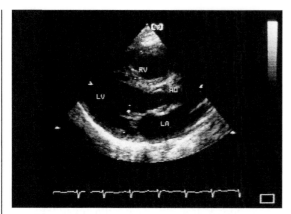

Fig. 1.5.3 Parasternal long-axis view with M-mode cursor in position. The interrogating line passes through the tips of the mitral valve. In this systolic frame, the mitral valve is closed and the aortic valve is open. This infant was 3.5 hours old, and the right ventricle is still large, making it difficult to obtain the perfect 'horizontal' interventricular septum for M-mode images of the left ventricle.

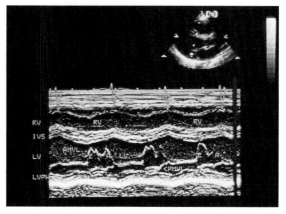

Fig. 1.5.4 Mitral valve leaflets are labelled: anterior, AMVL; posterior, PMVL. The passive filling (E) phase first causes mitral valve opening. There follows partial closure, where the leaflets come together, and then the active part of ventricular filling due to atrial contraction or the A phase. The anterior leaflet has greater excursion than the posterior leaflet.

hypertrophic cardiomyopathy or in infants of diabetic mothers or infants receiving steroids. The movement of the portion near the aortic valve parallels the aortic root moving anteriorly in systole. The septum below the mitral valve normally moves posteriorly in systole (i.e. the septum and posterior walls of the left ventricle move towards each other in systole).*

The **left ventricular cavity** is limited anteriorly by the interventricular septum and posteriorly by the left ventricular posterior wall. Its size reduces in systole as the septal and posterior walls come together with ejection. In late systole both posterior wall and septum move anteriorly.

The **mitral valve** is easily identified within the left ventricular cavity and has characteristic movements. Valves are usually thin membranous structures and cast thin echoes. Similarly, flow through valves should not be excessively turbulent and thus valve echoes should be clearly defined, not blurred. Cross-sectional echocardiography is more useful to assess both of the atrioventricular valves, but some signs are helpful. For example, in mitral stenosis, the anterior and posterior echoes fail to

separate normally during diastole and the leaflets often appear thickened.

The anterior and posterior mitral valve leaflets meet in systole (the C point) and move forward slightly in systole before separating at the beginning of diastole (the D point). After opening rapidly (D to E) they move together (E to F) before opening again with atrial contraction (A wave) and closing as systole begins again. The amplitude of excursion reflects blood flow through the valve and is less in smaller infants. Similarly the rate of diastolic closure (the E to F slope) decreases with decreasing size. The E to F slope is, in effect, a function of diastolic valve closure; flow through the mitral orifice is defined in terms of the gradient of the slope generated by a line taken across the E and F points of the valve in mm/s. A normal E:F slope in a neonate is around 40–80 mm/s. As well as decreasing with decreasing size it varies with LV end diastolic pressure and heart rate. A significant reduction in the E:F slope might suggest impaired opening such as with mitral stenosis.

The **pericardium**, anterior to the RV or behind the LV posterior wall, is usually only seen as a single line. However, in pericardial effusion an echo-free space may be present.

ASSESSING LEFT VENTRICULAR FUNCTION

Three measurements of LV function need to be discussed:

In infants with PPHN the septum may remain flat during systole or even move in the opposite direction because the right ventricle, rather than the left ventricle, is dominant. This is known as 'paradoxical septal motion', and makes accurate assessment of LV function difficult in these infants (see Chapters 4 and 9.2).

1. fractional shortening (FS) – this is by far the most useful and important single measure of LV function;
2. ejection fraction (EF);
3. velocity of circumferential fibre shortening (Vcf).

In assessing left ventricular size and function (see also Chapter 4), end diastole and and systole can be defined in different ways. The method we prefer is to use the excursion of the LV posterior wall (LVPW) to indicate the site of measurement; i.e. maximum posterior excursion of the LVPW defines end diastole and maximal anterior excursion of the LVPW defines end systole. In adults the septum can be used to time events, but the RV dominance in the newborn can make this less reliable. An alternative is (respectively) to use the R wave on the ECG (Fig. 1.5.5) and the point where the mitral valve begins to open (Fig. 1.5.6).

Left ventricular chamber measurements can be roughly related to volume by virtue of the shape of the cavity – an ellipsoid of revolution. (The same cannot be said of the right ventricle.)

Fractional shortening (FS)

Dynamic function of the left ventricle is most easily assessed using FS, which is the percentage change in LV diameter during systole.

$$FS\ \% = \left(\frac{LVEDD - LVESD}{LVEDD}\right) \times 100\%$$

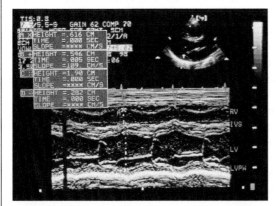

Fig. 1.5.5 Measurements made with on-line computer softwear during diastole (at the R wave on the ECG). Each measurement has a 'height', i.e. the distance between the two points; 'time', the time between the two points, which should be zero; and 'slope', which is only of relevance when measuring two points at different times. Here, A is RV dimension (0.62 cm), B is interventricular septal thickness (0.55 cm), C is LV end-diastolic dimension (or LVEDD, 1.90 cm) and D is LV posterior wall dimension (0.28 cm).

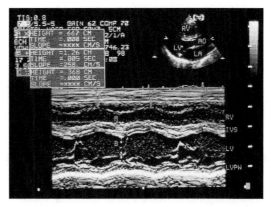

Fig. 1.5.6 Measurements at end systole (just before the opening of the mitral valve). A, interventricular septum (0.67 cm); B, LV (end-systolic) dimension (LVESD, 1.26 cm); C, LV posterior wall (0.37 cm). Fractional shortening of the left ventricle is therefore (1.90 – 1.26)/1.90 × 100 = 34%.

where LVEDD is the left ventricular end-diastolic diameter (sometimes abbreviated as LVIDd, LV internal diameter in diastole); and LVESD is the left ventricular end-systolic diameter (or LVIDs).

Normally the LV diameter decreases by around one third in systole such that fractional shortening is normally greater than 25% in the healthy newborn (and less than 41%) and greater than 28% in the older child.[2] (Lower values down to 20% are occasionally seen in healthy infants in the first day or two – probably due to the RV dominance discussed earlier.) This measurement is highly repeatable, and sequential measurement is particularly useful in the shocked infant. It is largely independent of heart rate and age but it is dependent on preload and afterload (see Chapter 4).

Ejection fraction (EF)

EF can be also derived from LVEDD and LVESD measurements but depends on assumptions about LV shape and involves cubing both measurements. Errors therefore multiply, and since the LV shape varies a lot, particularly with the RV dominance seen in the newborn, we prefer not to derive ejection fraction at all in the newborn. The equation is:

$$EF\ \% = \left(\frac{LVEDD^3 - LVESD^3}{LVEDD^3}\right) \times 100\%$$

Velocity of circumferential fibre shortening (Vcf)

Mean Vcf describes the *rate* of shortening of the V rather than the extent. It is calculated by:

$$\text{mean Vcf} = \left(\frac{\text{LVEDD} - \text{LVESD}}{\text{LVEDD}}\right) \times \text{LVET}$$

LVET is the left ventricular ejection time, usually measured from the opening and closure of the aortic valve on the M-mode trace. The normal value is 1.5 ± 0.04 circumferences/s in preterm and term infants.[3] This is further discussed in Chapter 4.

M-MODE AT THE LEVEL OF THE AORTIC VALVE

Using the same parasternal long-axis view, the cursor is aligned with the root of the aortic valve (Fig. 1.5.7). In this image the M-mode demonstrates the anterior wall of the aorta, aortic valve opening and closing with anterior and posterior leaflets meeting in diastole and opening in systole, posterior wall of the aorta, left atrium and posterior atrial wall.

The **aortic root** diameter is the distance between the parallel echoes of the anterior and posterior wall of the ascending aorta. The **aortic valve** can be seen within the aortic root which moves anteriorly during systole, and posteriorly during diastole. In diastole the aortic leaflets are together and appear as a single line. In systole the line separates into anterior and posterior leaflets before closing again. The period when the valve is open has a 'box-like' appearance (Fig. 1.5.8). In aortic stenosis, this box is reduced in depth and often has thickened edges from the echogenic dysplastic valve. With aortic incompetence the leaflets may

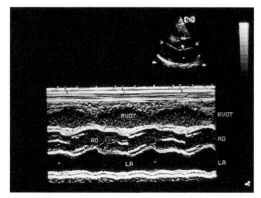

Fig. 1.5.8 The M-mode image generated. Note the large right ventricular outflow tract (RVOT) typical at this age (3.5 hours). Within the aorta (AO) the aortic valve leaflets open during systole and then close to form a 'box-like' appearance. The left atrium (LA) lies behind. Left atrial dimension is similar to that of the aortic root (see Chapter 7 to compare this appearance with that seen with a large left-to-right ductal shunt).

not appose in diastole and there may be visible vibration of the anterior leaflet of the mitral valve (on the lower cut) due to high-velocity blood flowing back into the left ventricle during diastole. In hypertrophic cardiomyopathy there may be abnormal mid systolic closure of the leaflets and abnormal systolic anterior motion of the mitral valve (known as 'SAM' among cardiomyopathy experts!).

This cut also allows the diameter of the **left atrium** to be assessed. This is useful since the left atrium dilates with increased pulmonary venous return such as with left-to-right ductal shunting. Left atrial dimension is typically measured at the end of systole (at its biggest) and is often compared with the diameter of the aortic root at the same time to create a ratio. This allows comparison between infants of different size. An increase in the LA:aortic root diameter ratio to above 1.4:1 is taken as circumstantial evidence of the presence of a large left-to-right ductal shunt in the preterm.* Table 1.5.1 lists normal values in M-mode echocardiography in newborns in the first 48 hours of life.

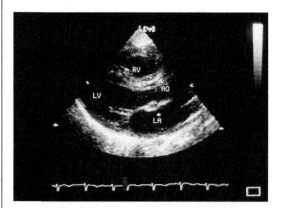

Fig. 1.5.7 Parasternal long-axis image demonstrating the position required to generate an M-mode image of the aortic root and left atrium. The interrogating line passes through the right ventricle before it passes through the aortic root at the level of the sinus of Valsava (this is the widening beyond the aortic valve from which the coronary arteries arise). The aortic valve leaflets are transected.

Such left atrial dilation might also occur with mitral regurgitation, mitral stenosis or LV dysfunction, and left atrial dilation is less marked when there is a large oval foramen and during dehydration, so this ratio should not be relied upon on its own to assess ductal shunting (see Chapter 7).

Table 1.5.1 Normal values in M-mode echocardiography in newborns in the first 48 hours of life

Cardiac dimension	Birth weight (g)					Gestation	
	600[1]	1400[1]	2300[2]	3200[2]	4500[2]	28/40[3]	Term[4] (2.7–4.6 kg)
RVAWD (mm)			2.0 (1.1–2.9)	2.5 (1.6–3.4)	3.2 (2.3–4.1)		3.0 (2.0–4.7)
RVEDD (mm)			12.5 (10.4–14.6)	13.7 (11.6–15.8)	15.6 (13.5–17.7)		11.4 (6.1–15.0)
IVSD (mm)			2.7 (2.1–3.3)	3.2 (2.6–3.8)	3.9 (3.3–4.5)		2.7 (1.8–4.0)
LVPWD (mm)			2.7 (2.0–3.4)	3.2 (2.5–3.9)	3.9 (3.2–4.6)		2.6 (1.6–3.7)
LVEDD (mm)			18.9 (16.1–21.7)	19.8 (17.0–22.6)	21.3 (18.5–24.1)	12.6	18.7 (12.0–23.3)
LVESD (mm)						7.8	13.3 (8.0–18.6)
Aortic root (mm)	0.52 (0.4–0.65)	0.63 (0.5–0.77)	10.3 (9.3–11.3)	11.2 (10.2–12.2)	12.6 (11.6–13.6)	5.6 (5.3–6.2)*	10 (8.1–12.0)
LA diameter (mm)			8.7 (6.8–10.5)	11.7 (9.8–13.5)	11.7 (9.8–13.5)		7.0 (5.0–10.0)
LV fractional shortening (%)	{----------33.5 (26.5–40.5)[5]-----------}					38 (36–40)*	35[6]
Mitral E:F slope (mm/sec)							40

All measurements quoted as mean (2 standard deviations) except* = (25th–75th quartile).

1. Reller MD, Meyer RA, Kaplan S. Normal aortic root dimensions in premature infants. *Journal of Clinical Ultrasound* 1983;11:203–205.
2. Solinger R, Elbl F, Minhas K.. *Echocardiography in the Normal Neonate Circulation* 1973;47(1):108–118.
3. Gill AB, Weindling AM. Echocardiographic assessment of cardiac function in shocked very low birthweight infants. *Archives of Disease in Childhood* 1993;68:17–21.
4. Hagan AD, Deely WJ, Sahn D, Friedman WF. Echocardiographic criteria for normal newborn infants. *Circulation* 1973;48(12):1221–1226.
5. Baylen B, Meyer RA, Korfhagen J, Benzing G, Bubb Me, Kaplan S. Left ventricular performance in the critically ill premature infant with patent ductus arteriosus and pulmonary disease. *Circulation* 1977;55:182–18.
6. Skinner JR (ed). LV fractional shortening data from personal series of infants during first three days of life. 17 healthy preterms (28–37 weeks), 37 healthy term infants.

REFERENCES

1. Sahn DJ, DeMaria A, Kisslo J, Weyman A. Recommendations regarding quantitation in M-mode echocardiography: results of a survey of echocardiographic measurements. *Circulation* 1978;6:1072–1083.

2. Gutgessell HP, Paquet M, Duff DF *et al.* Evaluation of left ventricular size and function by echocardiography. Results in normal children. *Circulation* 1977;56:457–462.

3. Sahn DJ, Deely WJ, Hagen AD *et al.* Echocardiographic assessment of left ventricular performance in normal newborns. *Circulation* 1974;49:232–236.

The Doppler effect and its applications in echocardiography

TA Whittingham

THE DOPPLER EFFECT

The Doppler effect is the change in the frequency of a wave experienced by a receiver when there is relative movement between the receiver and wave transmitter, towards or away from each other.

A commonly quoted example is the change in pitch of a train whistle from high to low as it passes an observer beside the railway track. Here the pitch (frequency) of the sound wave (whistle) reaching the observer is increased as the train approaches and decreased as it recedes, while to the train driver the pitch would remain constant throughout. If, instead, there was a whistle fixed beside the track, the train driver would hear a higher pitch as he approached it and a lower pitch after he passed it. Thus either the source or the receiver can be moving. The effect occurs for all types of waves. Some of many diverse examples include the 'red-shift' in the light received from receding stars, traffic speed detectors (which use radio waves) and ultrasonic intruder detectors.

The nature of the Doppler effect may be illustrated by means of an example involving water waves. Imagine that small waves are being generated by moving a stick up and down in the water. Once created, each wave crest (and trough) will travel across the lake at a fixed speed (c). Figure 2.1.1 shows the situations when this wave generator is on the shore (stationary transmitter) and Figure 2.1.2 shows the situation when it is in a boat (moving transmitter).

In clinical applications of the Doppler effect involving blood flow, both the transmitter and receiver are ultrasound transducers, usually housed in a single probe outside the body. The Doppler effect is here produced by the motion of scattering blood cells towards or away from the probe. Figure 2.1.3 represents a blood cell moving towards the probe.

In effect, the movement of the blood cell produces two Doppler shifts. First the cell acts as a moving receiver, experiencing a higher frequency (f_B) than that transmitted at the body surface (f_T). The cell then scatters a wave of this frequency (f_B) in all directions, including back to the receiving transducer. However, the cell is now acting as a moving transmitter, and thus the frequency (f_R) of the wave arriving back at the receiving transducer is Doppler shifted upwards again. This double action is why there is a '2' in the Doppler equation in the next section.

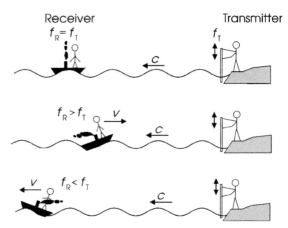

Fig. 2.1.1 The Doppler effect involving a moving receiver. If the boat is anchored, the frequency (f_R) with which the observer experiences the waves will be same as that (f_T) at which they are transmitted from the shore. If the boat steams towards the shore (at a speed v), it will meet each wave earlier and the observer will experience waves at a higher frequency. If the boat moves away from the shore, each wave will take longer to catch up with the boat and the observer will experience waves at a lower frequency.

If the blood cell had been moving away from the probe, both Doppler shifts would have contributed to a received frequency that was less than the transmitted frequency.

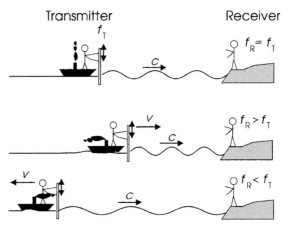

Fig. 2.1.2 The Doppler effect involving a moving transmitter. The wave generator is now mounted on the boat and the observer is stationary on the shore. If the boat steams towards the shore, the distance it moves between launching consecutive wave peaks means the distance between wave peaks is reduced. Thus more wave peaks will reach the observer in a given time, i.e. the received frequency is increased. If the boat steams away from the observer, the distance between peaks is increased and the number reaching the observer in a given time will be less, i.e. the observed frequency is reduced.

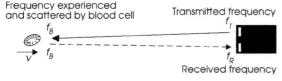

Frequency experienced and scattered by blood cell
f_B
f_B
v
Transmitted frequency
f_T
Received frequency
f_R

Fig. 2.1.3 A blood cell moving towards a Doppler probe.

THE DOPPLER SHIFT AND THE DOPPLER EQUATION

The difference (f_D) between the actual transmitted frequency (f_T) and that observed by the receiver (f_R) is called the Doppler shift frequency, or simply the Doppler shift or the Doppler frequency:

$$f_D = f_R - f_T$$

Note that f_D is positive if $f_R > f_T$, and negative if $f_R < f_T$. If the target were to move directly towards or away from the probe, the Doppler shift would be proportional both to the velocity (v) of the moving scatterer, expressed as a fraction of the speed of sound (c), and to the transmitted frequency (f_T):

$$f_D = 2\ (v/c)\ f_T$$

Thus if v is 1% of the speed of sound (c), f_D will be 2% of the transmitted frequency (f_T).

In general, blood cells will travel at some angle (θ) to the probe axis (Fig. 2.1.4). Since it is motion along the probe axis that is responsible for the Doppler effect, it is not simply the speed (v), but the component of the velocity which is directly in line with the probe axis that is relevant.

Hence, $v \cos \theta$ must replace v and the more general **Doppler equation** becomes:

$$f_D = 2\ (v \cos \theta/c)\ f_T$$

Blood cells and all moving structures in the body have speeds of no more than a few metres per

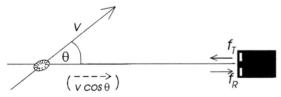

v
θ
$(v \cos\theta)$
f_T
f_R

Fig. 2.1.4 The figure represents a blood cell moving with a speed v at an angle θ to the probe axis. The velocity which will determine the Doppler shift is the rate at which the distance between the blood cell and the probe is changing. This will be less than v itself, depending on the angle θ; if θ were 0° it would be v and if θ were 90° it would be zero. In general, the component of v in line with the probe axis is $v \cos \theta$.

second, i.e. about 0.1% of the speed of sound. Consequently Doppler shifts using typical transmitted frequencies of a few megahertz will be a few kilohertz or less.

In clinical applications of the Doppler effect we are interested in finding out about v, having measured f_D, and for this it is more useful to rearrange the equation to:

$$v = (c/2)\ (f_D/f_T)\ (1/\cos \theta)$$

If θ is known (as it is when duplex equipment is used), it is possible to find the blood speed (v), since the speed of sound in blood can be substituted for c, and f_T is known. If θ is not known, an absolute value for v cannot be obtained. However, as long as the probe is held at a constant angle to the blood flow, there is a fixed proportionality between v and f_D. It is often sufficient simply to know the ratio of the values of v at different times in the cardiac cycle or at closely situated sites, and this can be found from the ratio of the corresponding values of f_D.

THE DOPPLER SIGNAL AND THE DOPPLER SPECTRUM

The function of a Doppler device is to present a 'Doppler signal' to the operator, indicating the speed(s) with which blood in a particular region is moving and, in relative terms, how much blood is moving at each velocity towards or away from the probe.

Every moving blood cell or clump of blood cells can be considered to be a target generating its own Doppler signal. The Doppler signal generated by the scattered wave from each cell is a sinusoidal signal with:

1. a frequency equal to the Doppler shift in the ultrasound wave scattered back to the probe by the target;
2. an amplitude proportional to the amplitude of the ultrasound wave scattered back to the probe by the target.

Since the Doppler shift produced by moving blood cells is never more than a few kHz, applying the Doppler signal to a loudspeaker will produce an audible signal. The frequency (pitch) of this audible signal is equal to the Doppler shift, and the loudness indicates the strength of the scattered wave.

For a group of blood cells, all moving at the same speed, the audible Doppler signal would be a

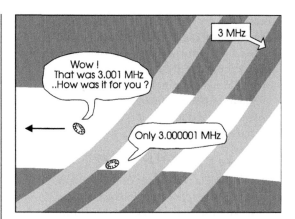

The slower the cell, the smaller the Doppler shift experienced due to it acting as a moving receiver. It also produces a smaller Doppler shift as it scatters the wave back to the probe, acting then as a moving transmitter.

pure note or whistle with a frequency (i.e. pitch) equal to the corresponding Doppler shift f_D. A high-frequency note would thus indicate high-speed cells producing a large Doppler shift, while a low-frequency note would indicate low-speed cells producing a small Doppler shift.

In practice, the region examined by a Doppler device will include millions of cells moving at a range of speeds, and possibly in many directions. The Doppler signal will thus be the sum of millions of weak sinusoidal signals and the audible version will be made up of a spectrum of notes. Just as, when listening to music, the ear and brain of the observer analyse this spectrum, to give an appreciation of which frequencies are present, and with what relative loudness. These frequencies correspond to the speeds of the blood cells, and their relative loudnesses correspond to the relative numbers of cells with those speeds.

There are generally more high-frequency notes than low-frequency ones since relatively few blood cells are close to the vessel wall and therefore moving slowly. Doppler signals from blood therefore have a 'swishy' sound rather than being the pure note or whistle that a single target would produce. The experienced operator soon recognizes turbulence since it creates a much broader spectrum of noises. Stenoses cause acceleration of blood and thus high frequency signals.

Spectral analysis

The Doppler signal may also be analysed electronically in terms of frequency and power and presented as a visible signal (as well as the audible one) on a TV screen or a paper record. Such 'spectral analysis' can give quantified information about the distribution of velocities in a blood vessel and, if the angle θ is known, their absolute values.*

In the representation shown in Figure 2.1.5, (a) represents a high-power Doppler signal from a single, strongly reflecting target moving towards the probe, decreasing its speed in a series of steps; (b) represents a low-power Doppler signal from a single, weakly reflecting target continuously oscillating alternately towards and away from the source; while (c) represents the spectrum of Doppler signals that might be obtained from within a blood vessel in which the flow is constant and away from the probe. The fact that the signal strength is greatest for the higher (−ve) frequencies indicates that the fast-moving blood cells are greater in number (and hence scatter more power) than the slow-moving cells. The narrow band of missing signal on each side of the central line ($f_D = 0$) is due to the suppression of low frequencies by the wall thump filter (see below).

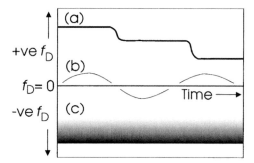

Fig. 2.1.5 Spectral analyser display. Distance above or below the baseline indicates the frequency of the Doppler signal. The grey level indicates the power of the Doppler signal. The break in the signal near the baseline ($f_D = 0$) is due to the 'wall thump' filter.

CONTINUOUS WAVE (CW) DOPPLER

The simplest form of Doppler instrument is a 'continuous wave (CW)' device. In its simplest form

---

Note that many spectrum analysers label the vertical axis directly as speed, with units of cm/s, instead of as frequency, with units of kHz. Operators should be aware that, unless they have specifically 'told' the machine the value of the angle θ (as is possible for duplex scanners, see later), then the machine has assumed a value of $\theta = 0°$. The speed scale will then only be accurate if the direction of blood flow is in line with the probe axis.

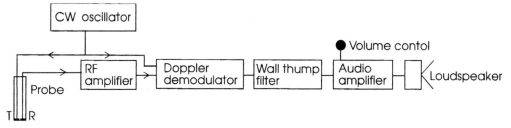

Fig. 2.1.6 Block diagram of a non-directional CW Doppler system.

this produces an audible Doppler signal, but more advanced models may incorporate paper chart outputs or display screens showing a spectrum analysis of the signal.

Figure 2.1.6 illustrates the functioning of a 'non-directional' device. A directional system, producing separate signals for forward and reverse flow (towards or away from the probe respectively) requires a special demodulator that can sense whether f_D is positive or negative, followed by two separate channels, each with its own wall thump filter, amplifier and loudspeaker.

A CW probe contains two transducers, one that continuously transmits and one that continuously receives (Fig. 2.1.7). Each is similar to the transducers used for imaging, except that there is no absorbing backing layer, since short pulses are not required, and the energy absorbed by a backing layer reduces sensitivity. Another difference is that there is usually no lens. The radiating faces of the transducers are usually either rectangular or in the form of back-to-back 'D' shapes, to make maximum use of the available area.

The **crossover region**, common to both the transmission and reception beams, defines the volume in which a moving target must be in order for it to cause the instrument to generate a Doppler signal (Fig. 2.1.8). The shape and size of the crossover region depends on the size and shape of the transmission and reception beams, and on the

relative inclination of each to the principal axis of the probe. The greater the inclination, the more superficial the crossover region. The operating frequency is also relevant – high frequencies restrict penetration due to attenuation, as well as generating narrower beams and thus smaller crossover regions.

The electronic circuit that produces the Doppler signal is known as a **Doppler demodulator**. There are a variety of types, but the commonest approach is to multiply the received signal by the electrical signal (frequency f_T) driving the transmission transducer. For a single moving target the received signal would be a weak sinusoid (frequency f_R) and the product would be a high-frequency $(f_R + f_T)$ sinusoidal ripple riding on a low-frequency $(f_R - f_T)$ sinusoid, as shown in Figure 2.1.9. The amplitude of both high- and low-frequency sinusoids is proportional to that of the received signal. Thus, extracting the low-frequency $(f_R - f_T)$ signal by suitable low-pass filters provides a signal with the desired frequency (f_D) and amplitude characteristics of the Doppler signal.

Once formed, the Doppler signal can be amplified by an audio amplifier and applied to a loudspeaker. In practice, one further stage is included before this. This is a **wall thump filter**, designed to reject Doppler signals with frequencies lower than around 100 Hz. This is necessary because there are a number of slow-moving

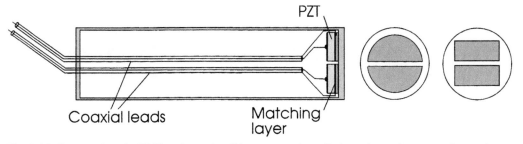

Fig. 2.1.7 Construction of a CW Doppler probe. Either rectangular or D-shaped transducers may be used.

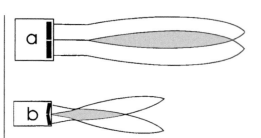

Fig. 2.1.8 The crossover region. (a) Low frequency, no inclination. Suitable for blood flow at a range of depths. (b) High frequency, slight inclination. Suitable for superficial blood flow.

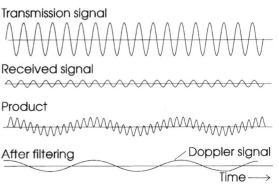

Fig. 2.1.9 Doppler demodulation by multiplication of the received signal with the transmitted drive signal.

interfaces in the body that reflect ultrasonic waves with much greater amplitude than that of the very weak waves scattered from blood cells. Heart chamber or arterial walls are important examples. The Doppler signals from such interfaces would have very much greater amplitude than those from moving blood cells. Before the amplification could be increased sufficiently to hear the blood Doppler signal, these larger signals would drive the amplifier into saturation. Fortunately the low speed of such interfaces means they produce Doppler frequencies that are low compared with most blood flow signals, and so they can blocked by the high-pass wall thump filter. Nevertheless, this does involve the sacrifice of the signal from the slowest blood cells, and produces a blank region near the f_D = 0 axis on the spectrum analyser display, as indicated in Figure 2.1.5.

PULSED DOPPLER (DUPLEX)

There are many occasions when it is desired to investigate the blood flow in a particular part of the heart or in a particular blood vessel. A CW Doppler device is of limited use in such cases as it will

produce Doppler signals from moving targets anywhere in the crossover region of the transmission and reception beams, irrespective of their ranges. A pulsed Doppler system solves the problem by pulsing the ultrasound transmissions, and presenting a Doppler signal only from those echo pulses that arrive over a time interval corresponding to the required depth range. The small region of tissue for which Doppler signals are presented is known as the **sample volume**.

At their simplest, pulsed Doppler instruments can be stand-alone devices, of the same general size as a CW Doppler device, but with the addition of controls to set the required depth interval. More usually, they form part of a **duplex scanner** (Fig. 2.1.10), which is simply a B-mode (cross-sectional) scanner with pulsed Doppler facilities built-in. A duplex scanner allows the operator to see the sample volume superimposed on a B-mode scan, thereby greatly facilitating its correct placement (Fig. 2.1.11). The **Doppler line**, representing the axis of the **Doppler beam**, may be placed as desired. A **Doppler cursor** (sample volume cursor or **range**

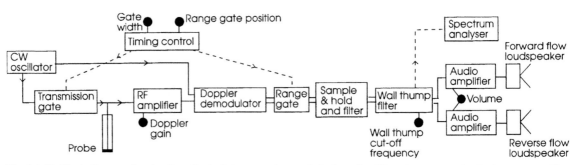

Fig. 2.1.10 Block diagram showing the principal stages and controls in the pulsed Doppler system of a duplex scanner. The double line between the audio stages indicates that there are two channels, one for forward flow and one for reverse flow. There are thus two sample and hold circuits, two low-pass filters, two wall thump filters, two audio amplifiers, etc.

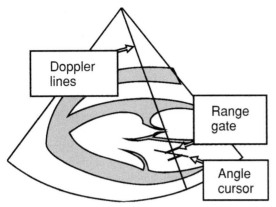

Fig. 2.1.11 Duplex scanner display. The Doppler beam angle, range gate depth, range gate width and angle cursor can all be adjusted by the operator.

gate) consisting of a pair of markers may be set to define the beginning and end of the sample volume. The separation of these markers defines the axial extent of the sample volume (**gate width**). A further valuable feature of a duplex display is that the operator can rotate an **angle cursor** so that it is parallel to the estimated direction of the blood flow, thereby giving the machine the angle θ needed to convert measurements of f_D into values of v, using the Doppler equation.

A pulsed Doppler system is similar to a CW Doppler system, except that the transmitted (and hence the returning) waves are in the form of

pulses. The transmitted pulses can be considered as being fragments of a CW transmission and the returning echoes can be considered as fragments of the received continuous wave signal that such a CW transmission would produce. Figure 2.1.12 illustrates the situation for a single moving target. The dashed waveforms represent how the transmitted (T) and received (R) signals would be if the transmission were continuous. Demodulation by multiplication of T with R would produce the continuous Doppler signal shown as a dashed line. Because only parts (bold) of the T signal are actually transmitted, only the corresponding sections (bold) of the R signal are actually produced and received as echo pulses. Although the dashed waveform T is not continuously transmitted, it is available as a reference signal, so that the corresponding sections of the Doppler signal are generated by multiplying T with the received echo pulses.

The amplitude of the Doppler signal is zero between each returning echo, and so the Doppler signal from a single target would consist of a sequence of 'samples' of the corresponding CW Doppler signal, one for each transmitted pulse (Fig. 2.1.12). These samples would only occur when the echoes reached the transducer, at times after transmission corresponding to the two-way travel time between the probe and the target.

If there were other moving targets at other ranges, they too would produce a sampled form of

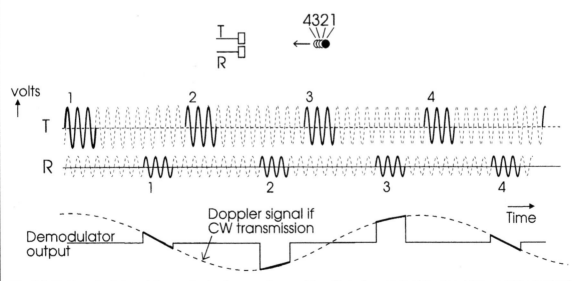

Fig. 2.1.12 For a single target, the received echoes can be considered to be fragments of the signal that would be received from a continuous transmission. Consequently only fragments (samples) of the Doppler signal are produced. Note that, in practice, the intervals between pulses would be hundreds of times longer than the pulses.

Doppler signal, but these samples would occur at different times to those of the first target. It is therefore possible to exclude Doppler signals from all targets except those in a desired range interval by having an electronic 'range gate' that only opens when echoes from that range are due back at the receiver (Fig. 2.1.13).

In the short time period represented in Figures 2.1.12 and 2.1.13, only four transmission pulses, and hence only four samples of the Doppler signal, were considered. Figure 2.1.14 shows a longer sequence of range-gated samples on a more compressed time scale. Although the signal consists only of samples, the amplitude and frequency of the signal is clear. A smooth continuous version of the Doppler signal is recovered by a 'sample and hold' circuit, which holds the signal steady between samples at the value of the previous sample. Further filtering removes the abrupt rises and falls at the sample times.

Pulsed Doppler systems are always directional, so once formed the Doppler signals are allocated to forward or reverse channels as appropriate. Each channel has a wall thump filter, audio amplifier and loudspeaker. The two channels are presented above and below the baseline ($f_D = 0$), respectively, of a spectrum analyser. The probe of a pulsed Doppler system contains just a single transducer that first acts as a transmitter and then as a receiver. Unlike a CW probe, this transducer has a backing layer, since reasonably short pulses are required (e.g. between 3 and 20 cycles, set by the 'gate width' control).

Summary of the principal controls on a duplex pulsed Doppler system

- **Range gate position.** This control(s) is used to position the sample volume at the desired place in the B-mode image. This may be a 2D tracker ball or, separate range and scan line select controls. The distance of the sample volume from the transducer defines the delay between transmission and the opening of the range gate.
- **Gate width.** This sets the duration for which the range gate is open, and hence the depth dimension of the sample volume.
- **Doppler gain.** The Doppler gain control allows the gain of the RF amplifier to be set just high enough to give a good signal, without amplifying the electronic noise any more than necessary.
- **Wall thump cut-off frequency.** This control allows the wall thump filter to be set to lose as little of the low-frequency Doppler signal (from slow-moving blood) as possible. One control affects both the wall thump filters in both channels equally.
- **Volume.** The volume control affects the audible sound level in both channels equally.

ALIASING IN PULSED DOPPLER SYSTEMS

The Nyquist upper limit for f_D

There is a penalty associated with the ability of a pulsed Doppler system to isolate a Doppler signal

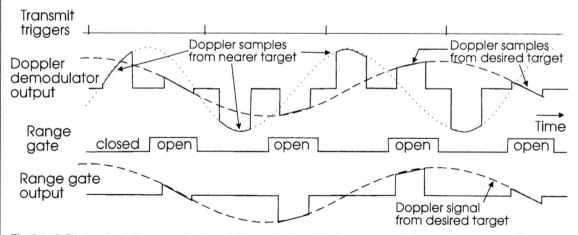

Fig. 2.1.13 The *two* dashed curves at the demodulator output show the Doppler signals that would be produced by *two* targets if continuous waves were transmitted. Since pulses are transmitted, only 'samples' of these signals will actually be produced, each sample lasting as long as the original pulse (and echo). A range gate that opens at a particular time after every transmission selects only those sections of the demodulator output that are produced by targets in a selected range interval.

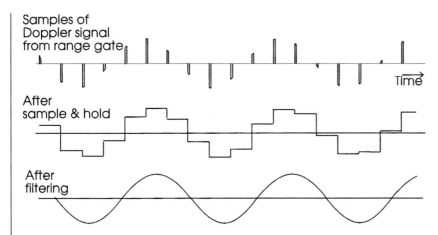

Fig. 2.1.14 The samples from the range gate are reconstituted into a continuous Doppler signal of the correct frequency.

from a specific range. Unlike a CW system, which can measure Doppler frequencies without any practical upper limit, pulsed Doppler systems have an upper limit (known as the Nyquist limit) to the Doppler frequency that can be measured.

In order to measure the frequency of any cyclic signal from a sampled version, the sampling frequency must be at least twice the frequency of the signal (Shannon's sampling theorem). In the case of pulsed Doppler, there is one sample for every transmitted pulse, so the number of transmitted pulses per second (the pulse repetition frequency, or simply prf) must be at least twice the frequency of the signal. In terms of the Doppler shift, the Doppler shift must lie between minus and plus half the prf:

$$f_{D\,max} = \pm\, prf/2$$

Figure 2.1.15 gives some insight into the problem and the reason for this limit. The prf is the same for the two signals (a) and (b), giving about 8 samples per cycle for the low-frequency signal (a), but less than two samples per cycle for the high-frequency signal (b). Whereas the sampled version of the

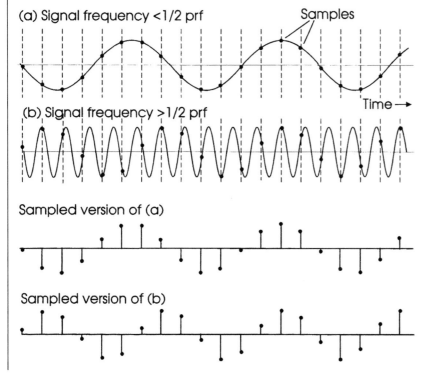

Fig. 2.1.15 The high frequency of sampled signal (b) means that the sampling frequency is less than twice the signal frequency. This leads to incorrect frequency measurement (aliasing).

lower frequency signal gives a clear indication of the true frequency, the sampled version of the higher frequency appears to have a frequency much less than in the original signal. The frequency in (b) exceeded the half prf limit, and so a false frequency measurement resulted. The production of false frequency estimates due to under-sampling is known as **aliasing**.

On a spectrum analyser display, nothing is shown outside the ±1/2 prf Nyquist frequency limits. If there are frequencies in the signal that are beyond the Nyquist limit (plus or minus), a spectrum analyser will add or subtract complete multiples of the prf to make it lie within the range ± 1/2 prf.

The spectrum (Fig. 2.1.16) appears as if the part of the spectrum beyond the upper or lower Nyquist limit has been 'wrapped around' behind the display to re-emerge and continue from the opposite limit.

What to do about aliasing

The Baseline shift. Control moves the $f_D=0$ baseline and the entire spectrum down the display. That part of the spectrum that is moved off one end of the display reappears at the opposite end. However, this is only a cosmetic operation which does not separate the aliased part of a signal from any genuine signal in the opposite direction which it may overlap.

Reduce the Doppler frequency. Reduce f_T (possibly meaning changing the probe), or increase the angle θ between the probe axis and the blood flow direction, in order to give a lower f_D. It is the Doppler shift f_D that has a limit, not the blood speed (v) itself.

Adjust the SCALE control. This control sets the maximum (full scale) Doppler frequency (positive and negative) that the spectrum display represents. Adjusting this will automatically increase the prf to twice the full scale Doppler frequency selected.

However, it will be found that the full scale Doppler frequency cannot be set above a certain limit, which will be inversely proportional to the depth to which the range gate is set. This follows from the requirement that the time between pulses must not be less than the time for the two-way trip to the sample volume. Thus setting a deep range gate means a low prf, and hence a low Nyquist limit and a low limit to the maximum SCALE setting.

Select HIGH PRF MODE. As mentioned above, the time between transmission pulses is normally made equal to or longer than the time needed for the pulse to make the two-way trip to the sample volume and back. This ensures there can be no doubt about which transmission pulse was responsible for any particular echo. In 'high pulse repetition frequency (high prf)' mode, the prf is increased to double or triple this normal limit. This increases the Nyquist limit by the same factor, but at the cost of introducing uncertainty about which transmission pulse was responsible for a given echo, and therefore creating ambiguity about the range of the target.

Thus, if the prf is increased to twice the normal limit, it would be impossible to say if a particular echo was due to a near target responding to the last

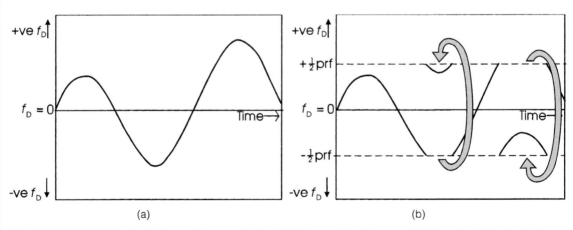

Fig. 2.1.16 (a) A CW Doppler device produces no aliasing. (b) The same target measured with a pulsed Doppler device. Aliasing occurs when the Doppler shift exceeds ± ½ prf.

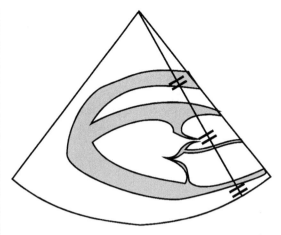

Fig. 2.1.17 Multiple sample volumes on a duplex scanner display when 'high prf' mode is selected.

transmission or a deeper target responding to the transmission before that.

Figure 2.1.17 illustrates the display on a duplex scanner where the prf is three times the normal limit. The Nyquist limit is trebled but three possible sample volumes are indicated. The ambiguity in range is not always a problem since it is often possible to eliminate all but one of the candidates for a particular Doppler signal. In this example, a high-frequency signal typical of a high-speed jet would only be likely to come from the middle sample volume (which is just above the aortic valve).

Switch to CW Doppler for the Doppler frequency measurement. The pulsed Doppler will have identified the location of the high-speed flow. Investigating this site with a CW probe or selecting CW Doppler on a duplex system (if available) will then allow the large Doppler frequency to be measured.

☞ *Practical Point*
- **To overcome aliasing with pulsed Doppler one can use a lower frequency probe, reduce the angle of insonance, increase the frequency scale, use high prf mode, or CW Doppler.**

ESTIMATION OF PRESSURE DIFFERENCES FROM DOPPLER MEASUREMENTS

The change in blood pressure across a constriction in a vessel, or a stenosed heart valve, can be estimated by comparing the blood speeds before and immediately after the constriction. This can be of enormous clinical value – examples are presented in Chapters 2.3 and 6.

The technique makes use of a simplified form of Bernoulli's equation for the gain in kinetic energy of liquid subject to acceleration due to a pressure gradient. The simplified equation assumes that there is steady flow, that hydrostatic pressure changes due to differences in elevation are negligible, and that the viscosity and compressibility of the liquid are negligible. These assumptions are satisfied for most applications to blood flow through stenosed cardiac valves.

Referring to Figure 2.1.18, and representing the density of blood as ρ, the blood pressure and maximum blood speed at the high pressure side of the constriction as p_1 and v_1, respectively, the pressure in the constriction (and hence in the vessel immediately downstream) as p_2 and the maximum blood speed in the constriction (and hence in the jet immediately beyond the constriction) as v_2, the equation is:

$$p_1 - p_2 = (1/2\rho v_{12}^2) - (1/2\rho v_1^2)$$

Since the relative change in speed across a stenosed heart valve is large ($v_2 > v_1$), the final term ($1/2\rho v_1^2$) is relatively small and can be ignored, leading to an even more simplified form of the equation:

$$p_1 - p_2 = 4\ v_2^2$$

where it is assumed that blood speed* is expressed in units of m/s and blood pressure is expressed in units of mmHg.

Important notes on the simplified Bernoulli equation in clinical pratice

- The pressure difference using the peak systolic speed is an *instantaneous* value. It should not be confused with the difference between peak pressure values measured (say by a pressure transducer) at opposite sides of a stenosed valve,

---

Frequently the jet speed is so high that aliasing prevents it from being measured using pulsed Doppler, even by selecting high prf mode or increasing the angle θ. It is then necessary to revert to CW Doppler. This task is much easier with some modern scanning systems that can generate a steerable CW crossover region as well as operate in imaging and pulsed Doppler modes, all with a single probe.

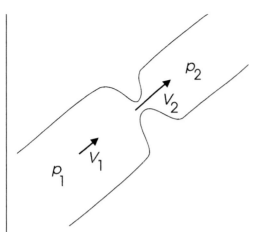

Fig. 2.1.18 Changes in pressure and velocity across a constriction are related by Bernoulli's equation.

which may occur at slightly different times and is often lower.

- One of the assumptions made in Bernoulli's equation is that there is steady blood flow. It cannot therefore be applied when the driving pressure is changing rapidly, for instance during early systole.
- The maximum speed (v_2) in the jet should be measured, close to the constriction, before the jet loses its identity and speed. If pulsed Doppler is being used, choose a large sample volume to reduce the chance of missing the maximum value and thus underestimating the pressure drop.
- The correct $\cos\theta$ correction should be made, bearing in mind that the jet is not always in line with the vessel axis. Care should be taken to record the highest velocity, ideally combining several approaches. Colour flow mapping (CFM), discussed in the next section, is useful for visualizing the orientation of eccentric jets.
- A pulsed Doppler check of the blood speed (v_1) in the region just upstream of a stenosis may be worthwhile. If the blood speed here is significant (such as aortic valve stenosis combined with subaortic stenosis), then the fourth term ($1/2\rho v_1^2$) should be included in the Bernoulli equation, i.e.

$$p_1 - p_2 = 4\left(v_2^2 - v_1^2\right)$$

COLOUR DOPPLER IMAGING

Introduction

This is a facility offered on some duplex scanners whereby a colour map of Doppler information is overlaid on a real-time cross-sectional image. Recalling that a Doppler signal from blood has two characteristics – frequency and power – it is possible to represent the value of either of these at a particular part of the image by a suitable choice of colour. If the frequency of the Doppler signal is used to determine the colour, it is called colour flow mapping (CFM) or colour flow imaging (CFI), whereas if the power of the Doppler signal is colour encoded, it is called power Doppler imaging.

Colour flow mapping (CFM)

Introduction

The operator defines a 'colour box' on the B-mode scan (Fig. 2.1.19). This is made up of Doppler interrogation lines emanating from the probe, each consisting of a column of **colour pixels**. Within the colour box, the grey levels of the B-mode image are replaced by colours representing *the mean Doppler shift within the volume corresponding to that colour pixel*. There is no universally agreed colour code, but a common arrangement is to have positive Doppler shifts shown in red and negative shifts shown in blue. Generally, the greater the frequency shift, the more saturated the colour.

Within each complete frame of the colour flow image, all the B-mode scan lines and all the Doppler lines must be interrogated. In order to prevent the Doppler measurements from slowing down the scanning rate excessively, the box is usually considerably smaller than the B-mode scan area and the colour pixels are larger than the grey-scale pixels of which the B-mode image is composed. The ultrasound beam completes a B-mode sweep and then a sweep through the colour box, making Doppler measurements down each Doppler line in turn.

There is a range gate and hence a sample volume for each colour pixel in the Doppler line. As for ordinary pulsed Doppler, each transmission–reception sequence results in one sample of the Doppler signal from targets in a sample volume. The same transmitted pulse interrogates all sample volumes along a single Doppler line, so each transmission provides one sample of Doppler signal for each colour pixel in the line. Successive samples from each sample volume are digitized and processed, by a device known as an autocorrelator, to provide an estimate of the mean frequency for

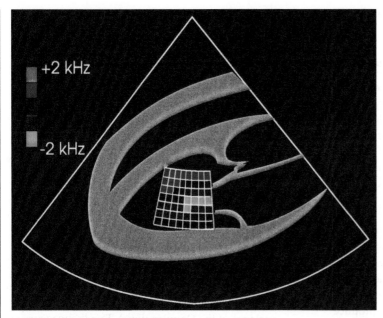
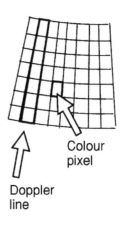

Fig. 2.1.19 Representation of a CFM scan. The boundaries of the colour box and of the individual colour pixels are shown in white – they would not be evident in a real scan.

that sample volume, and hence determine the colour of the corresponding colour pixel.

The lowest Doppler frequency and the accuracy of the frequency measurement is limited to the reciprocal of the time spent interrogating each Doppler line. Thus, for example, if samples of a Doppler signal were obtained over a period of 1 ms, the lowest Doppler frequency that could be measured would be 1 kHz (=1/(1 ms)) and the accuracy of the frequency measurements would be limited to 1 kHz.

If a useful level of accuracy and a reasonable lower frequency limit are to be achieved, it is therefore necessary to spend a few milliseconds on each Doppler line, giving time for several transmit–receive sequences along it.

If a lower Doppler frequency limit (and accuracy) of say 500 Hz and a colour box containing say 40 Doppler lines are required, then at least 80 ms (=40 × 2 ms) will be needed to perform the Doppler part of the scan. To this must be added another 20 ms or so for the B-mode part. Thus, frame rates may drop to as low as 10 frames/s (=1/100 ms) when colour Doppler is selected, as against say 50 frames/s in B-mode only. It is evident that the higher the frame rate, or the larger the colour box, the lower the accuracy of the mean frequency measurements and the faster

blood must travel before it will be shown in colour.

Some useful CFM controls (names may vary between machines)

- **Scale.** The **scale** control can be adjusted to set the positive and negative Doppler frequencies that corresponds to the extremes of the colour scales. There is an upper limit to the full scale frequency that can be selected, and this reduces as the maximum depth of the colour box increases. This is because the machine automatically tries to increase the prf to twice the full scale frequency in order to avoid aliasing, but, just as in normal pulsed Doppler, the prf is limited by the maximum depth.
- **Colour quality.** There may be a **colour quality** control which will determine the time spent on each Doppler line and hence the trade-off between the accuracy of each Doppler frequency measurement and frame rate. If low quality is selected, the frame rate will increase but there will considerable frame to frame, and pixel to pixel, variation in the colour of a region of blood, giving it a 'muddy' appearance.
- **Grey level priority.** This determines how dark the B-mode grey level has to be at each point in

the colour box before it is replaced by the appropriate Doppler colour.

Points to note when using CFM mode

- The colour of a pixel represents mean Doppler frequency, not blood speed directly. Recall that the constant in the Doppler equation relating Doppler shift to blood speed involves cos θ. Hence blood in a curved vessel might have the same speed everywhere, but it will produce a different Doppler shift, and therefore be shown in different colours, as its angle to the ultrasound Doppler lines changes.

- As in all forms of pulsed Doppler there is a maximum Doppler frequency (positive and negative) that can be measured (the Nyquist limit). If Doppler frequencies higher than this limit (corresponding to the extremes of the colour scale) are present, they will produce aliasing. Aliasing is shown by an abrupt change of colour from that representing full scale in one direction to that representing full scale in the other direction, e.g. from bright red to bright blue, or vice versa (Fig. 2.1.20). However, if the colour changes progressively with position from,

say, red through black to blue, then it represents a genuine reversal of direction (perhaps a local flow eddy) rather than aliasing.

- The slow frame rates of CFM mean that haemodynamic conditions can change between the start and end of a frame. This can result in misleading artifacts. Thus, for example, a frozen image may suggest that flow at one point of a vessel is to the right, but further along the vessel it is to the left. In reality, at any moment, the flow may well have been in the same direction throughout, but that at one end was captured when flow was in one direction and that at the other when the flow had reversed.

Showing turbulence as colour

As well as being able to calculate the mean frequency of a sampled signal, an autocorrelator can simultaneously measure a quantity known as the **variance** of the Doppler signal. This is a measure of the range (bandwidth) of frequencies in the Doppler signal. If the flow is turbulent there could be a wide range of speeds and directions in the flow within a certain pixel. Variance can therefore be a useful guide to the degree of turbulence present in the blood flow, and many CFM systems allow the operator to use the colour spectrum to show this instead of mean frequency. In some systems, provision is made for showing mean frequency and variance simultaneously, for example by using red and blue saturation to represent mean frequency as normal, but adding yellow or green in proportion to represent the variance.

Power Doppler imaging

This is similar to CFM, but now the colour represents the power of the Doppler signal for each colour pixel. The technique is better than CFM for simply demonstrating the presence of moving blood; it is useful for assessing perfusion of small vessels or outlining obstructions in larger vessels that are otherwise difficult to image. No information about Doppler shifts (and hence blood speed) is usually presented, though some systems code positive and negative shifts in different colours.

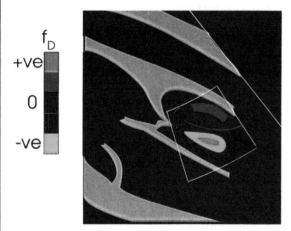

Fig. 2.1.20 The Doppler shift from the high-speed centre of the stenotic jet shows aliasing, changing abruptly from red to blue. The alias colour change does not pass through black, as it does in the larger eddy where the flow changes from forward to reverse (and vice versa) and is locally perpendicular to the Doppler lines.

Normal Doppler ultrasound measurements in the newborn

Jon Skinner

INTRODUCTION

While cross-sectional and M-mode echocardiography are of great value in the assessment of structure and function, Doppler ultrasound adds another dimension in the assessment of blood flow velocity. Normal patterns of flow within the heart and great vessels have been established, and identifying these should be part of the routine echocardiogram of the newborn infant. It is now possible to estimate pressure drop across stenoses, and also to assess volume of blood flow.

This chapter describes how to obtain Doppler tracings in the heart and great vessels in the newborn and describes their normal features. A brief introduction to the potential clinical uses and features of abnormal flow is given at each stage.

The examples are taken from an examination in a newborn term baby of the venous inflow to the branch pulmonary arteries and descending aorta. In practical terms, this is done by obtaining standard echocardiographic views and superimposing a pulsed Doppler sample at various sites from inflow to outflow. Colour Doppler images are obtained by placing the sampling window over the cross-sectional images.

Normal values for measurements made from Doppler studies in the preterm and term infant over the first few days of life are presented in Tables 2.2.1–2.2.3. Assessment of interatrial and ductal flow is discussed in Chapters 3 and 7.

BASIC PRINCIPLES

As stressed in Chapter 2.1, the ultrasound beam must be in line with flow (or less than 20° out of line) to minimize underestimation of blood velocity.

Table 2.2.2 Normal values for diastolic inflow in the preterm infant (28–36 weeks)

	1–10 days
TV E wave	46 ± 11
TV A wave	70 ± 14
TV E : A ratio	0.7 ± 0.1
MV E wave	55 ± 10
MV A wave	55 ± 13
MV E: A ratio	1.0 ± 0.1

These values are taken from Johnson et al.[11] Values are mean ± standard deviation.

Pulsed Doppler ultrasound is used for the lower velocities only because aliasing occurs at higher velocities. Velocities up to 2 m/s can often be measured without aliasing in the newborn owing to the short distance between the sampling gate and the probe. Continuous wave (CW) Doppler or high prf ultrasound must be used for higher velocities, though it needs to be remembered that both these modalities will record velocities from further along the ultrasound beam, and not just within a single sampling gate.

☞ *Practical Points*
- **Always align directly with the direction of blood flow.**
- **Use pulsed Doppler ultrasound to measure low velocities – do not measure when aliasing occurs.**
- **Use CW Doppler ultrasound to measure the higher velocities (typically 2 m/s and above in the preterm).**

Forward flow through the heart and large vessels is non-turbulent and low velocity (usually less than 1.5 m/s). Minor changes in velocity occur with

Table 2.2.1 Normal peak transvalvular velocities (cm/s) determined with pulsed Doppler in term infants during the early newborn period

	Fetal	<6 hours	6–24 hours	>24 hours
TV E wave	39 ± 11	33 ± 11	40 ± 10	35 ± 8
TV A wave	49 ± 10	44 ± 12	52 ± 13	46 ± 10
TV E : A ratio	0.8 ± 0.1	0.8 ± 0.1	0.8 ± 0.1	0.8 ± 0.1
MV E wave	34 ± 10	53 ± 11	50 ± 11	48 ± 8
MV A wave	40 ± 11	46 ± 14	46 ± 14	43 ± 9
MV E : A ratio	0.85 ± 0.02	1.2 ± 0.3	1.1 ± 0.2	1.1 ± 0.2
[a]Main pulmonary artery	66 ± 14	60 ± 9	61 ± 8	66 ± 12
(stroke dist, cm)		11.7 ± 2.4		14.6 ± 2.7
[a]Ascending aorta	78 ± 14	88 ± 14	74 ± 10	76 ± 8
(stroke dist, cm)		15 ± 3.4		14.7 ± 3.4

Stroke dist = stroke distance (flow velocity integral). Evaluation of stroke distance is important in volume calculations and is described further in Chapter 5.
[a] These data are from Takenaka et al.[10]; all other data from Wilson et al.[5] Other authors have reported values up to 20% higher.
Harada et al.[7] studied 20 healthy term infants at 2, 12 and 24 hours of age. Mitral inflow velocities were similar, but aortic stroke distance was lower with mean values of 12.2, 9.6 and 9.9 cm, respectively.

Table 2.2.3 Normal values for systolic outflow in the preterm infant (28–36 weeks)

	0–12 hours	13–36 hours	37–72 hours
PA (stroke dist, cm)	6.4 (3.9–9.6)	7.0 (4.9–10.1)	8.3 (6.2–12.1)
Ascending aorta (stroke dist, cm)	9.6 (7.2–10.7)	9.3 (7.3–11.3)	9.8 (7.2–11.5)

These values were taken from 17 preterm infants (28–35 weeks' gestation, 1165–2290 g) by the chapter author. Values are mean (10th–90th centile).

changes in cardiac output. Quantitative measurements of blood flow volume are possible when the cross-sectional area of the orifice through which the blood is travelling can be measured accurately, and flow is non-turbulent. For example, left ventricular output can be estimated from the ascending aortic velocity (measured with Doppler) and the diameter of the aortic root (determined from cross-sectional echocardiography). This is discussed further in Chapter 5.

Stenotic lesions cause an increase in velocity, but flow is then turbulent and velocities are usually higher, depending on the degree of obstruction. Determination of **pressure drop** across such a stenosis can be made by application of the modified Bernoulli equation to the velocity; this is discussed again in Chapter 2.3.

☞ *Practical Points*
- **Normal forward flow within the heart is not turbulent, thus pulsed Doppler traces are 'hollow' because all of the blood is travelling at much the same speed, at or just below peak velocity.**
- **Turbulent flow is seen as 'filled in' traces because a whole range of velocities are detected as well as the highest velocity.**

SYSTEMIC VENOUS RETURN

It is usually possible to record the pattern of flow in both the inferior and superior caval veins (abbreviated after with the better known 'IVC' and 'SVC' for inferior and superior vena cava). These measurements have not been extensively studied in neonates but is an area of active reseach. Velocities are low (<1.5 m/s) in the normal newborn and are best recorded with pulsed Doppler. The pattern of flow throughout the cardiac cycle is closely related to the central venous pressure waveform, so the flow velocities reflect the changing balance of intra- and extrathoracic pressure and the changes during the cardiac cycle. In the infant breathing

spontaneously the overall velocity increases during inspiration (while central venous pressure simultaneously decreases). In a vigorous healthy newborn, the peak velocity may reach 2 m/s during inspiration. During positive pressure ventilation, the velocity decreases during inspiration. Circulatory volume and diastolic right ventricular function are other factors influencing flow.

How to do it

The inferior and superior caval veins lie parallel to and to the right of the spine. They are thus not in the 'cardiac' axes described in Chapter 1.4. The best imaging axis for either of these veins is roughly straight up and down the body.

Start from the subcostal region, slightly to the patient's right of midline, with the cross-sectional image cutting straight up and down the body. The caval veins and right atrium are visualized. Alternatively, obtain a subcostal four-chamber view and angle anteriorly slightly. As the right pulmonary veins disappear the SVC comes into view; slight clockwise rotation may help stabilize the image, which may swing from the right pulmonary veins to the SVC with respiration.

Flow in the superior caval vein

Place the pulsed Doppler sample within the SVC. A typical recording is shown in Figure 2.2.1b.

Note that the highest velocity occurs during systole, following the QRS complex. The right atrium is filling while the tricuspid valve is closed (Fig. 2.2.2). The velocity then decreases almost to zero just before the tricuspid valve opens, resulting in passive filling of the right ventricle accompanied by a second phase of SVC flow into the right atrium during diastole. The peak velocity of the diastolic phase is lower than that of the systolic phase, and is influenced particularly by respiration. The diastolic peak of the second beat, which occurred during expiration, is lower than the other two beats. The velocity then falls to zero during right atrial contraction ('Active' filling of the right ventricle –

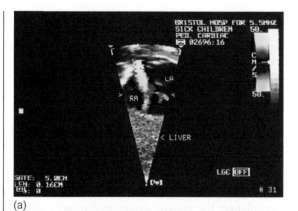

(a)

(b)

Fig. 2.2.1 (a) Subcostal image of the superior caval vein with colour Doppler flow.
(b) Pulsed Doppler recording of flow in the superior caval vein (SVC); flow is towards the subcostal probe. 'A' signifies the time of atrial contraction.

signified by the 'A' on the trace) and may be negative transiently before the next cycle begins.

Now place the colour Doppler window over the SVC – an example is shown in Figure 2.2.1a. There should be no turbulence, but a 'flare' of flow from the azygous vein into the back of the superior caval vein can often be seen with colour Doppler ultrasound.

Flow in the inferior caval vein

Now tilt the probe caudally, again along the imaging axis, to bring a long segment of the inferior caval vein into view. Place the Doppler sample within it. The pattern of flow should be similar to that from the SVC, but in the opposite direction. Alignment with flow is often as good from the mid-parasternal position, cutting along the same axis.

Interpreting the findings

Turbulence in the SVC is unusual and may signify the insertion of an anomalous pulmonary vein, or stenosis due to a central line or a thrombus. Elevated right atrial pressure results in reduced forward flow, particularly during the systolic (early) phase, so that this velocity is less than in the diastolic phase.[1] Right ventricular diastolic dysfunction causes exaggerated or prolonged retrograde flow during atrial contraction. On the other hand severe hypovolaemia causes the inferior caval vein to collapse during inspiration (particularly during positive pressure ventilation) and the diastolic velocity is very much reduced in comparison with the systolic velocity.

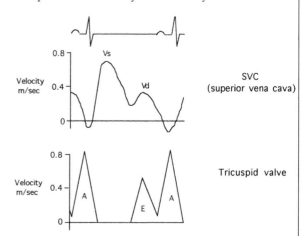

Fig. 2.2.2 This diagram shows the relationship of flow in the SVC to flow through the tricuspid valve. The fastest velocity in the SVC occurs when the tricuspid valve is closed, during systole (Vs). The second peak (Vd, velocity in diastole) coincides with passive filling of the right ventricle (the E wave of tricuspid flow). A brief period of retrograde flow occurs during right atrial contraction (the A wave of tricuspid flow).

PULMONARY VENOUS RETURN

It is important to exclude anomalous pulmonary venous connection in the cyanotic infant. Even the experienced paediatric cardiologist can find this difficult; a novice should always seek help with such patients. Nevertheless, recognition of normality is clearly the first step and colour Doppler ultrasound is particularly helpful.

How to do it

A number of views are useful. In the subcostal four-chamber view the probe is reasonably aligned with flow coming from the left-sided pulmonary veins. On colour Doppler blood is easily detected coming towards the probe and minor angulations will bring in the right-sided veins as well. An example is shown in Figure 2.2.3a. The pulsed Doppler sample can be placed within a vein as it enters the left atrium (Fig. 2.2.4). The apical four-chamber view is also useful (Fig. 2.2.3b).

A high parasternal/suprasternal coronal view of the left atrium may be useful. This shows the entry of the four major pulmonary veins best, but it is not always easy to obtain. The probe is placed at or just below the suprasternal notch, and is tilted back towards the heart, with the imaging cut going from left to right. The left atrium is cut along its back. The two upper veins are on either side of the top of the screen, nearest to the probe, and the lower two are at the other end of the atrium. An example is

shown in Figures 2.2.3c and 2.2.3d with colour Doppler ultrasound showing a flare from all four veins at the back of the left atrium.

Interpreting the signals

Normal flow

Normal pulmonary venous flow is low velocity (<1.5 m/s) and fluctuates markedly throughout the cardiac cycle and with respiration. Flow velocity is highest in the first hours after birth, with an average peak velocity of about 0.8 m/s, falling to 0.6 m/s by 24 hours. The higher velocity is probably related to left-to-right ductal shunting.[2] Flow dips towards zero or becomes transiently negative in late diastole (see Fig. 2.2.4a), coinciding with left atrial contraction.[3] Negative (retrograde) flow back into the pulmonary veins is brief – less than the duration

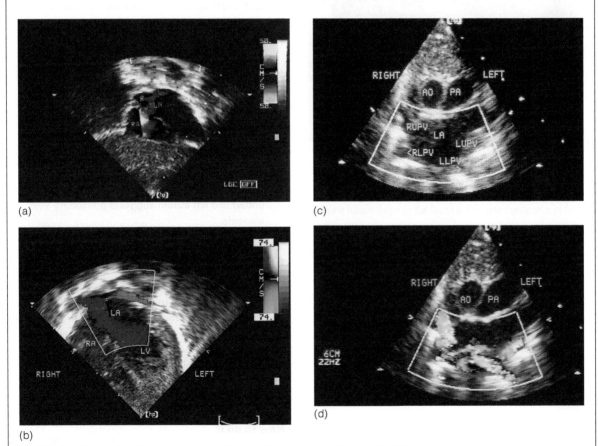

(a)

(b)

(c)

(d)

Fig. 2.2.3 (a) Subcostal view showing colour Doppler flow from the left- and right-sided pulmonary veins.
(b) An apical view of pulmonary venous flow, using a different colour map. Note that flow from the inferior left-sided veins is away from the probe (blue).
(c) Coronal view of four pulmonary veins (see text).
(d) Same coronal view with colour Doppler; blue highlights flow from the upper pulmonary veins (away from the probe), and orange from the lower pulmonary veins.

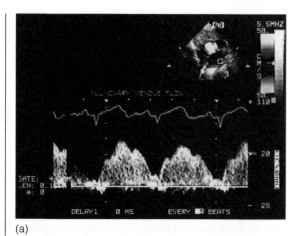

(a)

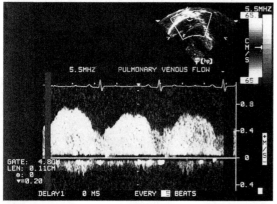

(b)

Fig. 2.2.4 Pulsed Doppler recording of flow at the entrance of the pulmonary veins in the left atrium.
(a) In a healthy baby without a ductal shunt.
(b) In a healthy baby with a small left-to-right ductal shunt.

of atrial contraction (judged from the A wave at the mitral valve; see below).

Note that in adults and older children there are typically three distinct phases of flow through the pulmonary veins, as with SVC and IVC flow, i.e. a systolic peak, a diastolic peak, and a sharp dip corresponding to atrial contraction in late diastole. In the newborn, the systolic and diastolic phases typically merge, as shown in Figure 2.2.4a. This is presumably due to the faster heart rates seen at this age.

Abnormal findings

A high velocity (greater than 1.5 m/s, up to 4 m/s) that fluctuates very little during the cardiac cycle and does not dip towards zero in late systole is suspicious of pulmonary venous stenosis. The flow pattern is 'filled-in', indicating turbulent flow. The

normally deep colours seen with colour Doppler are bright and a mosaic pattern of aliasing is present. (Be sure the velocity limit is set as high as possible on the colour map.) Infants with pulmonary venous stenosis typically have a small left atrium in association with pulmonary hypertension, and predominantly right-to-left flow across the oval foramen.

Broad colour Doppler jets arising from the veins with a velocity fluctuating with respiration are typically the result of increased pulmonary blood flow from a left-to-right ductal shunt. The flow remains non-turbulent. In these babies the left atrium is large, the pulmonary veins may be distended, and other features of a left-to-right ductal shunt are present (see Chapter 7). An example of pulmonary venous flow from a healthy infant at 24 hours with a small patent duct and left-to-right shunting is shown in Figure 2.2.4b; the velocity never approaches zero but still fluctuates during the cardiac cycle and with respiration.

Prolonged retrograde flow in late diastole and reduced overall velocity occurs with left atrial hypertension. This may be secondary to left ventricular diastolic dysfunction or to mitral stenosis.

☞ *Practical Point*
- **Continuous forward flow through the pulmonary veins with little alteration in velocity and an underfilled left atrium suggests pulmonary vein stenosis.**

ATRIOVENTRICULAR FLOW

The pattern of diastolic flow into the ventricles through the tricuspid and mitral valves reflects ventricular preload, the function of the atria and the atrioventricular valves, and the diastolic relaxation characteristics of the respective ventricle.

There are typically two flow waves with passive filling of the ventricle: the E wave, followed by that due to atrial contraction, the A wave.

How to do it

Pulsed Doppler ultrasound

Flow through the tricuspid and mitral valves during diastole is most easily recorded from the apical four-chamber view. The pulsed Doppler sample is placed at the tips and in the middle of the respective valves. An upward deflection on the Doppler trace represents flow towards the probe, through the valves. Two peaks are usually seen during diastolic flow causing an M-shaped profile, although they may blend into a single peak during tachycardia. Examples are shown in Figures 2.2.5 and 2.2.6.

Colour Doppler ultrasound

The sampling window is placed over the mitral or tricuspid valves in the four-chamber view from the apex. Flow is non-turbulent and the low velocities are represented as deep colours (see Fig. 2.2.7).

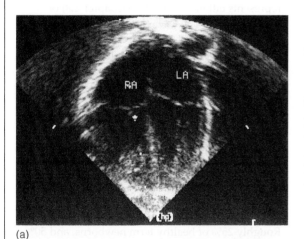

(a)

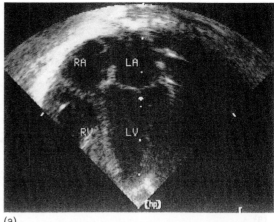

(a)

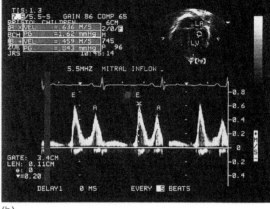

(b)

Fig. 2.2.6 (a, b) Pulsed Doppler recording of mitral valve inflow. The E wave is higher (0.64 m/s) than the A wave (0.46 m/s).

Interpreting the findings

Normal findings

The findings in the normal newborn are quite different from those in adults. In the adult, and in the child over one year of age, the E wave has typically a higher velocity, and a higher flow velocity integral (the mean velocity multiplied by the duration), than the A wave in both the tricuspid and mitral valves. In other words, passive filling contributes the majority of ventricular filling, and atrial contraction the minority. In the adult, the A wave is only higher than the E wave in pathological states with impaired diastolic relaxation. Hypertrophic cardiomyopathy is an example.

In the fetus, the pattern in both mitral and tricuspid valves tends to reverse, with the A wave being dominant or at least equal.[4]

(b)

Fig. 2.2.5 (a, b) Pulsed Doppler recording of tricuspid valve inflow. The A wave is higher (0.55 m/s) than the E wave (0.40 m/s). The measured value boxes also show pressure gradient (PG). This is an automatic feature on most echocardiography machines; the modified Bernoulli equation is applied to the measured velocity. This is neither useful nor appropriate at these low velocities.

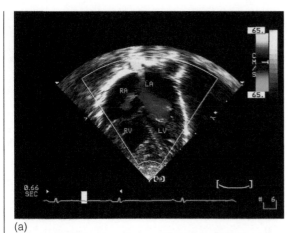

(a)

(b)

Fig. 2.2.7 Apical four-chamber view with colour flow during diastole across the atrioventricular valves.
(a) Early diastole. The mitral valve opens first, and flow is shown into the left ventricle.
(b) Mid diastole. Flow now occurs through both valves, and is a pure colour (orange) without any aliasing to suggest stenosis of either valve.

After birth, the tricuspid E wave is typically of lower velocity than the A wave, so that the E:A peak velocity ratio is on average 0.8:1.[5] The mitral E wave is typically slightly higher than the A wave. The average E:A ratio is between 1.1:1 and 1.2:1 over the first few days, and the A wave is higher than the E wave in many normal newborns. In preterm infants the E:A ratio is lower than in term infants due to a reduced E wave and increases linearly with increasing gestational age from 0.8:1 at 24 weeks to 1:1 at 30 weeks.[6] The ratio of these velocities gradually changes to the adult pattern over several months.

The reasons for these differences are not completely understood. However, the features suggest that diastolic relaxation of the ventricles in the newborn is transiently impaired which may be due to the greatly increased afterload faced by both ventricles after birth.

During tachycardia the E wave merges into the A wave so that there is only one phase of filling; there is less time for passive filling to occur before the atrium contracts.

Abnormal findings

A reduced E:A ratio on the right side may not indicate right ventricular pathology in the newborn and the E:A ratio must be greatly reduced on the left side to suggest pathology.

Increased velocity across the inflow valves represents either stenosis (see Chapter 2.3) or increased flow. The E wave in particular increases with increasing preload.[7] Thus a large interatrial shunt increases tricuspid valve flow, and a large ductal shunt increases mostly mitral valve flow. Peak velocities do not, even under these circumstances, usually exceed 1.2 m/s. Atrioventricular valve regurgitation also results in an increased E wave. Velocities above 1.5 m/s associated with turbulence suggest stenosis.

High-velocity aliasing retrograde flow in systole at either valve signifies regurgitation (see Chapter 6). Mild tricuspid valve regurgitation is the rule during hyaline membrane disease (over 90%).[8] Roughly 25% of healthy term newborns, and 50% of healthy preterm newborns, have trivial or mild tricuspid regurgitation in the first three days, but thereafter it is uncommon.[9] Mitral regurgitation is less common but trivial jets sometimes occur in healthy infants, and are more frequent during left-to-right ductal shunting.

☞ *Practical Point*
- **If you see low-velocity, non-turbulent retrograde flow at the mitral valve during systole, then it is likely that the Doppler sample has moved slightly from LV inflow and is detecting LV outflow below the aortic valve.**

VENTRICULOARTERIAL FLOW

The RVOT crosses in front of the LVOT, from right to the left, so it is not possible to align directly with both outflow tracts at the same time. For most purposes measurement of velocity within the main pulmonary artery and the ascending aorta is sufficient because if there is acceleration below the valves, then this will also be detected distal to them.

Right ventricular outflow tract and pulmonary arteries

How to do it

The pulmonary artery runs backwards from the third or fourth intercostal space; thus flow is from front to back. Measurements are best made by obtaining a standard precordial short-axis view and placing the pulsed Doppler sample in the centre of the main pulmonary artery, just beyond the tips of the pulmonary valve (Fig. 2.2.8); flow is away from the transducer. Best alignment with flow is often achieved by sliding the probe away from the left shoulder along the short axis while simultaneously angling towards the left shoulder, bringing the main pulmonary artery and valve into the centre of the image. The sample can be moved around the pulmonary artery, from below the valve onward into both branch pulmonary arteries.

Superimposing the colour sector onto the image produces a deep blue, representing low-velocity flow away from the probe, with some acceleration at the branch pulmonary arteries showing as a lighter blue (Fig. 2.2.9).

The right ventricular outflow tract is best interrogated from the subcostal position (Fig. 2.2.10). This view is obtained by tilting the probe anteriorly with slight clockwise rotation from a subcostal four-chamber view.

Interpreting the findings

Normal findings Normal flow in the main pulmonary artery should be low velocity (<1.0 m/s) and laminar, as seen in Figure 2.2.8. Over the first days of life the waveform representing pulmonary arterial pressure changes from a sharp pointed triangle, with a short time to peak velocity, to a smoother rounded shape by day five. This phenomenon reflects the falling pulmonary vascular resistance, and has been used to assess pulmonary arterial pressure non-invasively (Chapter 6).

At the origin of both pulmonary arteries there is a velocity increase due to relative (physiological)

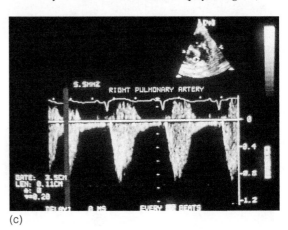

(a)

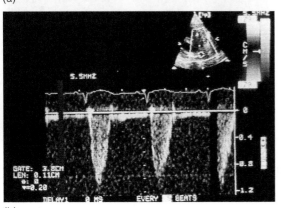

(b)

(c)

Fig. 2.2.8 (a) Pulsed Doppler recording from the main pulmonary artery (from the parasternal position). Flow is smooth and non-turbulent ('hollow' in appearance); peak velocity is less than 0.8 m/s.
(b) In the left pulmonary artery, flow accelerates to a peak velocity of 1.2 m/s and flow is turbulent ('filled-in').
(c) In the right pulmonary artery, flow is also turbulent but the peak velocity is a little lower than in the left. This may be because of relatively poor alignment with flow.

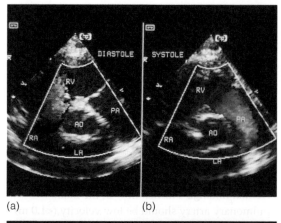

(a) (b)

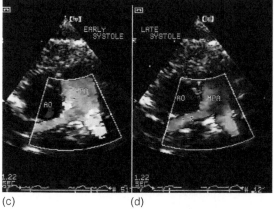

(c) (d)

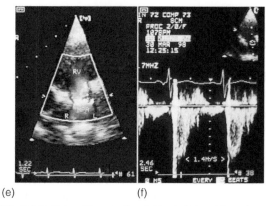

(e) (f)

Fig. 2.2.9 Colour Doppler flow in the right heart from the parasternal short-axis view in a normal heart (a–d) and in trivial pulmonary value stenosis (e–f).

(a) During diastole, orange flow demonstrates flow through the tricuspid valve into the right ventricle.

(b) During systole, with the ultrasound probe in the same position, blue colour shows flow away from the probe in the main pulmonary artery.

(c,d) In another subject, at the same phase of the cardiac cycle as (b), slight tilt of the probe away from the cardiac apex (towards the right shoulder) demonstrates the origin of the branch pulmonary arteries more clearly. Lighter blue at the origins demonstrates acceleration, and the yellow colour demonstrates aliasing at the origin of the left pulmonary artery. RA, right atrium; LA, left atrium, RV, right ventricle; PA, main pulmonary artery; AO, aorta.

(e) The acceleration of flow at the pulmonary valve due to trivial pulmonary valve stenosis, is seen on colour and is shown to be turbulent in figure (f) since the flow profile is filled in rather than hollow and the peak velocity is slightly high at 1.4m/sec.

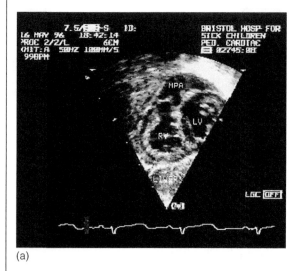

(a)

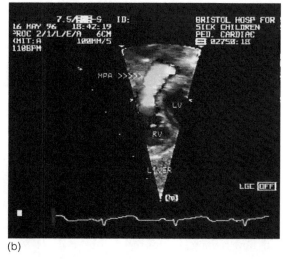

(b)

Fig. 2.2.10 (a) Subcostal view, tilted anteriorly to show the right ventricular (RV) outflow and main pulmonary artery (MPA). LV, left ventricle.
(b) Same view with colour Doppler superimposed. Yellow colour occurs due to aliasing at the origin of the left pulmonary artery.

branch stenosis, as shown in Figures 2.2.9c,d and 2.2.10b. This is typically most marked in the left pulmonary artery after ductal closure (but can affect the right), but is usually less than 2 m/s. A transient murmur may be caused (heard at the back), and the velocity can reach 3.5 m/s, with aliasing of the pulsed Doppler signal.[12] This should settle to less than 2 m/s by one month of age and gradually decrease thereafter.

Trivial pulmonary incompetence, detected as a tiny retrograde colour Doppler flare, is common in infants as at any age.

Turbulence within the main pulmonary artery in diastole usually indicates the presence of left-to-right ductal shunting. Some degree of ductal shunting is common in healthy term and preterm infants up to 4 days old. A bright retrograde flare of colour Doppler can be seen arising from the arterial duct at the distal end of the main pulmonary artery on the left of the screen (cranial and lateral). This is discussed, and examples are shown, in Chapter 7.

Abnormal findings An increase in right ventricular output will lead to mildly increased velocity with laminar flow in the main pulmonary artery (1–1.5 m/s). Turbulent flow, with a velocity over 2 m/s, signifies pulmonary valvar stenosis or RVOT obstruction. Retrograde flow in diastole proximal to the valve indicates pulmonary valve regurgitation. Very mild pulmonary valve stenosis may cause only slightly elevated velocity, but the flow profile indicates turbulent rather than laminar flow (see Fig. 2.2.9f).

☞ *Practical Point*
- **The only velocities higher than 2 m/s that occur in the *healthy* newborn arise from a closing arterial duct, trivial tricuspid valve regurgitation, or physiological branch pulmonary artery stenosis**

Left ventricular outflow tract and aorta

How to do it

Flow through the aortic valve in the newborn is usually best recorded from the suprasternal notch, with flow coming towards the probe, or from the apex, with flow going away from the probe. There is little space for an imaging probe in the suprasternal notch, so recordings are usually obtained with a non-imaging Doppler probe (either CW or pulsed Doppler ultrasound) – see Chapter 2.3 and Figure 5.1a.

From the apex, a long-axis view is obtained by rotating the probe slightly clockwise and tilting anteriorly from a standard apical four-chamber view. A pulsed Doppler sample can be placed anywhere along the outflow tract. To exclude aortic stenosis the sample is placed above the valve (Fig. 2.2.11), and reveals laminar flow. Colour Doppler images also demonstrate non-turbulent flow (see Fig. 2.2.11 and 2.2.12).

Flow in the aortic arch and descending aorta is assessed from the suprasternal notch after obtaining a view as described in Chapter 1.3. Colour Doppler detects the flow towards the probe in the ascending aorta and away from the probe in the descending aorta – shown as orange and blue colours in the systolic frame in Figure 2.2.12. The pulsed Doppler sample can be moved around the arch, taking care at each stage to align with the direction of flow.

Interpreting the findings

Ascending aorta Normally pulsed Doppler signals from the ascending aorta suggest laminar flow; the signal is 'hollow' rather than filled-in because all the blood is travelling at much the same speed. Minor velocity changes with laminar flow are mostly due to changes in volume of blood flow (this is explained further in Chapter 5). Reduced ascending aortic velocity occurs in low output states (low LV stroke volume) whereas moderately elevated peak velocity (1.0–1.5 m/s, with non-turbulent flow) signifies elevated LV stroke volume, most commonly secondary to left-to-right ductal shunting.

Velocity over 1.5 m/s with turbulent flow indicates valvar or subvalvar aortic stenosis.

ARCH AND DESCENDING AORTA

The flow velocity varies across the width of the arch as the blood travels round in systole, but does not usually exceed 1.5 m/s in the arch.[13] There is further acceleration at the isthmus in the region of the arterial duct. Velocities of 2 m/s are not uncommon in the term newborn, but higher than 2.5 m/s suggests aortic coarctation. Sometimes high velocities are obtained due to the sample detecting flow in the left pulmonary artery which crosses this area. Most importantly, the normal velocity of flow

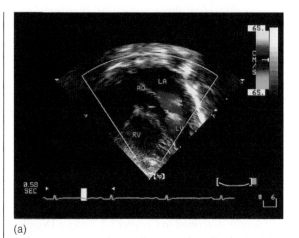

(a)

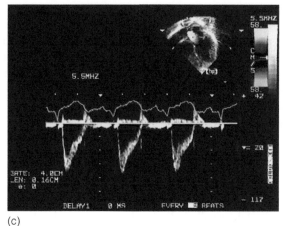

(c)

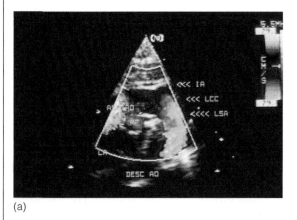

(b)

Fig. 2.2.11 Apical 'five-chamber' view showing the left heart.
(a) Orange colour Doppler flow across mitral valve in diastole.
(b) Blue flow, away from the probe in the LV outflow and ascending aorta. Note the absence of turbulence.
(c) Pulsed Doppler recording from just above the aortic valve. Note laminar ('hollow') flow profile.

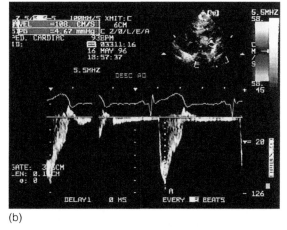

(a)

(b)

Fig. 2.2.12 (a) From the suprasternal position, the colour Doppler map shows ascending aortic flow (towards the probe) as orange, and descending aortic flow as blue. Ao, aortic valve; IA, innominate artery; LCC, left common carotid artery; LSA, left subclavian artery.
(b) Pulsed Doppler flow in the descending aorta; peak velocity is 1.1 m/s. Note that during early diastole there is retrograde flow briefly, before very low-velocity antegrade flow during the rest of diastole (due to the elasticity of the arch of the aorta forcing some forward flow).

---

in the descending aorta in **diastole** is very low, after being transiently slightly negative immediately after systole, as shown in Figure 2.2.12b. Continued forward flow in diastole in the descending aorta is classical of aortic coarctation (this is further discussed in Chapter 10.1). On the other hand, exaggerated retrograde flow in diastole in the descending aorta is a feature of a large left-to-right ductal shunt; blood is 'stolen' from the descending aorta into the pulmonary circulation via the duct during diastole (this is discussed further in Chapter 7).

☞ *Practical Points*
- **Reduced Doppler velocities with a non-turbulent profile are a sign of reduced cardiac output.**
- **Modestly elevated velocities with non-turbulent flow indicate increased volume of flow rather than stenosis.**

REFERENCES

1. Nagueh SF, Kopelen HA, Zoghbi WA. Relation of mean right atrial pressure to echocardiographic and Doppler parameters of right atrial and right ventricular function. *Circulation* 1996;93:1160–1169.
2. Agata Y, Hiraishi S, Oguchi K, Nowatari M, Hiura K, Yashiro K, Shimoda T. Changes in pulmonary venous flow pattern during early neonatal life. *British Heart Journal* 1994;71:2:186–6.
3. Rossvoll O, Hatle LK. Pulmonary venous flow velocities recorded by transthoracic Doppler ultrasound: relation to left ventricular diastolic pressures. *Journal of the American College of Cardiology* 1993;21:1687–1696.
4. Reed KL, Sahn DJ, Scagnelli S, Anderson CF, Shenker L. Doppler echocardiographic studies of diastolic function in the human fetal heart: changes during gestation. *Journal of the American College of Cardiology* 1986;13:700–705.
5. Wilson N, Reed K, Allen HD, Marx GR, Goldberg SJ. Doppler echocardiographic observations of pulmonary and transvalvar velocity changes after birth and during the early neonatal period. *American Heart Journal* 1987;113:750–758.
6. Harada K, Tamura M, Takahashi Y, Ishida A, Takada G. Role of gestational age and body weight on Doppler transmitral flow velocity pattern in very low birth weight infants. *Pediatric Cardiology* 1996;17:242–245.
7. Harada K, Shiota T, Takahashi Y, Tamura M, Toyono M, Takada G. Doppler echocardiographic evaluation of left ventricular output and left ventricular diastolic filling changes in the first day of life. *Pediatric Research* 1994;35:506–509.
8. Skinner JR, Boys RJ, Hunter S, Hey EN. Pulmonary and systemic arterial pressure in hyaline membrane disease. *Archives of Disease in Childhood* 1992;67:366–373.
9. Skinner JR, Boys RJ, Hunter S, Hey EN. Non-invasive determination of pulmonary arterial pressure in healthy neonates. *Archives of Disease in Childhood* 1991;66:386–390.
10. Takenaka K, Waffarn F, Dabestani A, Gardin JM, Henry WL. A pulsed Doppler echocardiographic study of the postnatal changes in pulmonary artery and ascending aortic flow in normal term newborns. *American Heart Journal* 1987;113:759–766.
11. Johnson GL, Moffet CB, Noonan JA. Doppler echocardiographic studies of diastolic ventricular filling in premature infants. *American Heart Journal* 1988;116:1568–1574.
12. So BH, Watanabe T, Shimizu M, Yanagisawa M. Doppler assessment of physiological stenosis of the main pulmonary artery: a cause of functional murmur in neonates *Biology of the Neonate* 1996;69.4:243–8.
13. Rahiala E, Tikanoja T. Non-invasive blood pressure measurements and aortic blood flow velocity in neonates. *Early Human Development* 1997;49.2:107–12.

Assessment of gradient and regurgitation

Jon Skinner

INTRODUCTION

This chapter describes how to assess pressure difference across cardiac orifices and stenotic valves using the modified Bernoulli equation, and also how to assess valvar regurgitation.

ASSESSMENT OF PRESSURE DROP

Doppler echocardiography became popular with clinicians when it was discovered that it could determine pressure drop across a cardiac valve non-invasively. In 1976, Holen *et al.* applied the simplified and modified Bernoulli equation (introduced in Chapter 2.1, $p = 4\,v^2$, where p = pressure drop (mmHg), and v = velocity (m/sec)) to the Doppler velocity across a stenosis mitral valve and derived a transvalvular pressure drop.[1] Values correlated closely with those from cardiac catheterization. The technique has since been validated at all the valves and is in daily use in clinical cardiology at all ages.

In paediatric cardiology the same technique has been used to determine pressure drop across ventricular septal defects,[2] the arterial duct,[3] and across vascular stenoses such as aortic coarctation.[4,5] An important application in neonatology is the determination of peak right ventricular pressure (and hence peak pulmonary arterial pressure) through measurement of the peak velocity of tricuspid regurgitation.[6]

In screening for valvar stenosis as part of the routine examination, a high, turbulent aliasing velocity through a valve on pulsed Doppler or colour Doppler examination indicates that the valve is stenotic. The pressure drop across the valve can normally be assessed reliably with continuous wave (CW) Doppler as part of the overall echocardiographic assessment.

This extremely useful technique has potential pitfalls. These are explained in this chapter with some examples of its use in congenital heart disease. Determination of pulmonary arterial pressure from tricuspid regurgitation and from ductal flow velocity is discussed in more detail in Chapter 6.

How to do it

Since the velocities recorded are high, CW Doppler (or high prf) rather than pulsed wave Doppler is used.

The single most critical factor in accurate measurement is to align accurately with the jet being interrogated. *Failure to align correctly results in underestimation of the true pressure drop.* In practice correct alignment is achieved by obtaining the highest recordable velocity from a number of different projections. Provided the alignment is within ± 20°, underestimation will be minimal.

Studies of repeatability have shown that it is better to take the highest recorded velocity rather than the mean of several peak values.

Use of 'in-line' CW Doppler ultrasound

If the ultrasound machine has in-line CW Doppler ultrasound (i.e. the CW beam can be placed over the image), then an image should be obtained first. The approximate direction of the jet is seen with colour Doppler, and the line representing the CW beam can be placed appropriately on-screen. Further fine manipulation is then required to achieve the highest velocity on the CW Doppler trace. It is not sufficient merely to align with the colour Doppler jet; the heart is a three-dimensional structure and the jet may be angled into or out of the cross-sectional image, i.e. into or out of the screen.

☞ *Practical Points*
- **Failure to align correctly with flow results in underestimation of the pressure drop.**
- **Do not rely entirely on the colour Doppler jet for correct alignment of the CW Doppler beam. Instead use this as an initial guide, and then seek the highest recordable velocity by further fine manipulation.**

Use of non-imaging CW Doppler ultrasound probe

The non-imaging CW Doppler probe has the advantage that it is smaller and easier to manipulate, particularly in obtaining ascending aortic velocity from the suprasternal notch. The operator needs to keep the orientation of the heart in mind, and remember which way blood is flowing through the heart and great vessels. It is not as difficult as it may at first sound; the gradual acquisition of such a three-dimensional picture is part of becoming an echocardiographer. For example, it is clear from the standard short-axis view that blood in the pulmonary artery travels from the anterior pulmonary valve towards the back. A probe placed at the left parasternal edge at about the third intercostal space will detect this flow if the beam is directed posteriorly (see Fig. 2.3.3a). The Doppler trace shows downward deflection, representing flow away from the probe (Fig. 2.3.3b). Similarly, if the probe is in the suprasternal notch (Fig. 2.3.2b), anterior tilt detects flow towards the probe (above zero on the trace) coming up the ascending aorta, and posterior tilt detects flow away from the probe (below zero on the trace) going down the descending aorta.

Valvar stenoses

Figures 2.3.1–2.3.3 give examples of the determination of pressure drop across the mitral, aortic and pulmonary valves. Pressure drop across

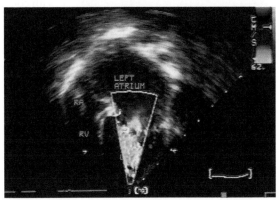

(a)

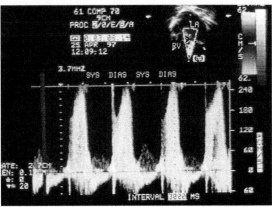

(b)

Fig. 2.3.1 Severe mitral stenosis.
(a) From an apical four-chamber view, low-velocity orange flow (towards the probe) above the mitral valve accelerates, first changing to lighter yellow before aliasing causes a mosaic pattern, identifying the site of stenosis. The left atrium is greatly enlarged.
(b) In-line CW Doppler reveals a peak velocity of over 2.4 m/s. Applying $p=4v^2$ gives a pressure drop of 23 mmHg.

the tricuspid valve is determined in the same way as across the mitral valve.

Ventricular septal defects

Figure 2.3.4 shows a subject with a small ventricular septal defect (VSD). The colour Doppler jet across the small defect is narrow, and the jet is always left-to-right. A high velocity such as this demonstrates that the right ventricular pressure is much lower than that in the left ventricle, and therefore helps to exclude significant pulmonary hypertension. The peak velocity between the left ventricle and right ventricle is 5 m/s. Applying the modified Bernoulli equation ($p=4\,v^2$), the pressure in the right ventricle must be approximately 100 mmHg less than in the left ventricle.

It can be difficult to align accurately with VSD jets, and validatory studies have shown that the derived pressure drops may not always closely relate to those from catheterization.[2] Nevertheless, the technique remains a useful clinical guide. A useful rule of thumb is that a left-to-right peak velocity greater than 4 m/s almost always indicates a normal pulmonary arterial pressure in the infant, whereas a velocity less than 3 m/s indicates elevated pulmonary arterial pressure.

Several examples of the further use of the simplified and modified Bernoulli equation occur later in the book, but some of the important limitations and necessary precautions are outlined below.

Limitations and precautions

There are several important points that need to be considered when assessing a pressure drop using the modified Bernoulli equation.

1. It is relatively easy to measure the wrong velocity.
2. The Doppler-derived pressure drop is the maximal *instantaneous* drop, which is often not the same as the *peak-to-peak* drop typically reported after cardiac catheterization.
3. If the orifice is too narrow, the velocity-derived pressure drop will underestimate the pressure gradient because of loss of energy as viscous friction.
4. Underestimation of the degree of valvar stenosis by Doppler is common in low output states.
5. Some types of stenoses are commonly known to give misleading results, or results that are very

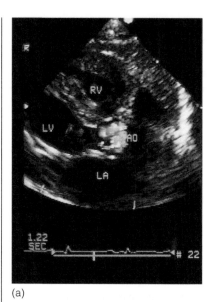

(a)

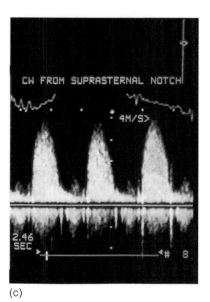

(c)

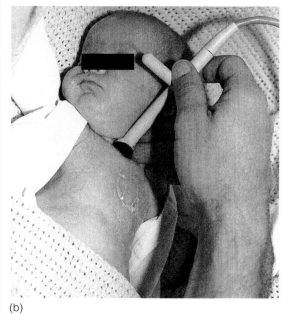

(b)

Fig. 2.3.2 Aortic stenosis.
(a) A parasternal long-axis view demonstrates aliasing at the site of the aortic valve.
(b) Best alignment with the flow is often obtained from the suprasternal notch using the 'blind' CW Doppler pencil probe.
(c) The peak velocity is over 4 m/s, suggesting a maximal instantaneous pressure drop of over 64 mmHg.

different from those obtained from simultaneous catheterization.

6. The method may be less accurate in assessing pressure drop across the arterial duct and some VSDs.

Measuring the wrong velocity

It needs to be remembered that a CW ultrasound beam detects velocities all the way along its path, not just those which may be nearest to the probe. The highest velocity along its path produces the highest velocity on the trace.

For example, when measuring velocity through the pulmonary valve, the beam may also pass through the origin of a branch pulmonary artery. If an elevated velocity is detected, the examiner may believe that there is pulmonary valve stenosis, instead of left pulmonary artery origin stenosis, which is a common transient phenomenon after ductal closure in the preterm.

Similarly, blood flow in the ascending aorta is travelling away from the apex of the heart, as might mitral regurgitation, for example. Thus if mitral regurgitation is present this can be detected from

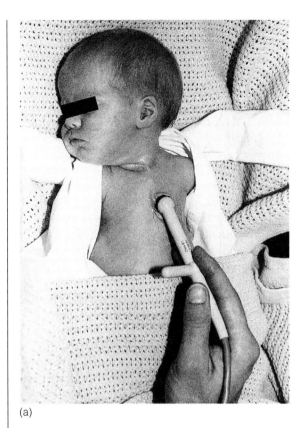

(a)

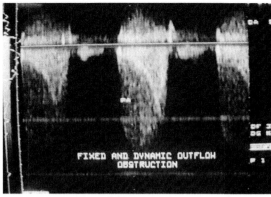

(b)

Fig. 2.3.3 Pulmonary stenosis.
(a) Position of the CW Doppler probe when assessing peak velocity through the pulmonary valve, and also for assessing left-to-right velocity through a patent arterial duct. The ultrasound beam is directed almost directly towards the back, often with a slight tilt towards the head.
(b) This patient (with tetralogy of Fallot) had both a fixed and dynamic obstruction to the right ventricular outflow. The narrow pulmonary valve causes a constant obstruction and velocity peaks in early–mid systole. Within the flow profile there is a second curve due to a gradually increasing obstruction during systole from the muscular infundibulum of the right ventricle as it narrows during ejection.

the suprasternal notch as velocity above the zero line occurring during systole, like ascending aortic flow. Mitral regurgitation is always a high-velocity jet because it is caused by the pressure difference between the left ventricle and left atrium in systole.

If such a high velocity were truly present in the ascending aorta, then this would indicate severe aortic stenosis.

It is usually possible to solve such problems by assessing all potential sites of increased velocity

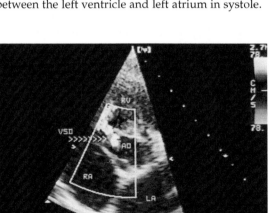

(a)

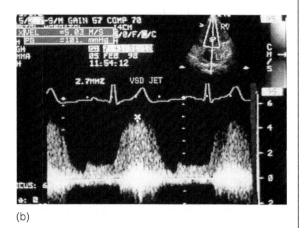

(b)

Fig. 2.3.4 Ventricular septal defect.
(a) Colour flow Doppler in a standard parasternal short-axis view demonstrates a narrow aliasing bright orange jet passing from the LVOT into the right ventricle. Ao, aorta.
(b) Alignment with this jet using 'in-line' CW Doppler reveals a peak left-to-right velocity of 5 m/s (demonstrating an approximate peak L–R pressure drop of 100 mmHg).

with pulsed wave Doppler. In practice, one has usually located an area of acceleration first with pulsed and colour Doppler ultrasound, and then afterwards the peak velocity is measured with CW. Thus when measuring velocity through the pulmonary valve, both the pulmonary valve and pulmonary artery origins are interrogated with pulsed Doppler and the site of acceleration can be found. When trying to assess mitral regurgitation, the mitral and aortic valves are independently interrogated with pulsed and colour Doppler from the apex. In-line CW can also be placed over the respective valves during imaging.

Overestimation of derived pressure drop with respect to peak-to-peak drop at cardiac catheterization

Doppler-derived values of pressure drop across the aortic and pulmonary valves are higher than those reported at cardiac catheterization. The reason for the difference is a phase delay between peak velocities and great artery systolic pressure, as illustrated in Figure 2.3.5. The largest pressure drop between the LV and the aorta during the cardiac cycle (*A*) is significantly greater than the peak-to-peak drop (*B*).

This does not mean that the non-invasive method is wrong, just that one should not directly

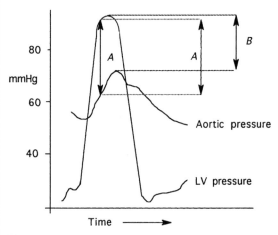

Fig. 2.3.5 Comparison of 'peak-to-peak' and instantaneous pressure drop. Schematic representation of pressure tracings from the left ventricle and the aorta during one cardiac cycle in an infant with aortic stenosis. *A* is the maximal *instantaneous* pressure drop during systole; this gives rise to the peak velocity on Doppler ultrasound. *B* is the *peak-to-peak* pressure drop, normally reported from cardiac catheterization. *A* is about 20% greater than *B* in this example.

compare echocardiographic and catheter-derived peak-to-peak values for pressure drop when describing severity of valvar stenosis. Most of the studies of the treatment of valvar stenosis by surgery or balloon valvotomy are based on catheter peak-to-peak gradients and not Doppler estimates.

With this problem in mind, some cardiologists now prefer to report the velocity rather than the derived pressure gradient. Severity of aortic stenosis can be divided into groups according to measured peak ascending aortic velocity, e.g. mild, less than 3 m/s; moderate, 3–4.5 m/s; and severe, greater than 4.5 m/s. This also has the advantage of eliminating the multiplication factors needed to derive pressure drop (avoiding 'multiplying the error' of measurement).

In adults it has been shown that Doppler assessment of mean rather than maximal pressure gradient across the aortic valve is more closely related to mean aortic gradient from cardiac catheterization. Also, inclusion of the subaortic velocity in the fuller form of the modified Bernoulli equation ($p = 4(v_2^2 - v_1^2)$) also improves correlation if there is a narrow LV outflow tract (v_1=subaortic velocity, v_2 =ascending aortic velocity). Such refinements are not of real importance to the neonatologist.

Underestimation of pressure gradient because the orifice is too narrow

Holen *et al.*'s original in vitro experiments[1] demonstrated that significant underestimation of the pressure drop occurred with velocities below 3 m/s and an effective orifice less than 3.5 mm diameter.

The orifice diameter can in fact probably be much less than this before the results become too misleading. Taking assessment of pressure across the arterial duct as an example, low birth weight preterm babies with a huge left-to-right shunt rarely have ducts with an internal diameter above 2.5 mm. Assessment of pressure gradient across such ducts is usually reasonably accurate.[3] The impression from our own studies is that the duct must be tightly constricted, probably less than 1 mm diameter, before significant underestimation occurs.[7]

Very high packed cell volume and high blood viscosity might theoretically cause some underestimation due to energy lost as viscous friction, but in vitro experiments[8] suggest that this is not the case for haematocrits in the physiological range (below 80%).

Underestimation of the degree of valvar stenosis in low output states

A failing myocardium may be simply unable to generate the energy required to force blood through a tight stenosis. In the case of a newborn with critical pulmonary stenosis, blood can off-load through the oval foramen, and pulmonary perfusion is maintained by the arterial duct. Very little blood passes through the pulmonary valve at all. The situation is similar with critical aortic stenosis. It is common for velocity through the stenotic valve to increase after successful valvotomy. This increase is related to the elevated left ventricular output, combined with a reduced valvar narrowing.

The cross-sectional echocardiographic features of these conditions are striking, and thus fortunately we do not have to rely on the flow velocities to make the initial diagnosis. These features are discussed further in the sections on congenital heart disease (Chapters 9.1 and 10.1).

Misleading results

Holen et al.'s original work with the modified Bernoulli equation used a discrete orifice. Vascular stenosis, such as coarctation of the aorta, and supravalvar aortic stenosis are irregular and are certainly not sharply defined orifices. Other in vitro work with irregular and tunnel-like obstructions[9] suggested that the equation should remain valid in most settings unless the cross-sectional area is less than 0.25 cm², but clinical experience has shown that in some cases the results are misleading.

Aortic coarctation is an important example. With neonatal coarctation the *pattern* of flow through the coarctation measured with CW in the descending aorta is characteristic, with continued high velocity throughout diastole, rather than returning to zero as normal (see Chapter 10.1). However, the peak velocity in the descending aorta, at all ages, has a poor correlation with true pressure gradient, even when the velocity before the obstruction is included in the equation.[4,5] The reason is unclear and is probably multifactorial. In the neonate, clinical evaluation of the femoral pulses and right arm-to-leg blood pressure differential remain very important.

Can Doppler measurements overestimate pressure drop?

Supravalvar and muscular subaortic stenosis are interesting examples of where the Doppler echocardiographically derived pressure drop is often much higher than that measured by catheterization. It had been recognized for some time that such patients often have a high ascending aortic velocity (often over 6 m/s) and a catheter-determined gradient of *much* less. This may be because Doppler echocardiography is usually done in an unsedated patient in outpatients, whereas cardiac catheterization is not. However, simultaneous studies showed similar differences.

> ☞ *Practical Points*
>
> **Procedure in the assessment of valvar gradient:**
> - **First, clarify with cross-sectional, pulsed and colour Doppler study where the abnormality or abnormalities are. Observe associated features such as ventricular hypertrophy and valvar morphology.**
> - **Measure the peak velocity with CW Doppler, ensuring that the beam does not pass through another region with high velocity.**
> - **Apply the modified Bernoulli equation to the highest velocity (v_2).**
> - **If there is acceleration beneath the valve (velocity > 1 m/s), measure this velocity (v_1) with pulsed wave Doppler and allow for this in the calculation ($p = 4(v_2^2 - v_1^2)$.**

This apparent paradox has been explained by in vitro studies[10] which described a phenomenon familiar to fluid engineers as 'pressure recovery' after a stenosis (see p. 94).* It seems that the Doppler measurements may be more closely related to severity, and the catheter measurements may be misleading.

ASSESSING VALVAR REGURGITATION

Equally important in the assessment of valvar function is the assessment of regurgitation. Colour Doppler is most useful, but it should be combined with other echocardiographic modalities. Attempts to quantify regurgitation volumetrically have been largely unsuccessful. At best one can hope to grade regurgitation into absent, trivial, mild, moderate and severe.

Doppler echocardiographic modalities are more sensitive for detecting regurgitation than the human ear and a stethoscope! Detection of trivial regurgitation at all valves is common among normal subjects at any age (although aortic regurgitation is very rare in the healthy newborn). It is particularly common at the tricuspid valve in the preterm with respiratory failure, and at the pulmonary valve in all groups. Mild to moderate regurgitation is common at both atrioventricular valves following perinatal asphyxia. However, even trivial regurgitation at the aortic valve suggests valvar pathology; such patients should be reviewed by a paediatric cardiologist.

☞ *Practical Point*

- **Mild regurgitation at the tricuspid, mitral and pulmonary valves is relatively common in functional cardiac disease, but mild aortic regurgitation in the newborn is likely to signify valvar pathology.**

Assessing severity of regurgitation

Basic principles

Severity of regurgitation is graded by combining all echocardiographic modalities, but colour Doppler echocardiography is particularly helpful. The aim is to classify severity into trivial, mild, moderate or severe.

Before going further, there is an important point to clarify. We have found that beginners with echocardiography often confuse measurement of the *severity* of regurgitation with measurement of the

---

*The basic physical principle is that energy is conserved as blood passes through a constriction. If no energy is lost to turbulence or viscous friction, then there must be complete pressure recovery distal to the obstruction, i.e. no change in pressure at all, and velocity returns back to pre-stenosis values. There is downstream recovery of kinetic energy as pressure. In this case a measuring catheter must be at the narrowest point (the 'vena contracta') where blood flow is fast and pressure high; after this the pressure recovers and no gradient is detected.

Half-way between these two cases is streamlined flow, where, after the vena contracta, the flow is gently guided back into the larger channel by gradual widening after the stenosis, minimizing turbulent interactions of the jet with the stagnant distal blood. Some pressure recovery occurs, such that if the measuring catheter is not exactly at the vena contracta, the pressure gradient will be underestimated.

Placement of the catheter tip reliably within the vena contracta may not be possible whereas CW Doppler always measures the highest velocity all the way along its beam. Therefore in this circumstance Doppler estimation of pressure drop may actually give a more reliable estimate of the load on the pumping chamber than that obtained from catheterisation.

---

velocity of regurgitation. It should be clear that a high regurgitant velocity does not imply a lot of regurgitation. Rather it implies that there is a high pressure gradient between the two chambers. To determine systolic right ventricular pressure, the modified Bernoulli equation can be applied to the velocity of regurgitation through the tricuspid valve (see Chapter 6). This regurgitation may be trivial or mild, and yet still have a high velocity if RV pressure is high. If there is very severe tricuspid valve regurgitation, regurgitant velocity is typically low; the right ventricle cannot generate a higher pressure because the blood is rapidly off-loaded back into the right atrium.

It is thus important to appreciate the difference between assessing the *volume* of regurgitation as opposed to the *speed* of regurgitation.

How to do it

The standard procedure for assessing regurgitation should follow the usual sequence of imaging, followed by colour and pulsed Doppler, and finally CW Doppler.

Tricuspid and mitral valve regurgitation

Cross-sectional echocardiography may indicate atrial dilatation with moderate and severe regurgitation but not with mild regurgitation (see Figs 2.3.6–2.3.8). The valve morphology and the size of the annulus are examined. The valve may be seen to close incompletely (failure of 'coaptation') due to stretching of the valve ring with severe myocardial dysfunction and ventricular dilatation. If the valve appears stiff or thickened, then clearly there is valvar pathology rather than a functional problem. In Ebstein's anomaly the tricuspid valve is displaced down towards the apex of the right ventricle, and is commonly severely regurgitant.

Colour and/or pulsed Doppler reveal high-velocity retrograde flow after valve closure. The operator can assess the width of the colour Doppler jet,[11] how far it travels, and its duration. Attention to gain settings is very important; increasing gain too high increases the apparent width of the jet. Consistency between studies is imperative; there can be considerable differences between ultrasound machines as well as between observers.

In the absence of colour Doppler, 'pulsed Doppler mapping' can be done by moving the

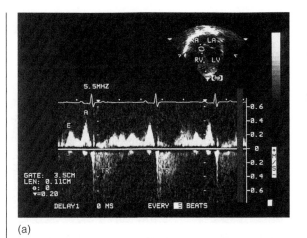

(a)

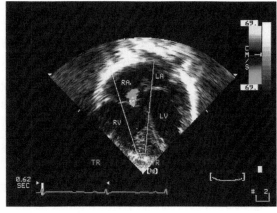

(b)

Fig. 2.3.6 Trivial tricuspid valve regurgitation (healthy term infant at 12 hours of age).
(a) Pulsed Doppler sample at the tricuspid valve reveals an aliasing signal during systole.
(b) Colour Doppler reveals a small blue flare of tricuspid regurgitation.

sample around the atrium and assessing how far retrograde flow penetrates into the atrium. Severe regurgitation causes retrograde flow into the

systemic or pulmonary veins, respectively. Pulsed Doppler assessment of forward flow through the valve typically reveals an elevated velocity overall

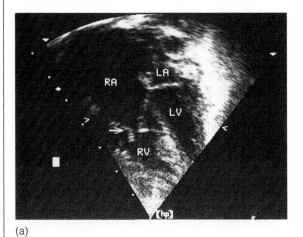

(a)

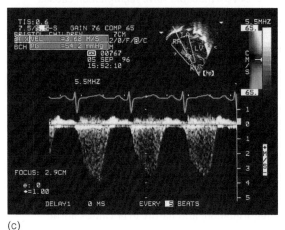

(c)

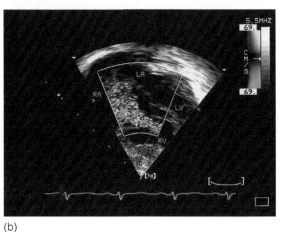

(b)

Fig. 2.3.7 Severe tricuspid valve regurgitation. This infant was cyanosed at birth and had a dysplastic tricuspid valve. As the pulmonary vascular resistance fell during day 2, the regurgitation remained moderately severe but the hypoxia resolved and he did well.
(a) Systolic frame from the apical four-chamber view showing failure of the tricuspid valve to coapt. The atrial septum bulges to the left.
(b) Colour Doppler shows a broad jet travelling well into the right atrium.
(c) The peak velocity of the regurgitant jet was high (3.68 m/s) owing to the concurrently elevated pulmonary vascular resistance. The regurgitation remained severe, but this velocity fell to 2.4 m/s by the next day as pulmonary arterial pressure fell (see text).

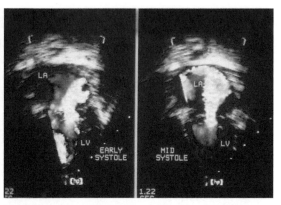

Fig. 2.3.8 Severe mitral regurgitation. There is a broad colour jet into the dilated left atrium which swings across the left atrium during systole and enters into the pulmonary veins.

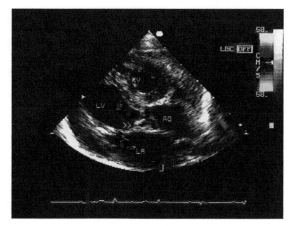

Fig. 2.3.9 Mild aortic regurgitation. The highlighted (arrowed) narrow blue flare in this long-axis view demonstrates trivial or mild aortic regurgitation. This infant had severe aortic stenosis, underlining the point that aortic regurgitation is usually pathological, and rarely a physiological phenomenon in the newborn.

and in particular an elevated E wave with moderate or severe regurgitation.

> ☞ *Practical Points*
> - *Severe tricuspid valve regurgitation causes systolic retrograde flow in the SVC and IVC which can be detected with pulsed Doppler.*
> - *Severe mitral regurgitation causes retrograde flow in the pulmonary veins.*

Pulmonary and aortic valve regurgitation

The principles are the same as for atrioventricular valves; some examples are shown in Figures 2.3.9 and 2.3.10. However, although tricuspid and mitral regurgitation are common features of myocardial dysfunction in the newborn, functional cardiac disease rarely contributes to pulmonary regurgitation, and hardly ever causes aortic

regurgitation. The assessment of arterial valve regurgitation is usually best left to the paediatric cardiologist.

Severe and moderate regurgitation cause ventricular dilatation, and the ventricular function often appears hyperdynamic. The width and extension of the retrograde colour jet are assessed. Pulsed Doppler evaluation of forward flow beyond the valves is also helpful; a sign of moderate to severe regurgitation is exaggerated retrograde flow during diastole in either the proximal pulmonary artery branches (with pulmonary regurgitation) or the aortic arch (with aortic regurgitation).

CW Doppler, aligned with flow as normal, detects the regurgitant jet and sounds similar to what is heard on auscultation. The velocity of the jet

Table 2.3.1 Atrioventricular valves: a rough clinical guide for the echocardiographic assessment of valvular regurgitation in the newborn

	Trivial	Mild	Moderate	Severe
Atrial dilatation	0	0	+	++
Coaptation of leaflets (appearance on cross-sectional echo)	normal	normal	normal/tiny gap	visible gap
Colour Doppler jet[a]:				
Width at the valve	linear	<1 mm	1–2 mm	2 mm+ to very broad
Duration	less than systole	pansystolic	pansystolic	pansystolic
Extent of jet[b]	<1/3 of atrium	1/3–2/3 of atrium	back of atrium	into IVC/SVC or pulm. veins and whorls forwards
Pulsed Doppler forward flow	normal	normal E wave	increased E wave	increased

[a] The regurgitant colour Doppler jet is usually a bright mosaic from high velocity and turbulence, but in severe regurgitation the colour may be deeper, representing lower velocity due to 'free' regurgitation.
[b] The direction of the jet varies between patients, and is also affected by the pressure gradient across the valve – thus the jet will travel further if ventricular pressure is high, although the width of the jet should not be markedly affected.
Examples of severe tricuspid valve regurgitation are shown in Fig. 2.3.7.

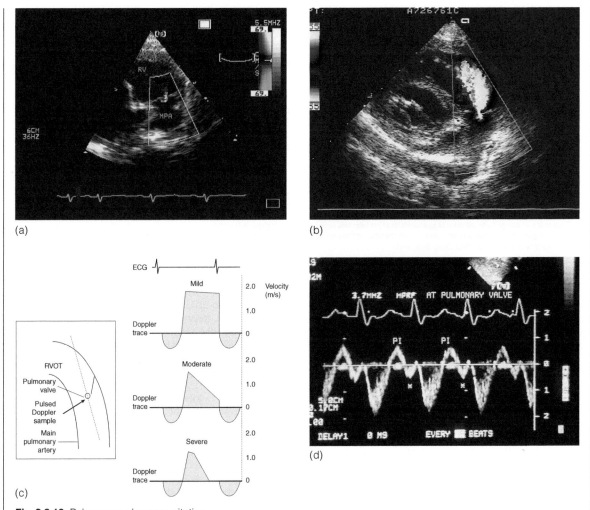

Fig. 2.3.10 Pulmonary valve regurgitation.
(a) This parasternal long-axis view of the pulmonary valve reveals mild pulmonary incompetence in an infant with pulmonary hypertension. This degree of incompetence is normal with or without pulmonary hypertension.
(b) This echocardiogram, in the same view as (a), is from an infant who also had pulmonary hypertension, but the pulmonary valve was slightly dysplastic, explaining the broader jet indicating moderate regurgitation.
(c) This schema shows the Doppler profile at the pulmonary valve in mild, moderate and severe pulmonary regurgitation. The severe form is most commonly seen in patients after outflow tract repair in tetralogy of Fallot and always indicates valvar pathology. The absence of flow at end diastole is due to equalization of the pressures between the right ventricle and pulmonary artery at this stage.
(d) An example of pulsed Doppler flow at the pulmonary valve with severe regurgitation. Regurgitation is brief and low velocity. (The asterisks indicate forward flow transmitted through the ventricle from right atrial contraction – a feature of a very stiff right ventricle.)

reflects the pressure drop between the artery and the ventricle during diastole. With mild regurgitation the velocity remains much the same throughout diastole, because the pressure differential between the artery and ventricle is maintained. With severe regurgitation, the pressure differential between artery and ventricle is not maintained; the end diastolic pressure in the artery is the same as in the ventricle, so the velocity reaches zero before the end of diastole. Tables 2.3.1 and 2.3.2 provide a practical clinical guide for all the cardiac valves.

Table 2.3.2 Arterial valves: a rough clinical guide for the echocardiographic assessment of valvular regurgitation in the newborn

	Trivial	Mild	Moderate	Severe
Ventricular dilatation	0	0	+	++
Coaptation of leaflets (appearance on cross-sectional echo without colour)	Normal	Normal	Normal/tiny gap	Visible gap
Colour Doppler jet:				
Width at the valve[c]	Linear	<1 mm	1–2 mm	2 mm +
Duration	Less than diastole	Pandiastolic	Pandiastolic	Pandiastolic[d]
Travel into ventricle	<Width aorta	1–2 × width aorta	Well down into ventricle	Reaches apex, swirls in ventricle
Pulsed Doppler forward flow	Normal	Normal	Increased velocity	Increased velocity
Retrograde flow in branch PAs or aortic arch	No	No	Slight	Marked
Speed of regurgitation (with CW Doppler)	High throughout	High throughout	Reduced at end systole	Zero at end systole

[c]These widths are a rough guide and would be appropriate for a term baby. Mild aortic regurgitation is shown in Fig. 2.3.9.

[d]In severe regurgitation, particularly on the pulmonary side, the retrograde flow may cease before the true end of diastole when the ventricle is full to capacity. The duration of regurgitation is then dictated by the relaxation characteristics of the ventricle.

REFERENCES

1. Holen J, Aaslid R, Landmark K, Simonsen S. Determination of pressure gradient in mitral stenosis with a non-invasive ultrasound Doppler technique. *Acta Medica Scandinavia* 1976;199:455–460.

2. Houston AB, Lim MK, Doig WB, Reid JM, Coleman EN. Doppler assessment of interventricular pressure drop in patients with ventricular septal defects. *British Heart Journal* 1988;60:50–56.

3. Musewe NN, Poppe D, Smallhorn JF *et al.* Doppler echocardiographic measurement of pulmonary artery pressure from ductal Doppler velocities in the newborn. *Journal of the American College of Cardiology* 1990;15:446–456.

4. Houston AB, Simpson IA, Pollock JCS, Jamieson MPG, Doig WB, Coleman EN. Doppler ultrasound in the assessment of severity of coarctation of the aorta and interruption of the aortic arch. *British Heart Journal* 1987;57:38–43.

5. Chan KC, Dickinson DF, Wharton GA, Gibbs JL. Continuous wave Doppler echocardiography after surgical repair of coarctation of the aorta. *British Heart Journal* 1992;68(2):192–194.

6. Skinner JR, Stuart AGS, O'Sullivan J, Heads A, Boys RJ, Hunter S. Validation of right heart pressure determination by Doppler in infants with tricuspid regurgitation. *Archives of Disease in Childhood* 1993;69:216–220.

7. Skinner JR. Relationship of pattern of ductal flow and flow velocities to systolic pulmonary: systemic arterial pressure ratio. In: Skinner JR, MD thesis, *Non-invasive determination of pulmonary arterial pressure in the newborn*, ch 13, pp 185–216. University of Leicester, UK 1993.

8. Vasko SD, Goldberg SJ, Requarth JA, Allen HD. Factors affecting accuracy of in vitro valvar pressure gradient estimates by Doppler ultrasound. *American Journal of Cardiology* 1984;54:893–896.

9. Teirstein PS, Yock PG, Popp RL. The accuracy of Doppler ultrasound measurement of pressure gradients across irregular, dual and tunnellike obstructions to blood flow. *Circulation* 1985;72:577–584.

10. Levine RA, Jimoh A, Cape EG, McMillan S, Yoganathan AP, Weyman AE. Pressure recovery distal to a stenosis: potential cause of gradient 'overestimation' by Doppler echocardiography. *Journal of the American College of Cardiology* 1989;13:706–715.

11. Rivera JM, Vandervoort P, Mele D, Weyman A, Thomas D. Value of proximal regurgitant jet size in tricuspid regurgitation. *American Heart Journal* 1996;131:742–747.

Haemodynamic Assessment

CHAPTER 3

Assessment of interatrial shunting

Nick Evans

INTRODUCTION

Just as the oval foramen (or 'foramen ovale') plays an important role in the fetal circulation, its presence is important to newborn infants not only as a site for right-to-left shunting in babies with pulmonary hypertension but, more commonly, as a site for left-to-right shunting. In the early postnatal period, small left-to-right shunts through an incompetent oval foramen are a common finding in healthy term infants. In preterm infants these shunts can be of haemodynamic importance, particularly when associated with a ductal shunt.[1,2] Doppler echocardiography allows both quantitative assessment of the direction of atrial shunting through the cardiac cycle and also, with colour Doppler, semiquantitative assessment of the degree of this shunting.

EMBRYOLOGY AND ANATOMY OF THE OVAL FORAMEN

The oval foramen, like the rest of heart, undergoes important structural changes in the last trimester. These occur in preparation for the change from the antenatal role of allowing the oxygenated placental venous return to pass through to the left side of the heart and hence to the head and neck, to the postnatal role of separating the pulmonary and systemic circulations. There are two components to the oval foramen: the oval fossa, a muscular rimmed rounded hole in the secondary septum, and the thin foraminal valve that hangs like a curtain on the left side of the oval fossa. In utero, this foraminal valve tissue has excessive fullness and balloons into the left atrium, allowing an anterior opening for blood to shunt from right-to-left. The relative size of this anterior opening reduces through pregnancy, particularly in the last trimester. In relation to the inferior caval vein, at 9 weeks' gestation it is the same size, reducing to roughly 55% in preterm infants and to 40% at term.[3]

After birth, the increased pulmonary venous return and higher left atrial pressure push the valve tissue back to the right against the rim of the oval fossa. Echocardiographically it is possible to see that it often prolapses through into the right atrium in the early postnatal period; this is the reason why left-to-right shunting occurs. Gradually the slackness disappears and the orifice is functionally sealed. The oval foramen does not always

structurally seal and is often found to be probe patent at adult autopsy.

NORMAL INTERATRIAL PRESSURE DIFFERENTIALS

An understanding of the normal pressure differential between the two atria through the cardiac cycle is fundamental to the interpretation of Doppler assessment of interatrial shunting. The shunt pattern in adults and children with atrial septal defects (ASDs) commonly includes, at the onset of ventricular contraction, a brief period where right atrial pressure exceeds left and so blood shunts from right-to-left. Right-to-left atrial shunting is also found in normal newborns, but at the onset of ventricular diastole. This is because the mitral valve opens before the tricuspid valve in newborns, in contrast to adults where the tricuspid valve opens first.[4] This delay in the opening of the tricuspid valve results in the left atrial pressure falling slightly before the right, and so blood shunts briefly from right-to-left. The relative pressures between the atria during the cardiac cycle are shown in Figure 3.1. It can be seen that at the onset of mitral flow, left atrial pressure falls relative to right until briefly right atrial pressure exceeds left. At the onset of atrial systolic flow, left atrial pressure rises relative to the right and exceeds it throughout ventricular systole. So some degree of right-to-left shunt is normal in newborn infants. This fact is vital to the interpretation of atrial shunt patterns in babies with pulmonary hypertension, which are described in more detail later in this chapter.

ECHOCARDIOGRAPHY OF THE ATRIAL SEPTUM

Cross sectional imaging

The atrial septum is best imaged from the subcostal four-chamber view, shown in Figure 3.2 (and 1.4.8). This view is obtained by placing the probe below the xiphisternum with the beam cutting a cross-section through the body. The beam is then angled anteriorly and pointed slightly towards the left shoulder and the view shown in Figure 3.2 will appear. For optimal views of the atrial septum, keep the probe as far below the xiphisternum as is compatible with getting a full view of the heart. If the ultrasound probe is placed too close to the

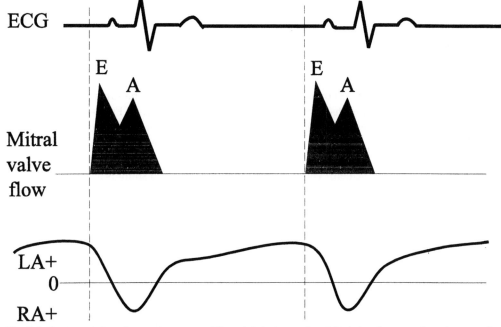

Fig. 3.1 Representation of normal pressure differentials between the atria during the normal newborn cardiac cycle. The top line represents the ECG. Below is a diagrammatic representation of the flow velocities through the mitral valve and below that is a graphical representation of the pressure differences between the atria with zero being equal pressure. LA+ means left atrial pressure exceeds right and RA+ means right atrial pressure exceeds left.

xiphisternum, the view of the atrial septum will be foreshortened. The transducer will need to be pressed down slightly on the upper abdomen to get the ultrasound beam underneath the rib cage.

Because of this it can be difficult to get good images unless the baby is relaxed. The convention for the subcostal views is that the screen is inverted and the left-hand side of the screen is the right-hand side of

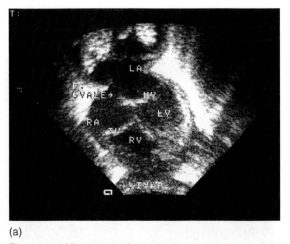

(a)

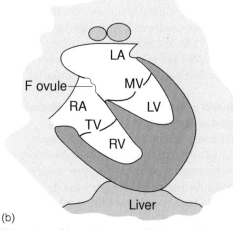

(b)

Fig. 3.2 (a) 2D subcostal four-chamber view to illustrate normal 2D imaging of the atrial septum. The beam initially cuts through the liver, behind which is the right ventricle (RV). Posteriorly and to the left (right on the screen) is the left ventricle (LV). The two atria (RA and LA) can be seen posteriorly and slightly to the right (left on the screen) of their respective ventricles connected by the atrioventricular valves (tricuspid valve, TV, and mitral valve, MV). The atrial septum is the thin membrane running from the septal insertion of the atrioventricular valves posteriorly and to the right (left of the screen). The oval foramen (F. ovale) is identified by the mobile foraminal valve tissue which moves in both directions through the cardiac cycle. (b) Line diagram showing the location of the structures described in (a).

the body, so the anatomical orientation of the heart on the screen is correct.

The beam initially cuts through the liver. Behind the liver and often partially hidden is the right ventricle. Posteriorly and to the left (right on the screen) is the left ventricle. The two atria can be seen posteriorly and slightly to the right (left on the screen) of their respective ventricles connected by the atrioventricular valves. The atrial septum is seen as a relatively thin membrane running from the septal insertion of the atrioventricular valves posteriorly and to the right (left of the screen). The oval foramen is identified by the thin and often very mobile foraminal valve tissue that can be seen moving in both directions through the cardiac cycle.

☞ *Practical Point*

- **For optimal views of the atrial septum, keep the probe as far below the xiphisternum as is compatible with getting a full view of the heart. If the ultrasound probe is placed too close to the xiphisternum, the view of the atrial septum will be foreshortened.**

It is possible to get some idea of the relative pressures between the two atria by the direction of bulge and movement of the atrial septum and foraminal valve tissue. In normal babies the valve tissue will move backwards and forwards. With high right-sided pressures the septum and the foraminal tissue will bulge towards the left atrium and the opposite will occur with high left-sided pressures. While this tells you about relative atrial pressure, it does not tell you whether there is a shunt – for that you need Doppler ultrasound.

Colour and pulsed Doppler assessment of presence and direction of atrial shunt

Optimal assessment of the size, position and direction of any atrial shunt (in either direction) is helped enormously by colour Doppler mapping. Using the subcostal four-chamber view described above, the colour Doppler window is placed over the oval foramen including a reasonable proportion of both atria. Because the velocities of atrial shunts are usually low, optimal images will be obtained by reducing the peak velocity of the colour Doppler scale to between 0.2 m/s and 0.5 m/s. Left-to-right atrial shunting can be seen as a coloured (orange in Fig. 3.3) jet coming towards the transducer and

right-to-left shunt as a coloured (blue in Fig. 3.4) jet directed away from the transducer. Often both colours can be seen at different times in the cardiac cycle in the same subject. One potential source of confusion with left-to-right atrial shunts is the venous flow coming down from the superior caval vein. The site of entry of the superior caval vein into the right atrium is shown in Figure 3.5. On colour Doppler this flow codes the same colour as any left-to-right atrial shunt, and as they can be anatomically quite closely related it is possible to confuse them. An atrial shunt is anterior and to the left (below and to the right on your screen) of the caval flow. Colour Doppler also allows some assessment of the diameter of the effective orifice of the oval foramen. As will be described later, this can be used as a semiquantitative measure of shunt volume.

☞ *Practical Point*

- **Because the velocity of interatrial shunting is usually low, optimal colour Doppler images are usually obtained by reducing the peak velocity of the colour Doppler scale to between 0.2 m/s and 0.5 m/s.**

Once the site of an atrial shunt has been identified, the pulsed Doppler range gate can be placed within it and the flow direction and velocity throughout the cardiac cycle can be recorded. Figure 3.6 shows a typical normal shunt pattern from a

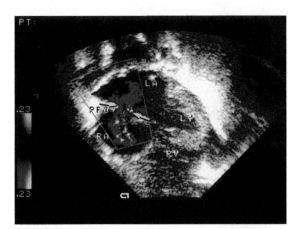

Fig. 3.3 Left-to-right atrial shunt on colour Doppler is shown by the orange jet coming through the oval foramen towards the transducer. The diameter of the shunt can be measured at the level of the atrial septum as marked by the arrows.

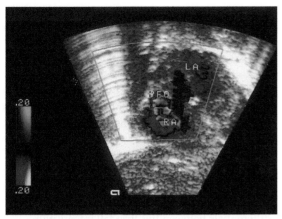

Fig. 3.4 Right-to-left atrial shunt on colour Doppler is shown by the blue jet going through the oval foramen away from the transducer.

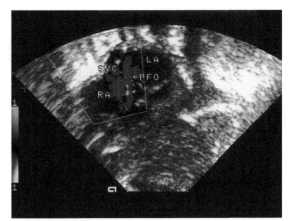

Fig. 3.5 The site of entry of the superior caval vein (SVC) with respect to the patent oval foramen (PFO). Their proximity and common direction of flow make them easy to confuse. The SVC is always posterior and to the right (left on the picture) of the oval foramen.

healthy newborn infant. The similarity to the relative pressure trace in Figure 3.1 is apparent with a short period of right-to-left shunting (negative Doppler signal) followed by left-to-right shunting (positive Doppler signal) through the rest of the cardiac cycle. Most atrial shunts are bidirectional, as shown in Figure 3.6, or pure left-to-right. Within the range of bidirectional shunts there is a varying degree of right-to-left shunt. Hiraishi *et al.*[5] described a method for measuring this variation quantitatively. As shown in Figure 3.7, this involves measuring the duration of right-to-left flow and

expressing this as a ratio of the length of the whole cardiac cycle. The mean for this ratio in healthy term newborns is 0.15:1 with a range up to 0.32:1.

Limitations of Doppler assessment of atrial shunting

Without colour Doppler, large atrial shunts can usually be detected by placing the pulsed Doppler range gate in the area of the oval foramen and recognizing and recording the typical flow pattern. It is, however, easy to miss smaller shunt jets using

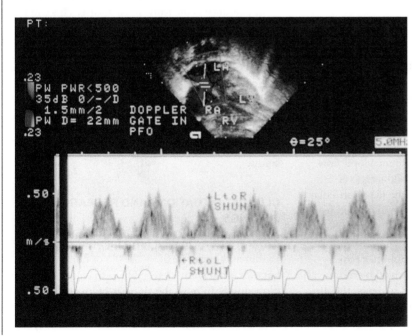

Fig. 3.6 The normal bidirectional pattern of newborn atrial shunting. The similarity with the relative pressure trace in Fig. 3.1 is apparent with a short period of right-to-left shunting (negative Doppler signal) followed by left-to-right shunting (positive Doppler signal) through the rest of the cardiac cycle.

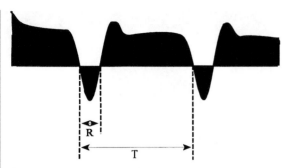

Fig. 3.7 Diagrammatic representation of an interatrial shunt Doppler flow pattern showing how the time of right-to-left shunt (R) can be expressed as a ratio of the time of the whole cardiac cycle (T).

this method. Pulsed Doppler assessment of atrial shunting is limited by two factors. First, the direction of the jet is unpredictable, making alignment with flow difficult, thus peak velocity measurements are of limited accuracy. This can be minimized using colour Doppler, but peak velocity measurements should be seen as approximate only. The second problem is that the flow tends to be turbulent, such that flow estimates derived from velocity time integrals cannot be done in the way they can from the laminar flow in the great vessels. Because of this, other indirect means of assessing atrial shunt volume such as relative ventricular outputs and colour Doppler diameter need to be used.

INDIRECT METHODS OF ASSESSING ATRIAL SHUNT VOLUMES

Doppler-derived pulmonary-to-systemic flow ratios

Left-to-right atrial shunting increases right ventricular output in relation to the left ventricular output. When the arterial duct is closed, RV output represents pulmonary blood flow (Qp) and left ventricular output represents systemic blood flow (Qs). The pulmonary-to-systemic flow ratio is derived by dividing the right by the left ventricular output.[1,2] Ventricular outputs can be measured using Doppler echocardiography, as described in (Chapter 5). Good correlation has been shown between this Doppler method of measuring pulmonary-to-systemic flow ratios and those derived by more invasive measures in catheterized patients. If both outputs can be measured accurately, this gives a good index of the size of the shunt provided there is

only a shunt at atrial level. The problem in preterm infants is that often there is also a left-to-right shunt at ductal level. This confounds this measurement because the ductal shunt into the pulmonary artery bypasses the right side of the heart and thus increases left rather than right ventricular output. This makes relative ventricular output inaccurate as a measure of shunting at either site.

Colour Doppler shunt diameter
The size of a shunt across any defect relates directly to both the size of the defect and the pressure differential across that defect. Because pressure differentials between the atria fall into quite a narrow range, it has been shown in people with ASDs that the colour Doppler diameter of an atrial shunt has a reasonable correlation with pulmonary to systemic flow ratios measured by invasive means.[6] While there are limits to the spatial resolution of colour Doppler, good correlations have been shown between the colour Doppler diameter of ventricular septal defects and that found at angiography or surgery.[7] Fundamental to this technique is the optimization of the colour Doppler mapping. Three factors are critical.

1. Minimize colour Doppler window size.
2. Reduce the peak velocity of the Doppler scale to 0.5 m/s or lower (atrial shunts are usually low-velocity shunts).
3. Optimize the colour Doppler gain such that the appearance is the same in each case. This can be done by increasing the gain as high as possible without causing spontaneous peripheral interference.

The colour Doppler diameter can then be measured at the level of the atrial septum during the left-to-right component of the shunt (marked by arrows in the Figure 3.3). The validation and use of this measurement in preterm infants are described below.

CLINICAL SITUATIONS AND RESEARCH FINDINGS

Atrial shunting in well term babies
Within an hour of birth, over 90% of normal babies have an atrial shunt detectable with colour Doppler ultrasound.[5] In most the shunt is bidirectional but the left-to-right component predominates. Roughly half still have a shunt detectable at 5 days of age.

This shunting disappears with time in almost all babies but can uncommonly still be detectable at 1 year of age.[8] The long-term implications of this are uncertain, but it has been suggested that the presence of valve tissue within the foramen is highly predictive of spontaneous closure.[9] This is in contrast to secundum ASDs, where the two edges of the defect are clearly demarcated and there is no valve tissue seen moving within the defect.

Atrial shunting in preterm infants

For some time atrial shunting in preterm infants has also been assumed to have little haemodynamic significance, being seen primarily as a marker of left-sided overload due to ductal shunting. Data recently published have questioned this assumption[1,2] and a summary of these data is presented below.

We used serial Doppler echocardiographic examination to assess patterns of atrial shunt and also to examine the effects of both ductal and atrial shunting on both right and left ventricular outputs in 51 ventilated preterm infants whose birth weight was less than 1500 g. Pulmonary-to-systemic flow ratios derived from relative ventricular outputs can only be used when there is shunting at just one site. We validated the use of colour Doppler diameter as a measure of atrial shunt size by analysing 297 echocardiograms on these 51 babies where the arterial duct was closed.

Direction of atrial shunting in the ventilated preterm

In the absence of any ductal shunt, the usual pattern of atrial shunting in ventilated preterm infants is bidirectional (75% of studies). In 23% of studies the shunt was pure left-to-right and pure right-to-left shunt was found in just 2% of studies. In those with a bidirectional shunt, the dominant direction was left-to-right; on average only 25% of the cardiac cycle was right-to-left. The degree of this right-to-left shunting did not increase significantly in studies when there were higher oxygen requirements ($FiO_2 > 0.6$). So predominantly right-to-left atrial shunts are the exception in ventilated preterm infants. They are seen in the sickest babies with very high ventilatory requirements but quite marked right-to-left atrial shunts sometimes occur in babies with really very minimal respiratory problems. For example in the group described above, one baby with pure right-to-left atrial shunt

was in 40% oxygen with minimal ventilation. As a general rule, though, it is left-to-right atrial shunting which is the dominant feature in the premature infant.

Validation of the assessment of atrial shunt diameter using colour Doppler ultrasound in preterm infants

Atrial shunt colour Doppler diameter and both right and left ventricular output were recorded in 297 studies on the 51 infants. A significant correlation was found between the pulmonary-to-systemic flow ratio and atrial shunt diameter (Fig. 3.8). Shunting was minimal when the diameter was less than 2 mm and gradually increased with diameter such that when it exceeded 4 mm, the average Qp:Qs ratio was 1.5:1. Thus in some preterm babies, significant amounts of blood can shunt back through the lungs at atrial level even when the duct is closed.

Incidence and natural history of atrial shunting in preterm infants

We then used this measure to describe the natural history of preterm atrial shunting on the 49 babies who survived. Thirty-three percent (16/49) of the babies had no clear atrial shunt seen at any time. A further 37% (18/49) had a small shunt (<3 mm in diameter) seen in the early postnatal period. This shunt resolved during the first 10 days in 7 of these 18 babies. In the others it persisted for the time we were able to follow the babies (average follow-up 37 days). The final 31% of the babies had large shunts (>3 mm in diameter). The shunt resolved in 9/15 of these on average by day 30. In the other 6 babies, it persisted for the duration of follow-up (average follow-up 45 days).

This presents a very different picture from that found in term babies, where most shunts are small and transient. While there was a lot of variation between premature babies, most had some atrial shunting, and in most of these, this shunt persisted through the early neonatal period. Although atrial shunt size may usually be smaller than that from ductal shunting, the fact that it persists for longer may mean that it has an important potential clinical impact. In the group of babies described above, those with an atrial shunt spent significantly longer in oxygen and had a significantly higher incidence of chronic lung disease than those with no or transient atrial shunts, even when other possible

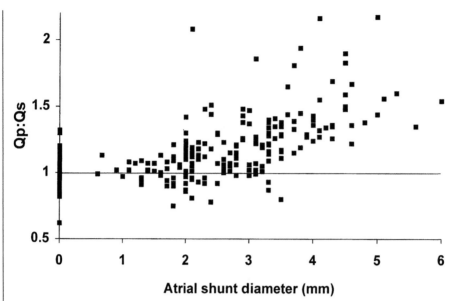

Fig. 3.8 Foramen diameter plotted against pulmonary to systemic flow ratio (Qp:Qs) in studies where the arterial duct was closed. There is a significant correlation, $r = 0.71$, $p < 0.001$ (reprinted with permission of Mosby Year Book Inc[1]).

confounding variables were controlled for. In the few babies we have followed beyond the newborn period the atrial shunt disappeared within the first 4 to 6 months.

The haemodynamic impact of atrial shunting when the atrial duct is patent

Ductal shunting places a volume load on the left side of the heart, stretching the left atrium and the oval foramen and encouraging left-to-right atrial shunting. So it is to be expected this shunting would be even more marked in the presence of a

large ductal shunt. Our studies confirmed this. In the presence of left-to-right ductal shunting, the atrial shunt pattern is more likely to be pure left-to-right throughout the cardiac cycle and the peak velocity of the interatrial to be higher than when the duct is closed.[2] The data suggested that the haemodynamic impact of this atrial shunting can be as much and sometimes more than that which occurs through the duct.

The extent of this haemodynamic impact can be seen in Figure 3.9, which plots ductal diameter (as measured by colour Doppler) against the ratio of

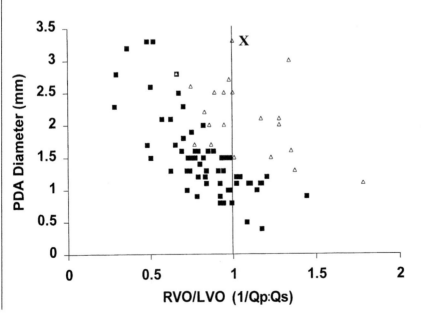

Fig. 3.9 Graph contrasting the relationship between ductal (patent ductus arteriosus, PDA) diameter and RVO/LVO (1/Qp:Qs). The closed squares mark studies with minimal associated atrial shunting. There is a significant correlation, $r = -0.80$, $p < 0.0001$. The open triangles mark studies where there was a large atrial shunt (>4 mm diameter). In these cases the plot is moved significantly to the right, representing the increase in RVO due to interatrial shunting (reprinted with permission of Mosby Year Book Inc[2]).

right-to-left ventricular output (RVO:LVO). The squares represent 69 studies where there was a patent duct and minimal or no atrial shunting. In these patients the relative ventricular output should be a quantitative measure of ductal shunting.*

It can be seen that there is a correlation between ductal diameter and the degree of shunting ($r = -0.8$), similar to that seen with diameter of the atrial defect and interatrial shunting. Contrast this plot with the triangles, which represent 18 studies where there was a patent duct and large atrial shunt (>4 mm in diameter). It can be seen that the plot is moved significantly to the right; in many cases RVO was more than the LVO.

To illustrate the haemodynamic importance of this, consider the point marked X on the graph where the RVO/LVO was almost 1. If there were no atrial shunt, this 3.4 mm diameter duct would result in a Qp:Qs in excess of 2:1 (RVO:LVO <0.5:1 or the LVO would be over twice the RVO). For the RVO to be the same as the LVO, the same volume of blood shunting left-to-right through the duct must also be shunting back to the right side of the heart through the oval foramen. Both shunts go through the lungs and so combine to increase the pulmonary blood flow to in excess of three times the systemic blood flow. When the RVO:LVO is more than 1:1, the atrial shunt must be larger than the ductal shunt.

☞ *Practical Points*
● A large left-to-right atrial shunt in the preterm is associated with:
1. Oval foramen diameter of greater than 4 mm determined with colour Doppler ultrasound.
2. Increased right ventricular volume on cross-sectional echocardiography.
3. Increased pulsed Doppler velocity at the pulmonary valve (typically 0.8–1.5 m/s) and increased RV stroke volume.
4. Paradoxical septal motion on M-mode echocardiography if ductal shunting is minimal.

In conclusion, left-to-right atrial shunting does occur in a significant number of preterm infants and

Since the duct is beyond the left ventricle, an increase in L–R ductal flow causes a rise in LV output. Therefore, in Figure 3.9 an RVO:LVO ratio of 0.5:1 means that LVO (representing pulmonary blood flow) is twice the RVO (representing systemic blood flow), i.e. there is a 2-to-1 shunt.

it exacerbates the effects of ductal shunting. It often persists for considerably longer than ductal shunting and so may have as much, if not more, impact on long-term respiratory outcomes. While we have no therapeutic means to control atrial shunting, a wider awareness of its potential haemodynamic effects will help to clarify its role in acute and chronic preterm respiratory problems.

RIGHT-TO-LEFT ATRIAL SHUNTING

High pulmonary vascular resistance is one of several factors which can lead to right-to-left atrial shunting. Right ventricular dysfunction (particularly impaired relaxation in diastole) is an important cause of right-to-left atrial shunting. Respiration influences venous return, and also therefore interatrial shunting. Spontaneous inspiration increases systemic return to the right atrium and reduces pulmonary venous return to the left atrium; it can therefore exacerbate right-to-left atrial shunting. Doppler patterns of interatrial shunting during spontaneous respiration are often very polymorphic, particularly if the right-sided pressures are raised. Inspiration during positive pressure ventilation has the reverse effect, exacerbating left-to-right shunting. Tricuspid incompetence may also increase right-to-left atrial shunt by reflecting right ventricular systolic pressures back into the right atrium. Generally, though, it is ventricular filling or diastolic pressures which will have more effect on atrial shunt patterns than systolic pressures. In pulmonary hypertension in the newborn, often pulmonary systolic pressures are suprasystemic but diastolic pressures are subsystemic. It is quite possible to have a predominantly right-to-left shunt at ductal level with a left-to-right shunt at atrial level.

It is only possible to make semiquantitative assessment of right-to-left atrial shunting. Three factors in particular should be taken into account.

1. The colour Doppler diameter of the oval foramen. While this has not been validated for right-to-left shunting, basic principles would dictate that this will also be an important factor for right-to-left shunt size. Right-to-left shunt velocities are often very low, so the maximum of colour Doppler velocity scale will need to be reduced to 0.2 m/s or less to optimize the image.

2. Duration of right-to-left shunt as a ratio to the whole cardiac cycle, as described above. This ratio can vary widely. In a study of normal term newborns,[5] the mean ratio when the atrial shunt is bidirectional was 0.15:1 with a range up to 0.32:1, whereas a small group of babies with idiopathic pulmonary hypertension almost all had ratios in excess of 0.3:1. In healthy preterm babies with minimal respiratory problems, we found a fairly similar range in those with bidirectional atrial shunts with a mean of 0.21:1 with a range up to 0.38:1. Thus, in the individual patient, the duration of right-to-left atrial shunt is probably abnormally long if it exceeds 30% of the cardiac cycle and it is definitely abnormal if it exceeds 40% (ratio 0.4:1). Figure 3.10 shows atrial shunt Doppler patterns with increasing degrees of right-to-left shunt, the normal bidirectional

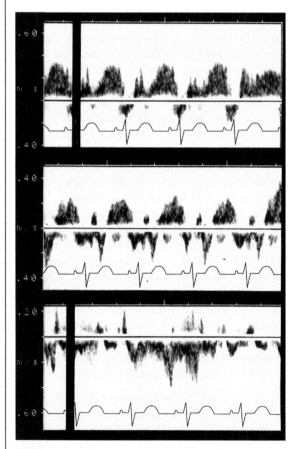

Fig. 3.10 Interatrial shunt Doppler patterns. The degree of right-to-left shunt increases from top to bottom. Top, the normal bidirectional pattern (right-to-left ratio 0.20:1); middle, an abnormal bidirectional pattern (right-to-left ratio 0.47:1); bottom, a pure right-to-left shunt.

pattern on the left (right-to-left ratio = 0.2), an abnormal bidirectional pattern in the middle (right-to-left ratio = 0.47) and a pure right-to-left shunt on the right.

3. Right-to-left velocity of the shunt. Notwithstanding the limitations of velocity assessment of atrial shunts described above, the degree of pressure differential will be reflected in the estimated right-to-left velocity of the shunt. It is unusual with normal bidirectional shunting for the maximum velocity of the right-to-left component to be over 0.2 m/s when insonating from the subcostal position. Usually velocities higher than this go together with longer duration of right-to-left shunt. However, it should be remembered that high velocities may indicate restriction of the oval foramen due to small size, and although high right-to-left velocities confirm that right atrial pressure is higher than left, quantifying flow directly is not possible.

☞ *Practical Points*
- **Echocardiographic features of a large right-to-left interatrial shunt are:**
1. **The interatrial septum bows to the left on subcostal or apical imaging.**
2. **The duration of right-to-left flow assessed by pulsed-Doppler ultrasound is greater than 40% of the cardiac cycle.**
3. **Pulsed Doppler velocities at the pulmonary valve are reduced (<0.4 m/s), as is right ventricular stroke volume.**

TERM INFANTS WITH RESPIRATORY FAILURE

In ventilated term babies with oxygen requirements greater than 80% (i.e. the group of babies who are commonly labelled as having pulmonary hypertension), there are three interesting anecdotal observations which have emerged from our experience.

1. Many babies, particularly those with primary respiratory problems, have predominantly left-to-right atrial shunting. This may reflect the fact that while pulmonary arterial pressure is high, it is often subsystemic (particularly during diastole). It may also suggest that pulmonary blood flow is adequate despite high pulmonary artery pressures and hypoxaemia.

2. Predominantly right-to-left atrial shunting is seen in two groups of babies: those with 'PFC' syndrome (i.e. hypoxaemia and elevated pulmonary vascular resistance with relatively normal lungs) particularly in the early postnatal period, and the very sickest of the babies with primary respiratory problems.

3. In almost all babies, the postnatal maturation of the oval foramen continues to occur despite their illness and it is unusual to see atrial shunts with large colour Doppler diameters after the first 3 to 4 postnatal days.

In general, atrial shunting is very difficult to assess from the clinical signs in any baby. This emphasizes the need for wider dissemination of and immediate access to echocardiographic skills within newborn intensive care units. It is to be hoped this will improve our understanding and the appropriateness of our therapy for these sick babies.

REFERENCES

1. Evans N, Iyer P. Incompetence of the foramen ovale in preterm infants supported by mechanical ventilation. *Journal of Pediatrics* 1994;125:786–792. Mosby Year Book Inc.

2. Evans N, Iyer P. Assessment of ductus arteriosus shunt in preterm infants supported by mechanical ventilation: effects of interatrial shunting. *Journal of Pediatrics* 1994;125:778–785. Mosby Year Book Inc.

3. Patten B, M. Closure of the foramen ovale. *American Journal of Anatomy* 1931;48:19–44.

4. Steinfeld L, Almeida OD, Rothfeld EL. Asynchronous atrioventricular valve opening as it relates to right to left interatrial shunting in the normal newborn. *Journal of the American College of Cardiology* 1988;12:712–718.

5. Hiraishi S, Agata Y, Saito K et al. Interatrial shunt flow profiles in newborn infants: a colour flow and pulsed Doppler echocardiographic study. *British Heart Journal* 1991;65:41–45.

6. Pollick C, Sullivan H, Cujec B, Wilansky S. Doppler color-flow imaging assessment of shunt size in atrial septal defect [published erratum appears in *Circulation* 1988 Oct; 78(4):1081]. *Circulation* 1988;78:522–528.

7. Hornberger LK, Sahn DJ, Krabill KA et al. Elucidation of the natural history of ventricular septal defects by serial Doppler color flow mapping studies. *Journal of the American College of Cardiology* 1989;13:1111–1118.

8. Hannu H, Pentti K, Henrik E, Markku S, Ilkka V. Patency of foramen ovale – does it influence haemodynamics in newborn infants? *Early Human Development* 1989;20:281–287.

9. Fukazawa M, Fukushige J, Ueda K. Atrial septal defects in neonates with reference to spontaneous closure. *American Heart Journal* 1988;116:123–127.

CHAPTER 4

Ventricular
function

Jonathan P Wyllie

BACKGROUND

Ventricular function may be depressed in neonatal disease processes such as hypoxia, sepsis, rhesus haemolytic disease, hyaline membrane disease, PPHN and transient tachypnoea.[1-6] In contrast to adult patients, little is known about the best way to assess ventricular function. Invasive monitoring of central venous pressure, capillary wedge pressure and cardiac output are seldom done in the neonate and especially the preterm. Usually heart rate and blood pressure are the only measured indices of cardiac function and they may be misleading. A dysfunctional heart may be tachycardic, bradycardic or have a normal rate. In hypotensive neonates cardiac function may be depressed, normal or even hyperdynamic.[1,4-6]

Therapeutic interventions may modify cardiac function or cardiac output intentionally or incidentally so an index of ventricular performance is needed to make sure that such interventions are appropriate. This is now possible by echocardiography. Serial measurements allow rapid assessment of the effectiveness of therapeutic interventions.

SYSTOLIC FUNCTION

Most of what is known about ventricular function in the neonate pertains to systole rather than diastole, although both are important. With regard to systolic function, the left ventricle is technically much easier to assess than the right, mainly due to its cavity shape.

Myocardial function and cardiac output

It is important to remember that ventricular function (or 'myocardial fibre shortening') and cardiac output are not the same thing. Cardiac output is a product of stroke volume and heart rate. Stroke volume is, in turn, determined by (1) ventricular size and (2) myocardial fibre shortening. The latter is determined by the ventricle's contractile state and its preload and afterload. Echocardiographic assessments of myocardial fibre shortening can therefore be normal with a low cardiac output – such as in hypovolaemia (low preload), where the treatment is volume replacement and not inotropes.

Contractility is affected by heart rate as well as by metabolic and pharmacological factors. Also, for a given level of contractility, ventricular function varies with preload (end-diastolic ventricular volume) and afterload (systemic resistance). The former is described by the Frank–Starling curve (Fig. 4.1). Stroke volume increases with increased end-diastolic volume up to a limit. Increased contractility will shift the curve up. Conversely, there is an inverse relationship between stroke volume and systemic resistance for a given level of contractility.

Ventricular function and cardiac output need to be measured and considered separately, and an assessment made of preload and afterload, to gain the whole haemodynamic picture.

Defining systole

Figure 4.2 summarizes the different phases of the cardiac cycle. In the left ventricle, systole may be defined as the period from the closure of the mitral valve to the closure of the aortic valve. However, if ECG leads are attached during echocardiography (as should be the rule), systole may also be defined as starting with ventricular depolarization (QRS complex). Whichever definition is used, mitral valve closure is followed by a period of isovolumic contraction (the 'pre-ejection period') during which pressure rises rapidly until it exceeds that in the aorta. When this occurs, the aortic valve opens and the ejection phase commences, during which ventricular volume decreases as blood flows into the aorta. Ventricular pressure exceeds aortic during the ejection phase resulting initially in acceleration of blood into the aorta. During the second part of ejection the pressure difference declines, resulting in deceleration of blood flow until the aortic valve closes.

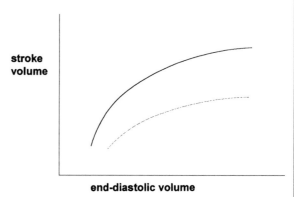

stroke volume

end-diastolic volume

Fig. 4.1 The relationship between stroke volume and end-diastolic volume for a normal and a failing ventricle.

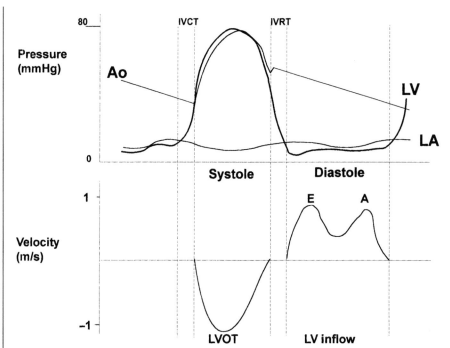

Fig. 4.2 The cardiac cycle. Left ventricular (LV), aortic (Ao) and left atrial (LA) pressures are shown with Doppler velocity curves from the left ventricular outflow and inflow. Isovolumic contraction time (IVCT) and isovolumic relaxation time (IVRT) are also shown.

Assessing left ventricular systolic function

Full assessment of left ventricular systolic function depends upon cross-sectional, M-mode and Doppler echocardiography.

Cross-sectional echocardiography

With experience, echocardiographers can learn to make a clinically useful subjective assessment of left ventricular function by 'eyeballing' parasternal long-axis and four-chamber views of the heart. Such an assessment of ventricular contractility, end-systolic and end-diastolic volumes can be used to classify function as 'hypercontractile', 'normal', 'mildly reduced' or 'poor'. This can be useful in patient management but has little place in research and is not desirable in monitoring interventions. Cross-sectional echocardiography also permits accurate positioning of an M-mode beam in the long-axis parasternal (see Fig. 1.5.1) or short-axis parasternal view (see Fig. 1.5.2) of the left ventricle. These measurements are the most useful.

M-mode echocardiography

Measurements are most commonly taken from the long-axis view, which profiles the left atrium, mitral valve, left ventricle and aortic valve (see Chapter 1.5). The M-mode beam is positioned just at the mitral leaflet tips, perpendicular to the long axis of the ventricle. In the short axis the M-mode should be centred. Measurements must be taken from standard and reproducible positions.[7,8]

Measurements are taken at end systole and end diastole of interventricular septal thickness (IVSS, IVSD), left ventricular internal diameter (LVEDD, LVESD) and posterior wall dimensions (PWDS, PWDD) (see Fig. 4.3).

From these measurements several parameters of ventricular function can be calculated.

Fractional shortening
Fractional shortening (FS) characterizes left ventricular contractility although

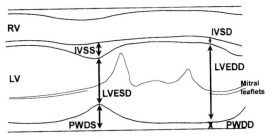

Fig. 4.3 M-mode of left ventricle at the level of the mitral valve leaflets. Measurements of LV internal diameter in systole (LVESD) and diastole (LVEDD), interventricular septum in systole (IVSS) and diastole (IVSD), posterior wall in systole (PWDS) and diastole (PWDD).

it is also affected by preload and afterload. It is calculated as

$$FS\ (\%) = \left(\frac{LVEDD - LVESD}{LVEDD}\right) \times 100\%$$

The normal range in adults is 25–45% (95% confidence limits) but the range in preterm babies is 23–40% and 25–41% in term babies (10th and 90th centiles). Fractional shortening is one of the most reproducible measurements of left ventricular function, but errors occur if the M-mode is not positioned accurately and overestimation of dimensions may occur if the beam is oblique. This can be minimized with cross-sectional positioning of the M-mode cursor.

☞ *Practical Point*
- **In measuring left ventricular fractional shortening, the M-mode beam must be perpendicular to the interventricular septum (parasternal long-axis view) and central within the left ventricle (parasternal short-axis view).**

Velocity of circumferential fibre shortening (Vcf)

Errors in fractional shortening estimation may occur in early preterm life due to distortion of the left ventricle and abnormal septal wall motion associated with neonatal right ventricular dominance.[9,10] Mean velocity of circumferential fibre shortening (Vcf) has been suggested as a simple alternative measurement of left ventricular contractility.[11,12] It is less sensitive to minor dimensional discrepancies and involves no assumptions about ventricular shape. It offers a reproducible measurement of neonatal ventricular contractility.

LVEDD and LVESD are measured as above and left ventricular ejection time (LVET) is usually measured from the closure to the opening of the mitral valve (taken from the M-mode trace; see Fig. 4.4).

$$Vcf = mean \left(\frac{LVEDD - LVESD}{LVEDD}\right) \times LVET$$

The units are circumferences per second.

The normal value was established by Sahn *et al.*[12] as 1.5 ± 0.04 circumferences/s in preterm and term infants. They reported no significant changes with age after the first 30 minutes of life (before this an increase was observed in seven babies studied serially).

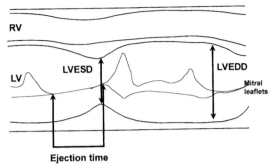

Fig. 4.4 M-mode of the LV at the level of the mitral valve leaflets showing LVEDD, LVESD and LVET (for calculation of velocity of Vcf).

Like fractional shortening, Vcf is influenced by left ventricular volume. It is usually higher in LV volume overload, particularly when afterload is also reduced, such as with a left-to-right ductal shunt. It is being used increasingly in haemodynamic research in the newborn (see Chapter 9.3). Correction for heart rate can be done by substituting LVET by LVETc, where LVETc is LVET divided by the square root of the R–R interval (the normal value is 0.98 ± 0.07 circumferences/s).

One should of course be very wary of such calculations which require so many measurements. In each factor measured there is measurement error, and these errors may multiply each other!

Stroke volume Stroke volume (SV) is most accurately determined using Doppler echocardiography, as described in Chapter 5, but it can be calculated from M-mode measurements. The calculation assumes that the left ventricle is an ellipsoid of revolution. This is often not the case in the newborn, however, due to right ventricular dominance distorting the shape of the left ventricle.

$$SV = LVEDD^3 - LVESD^3$$

Ventricular output can be calculated from this by multiplying the stroke volume by heart rate.

Ejection fraction Similarly, the proportion of ventricular contents which is ejected during systole, or the 'ejection fraction' (EF), can be calculated from:

$$EF = stroke\ volume/end\text{-}diastolic\ volume$$

Thus

$$EF\ (\%) = \left(\frac{LVEDD^3 - LVESD^3}{LVEDD^3}\right) \times 100\%$$

These measurements have been used a great deal in adult practice. However, the measurements made are cubed, and thus any errors in those measurements will be cubed. In adults with large hearts such errors are relatively small, but in neonates the errors tend to be larger. Any change in shape of the ventricular cavity also makes this method particularly unreliable. For these reasons we would recommend the use of fractional shortening rather than ejection fraction.

Left ventricular mass This can be calculated from the measurements, taken at end diastole, of interventricular septal thickness (IVSD), posterior wall dimensions (PWDD) and left ventricular internal diameter (LVEDD). This calculation also assumes that the ventricle is an ellipsoid of revolution. If leading edge to leading edge measurements are used, the formula is[8]:

$$\text{LV mass} = 0.8 \times 1.055 \times [(\text{IVSD}+\text{PWDD}+\text{LVEDD})^3 - \text{LVEDD}^3]$$

This has not been validated for use in the neonate, but is of some interest as a research tool (see Chapter 9.3).

Volume load assessment M-mode assessment of the left ventricle and atrial size provides information about changes in ventricular preload. The ratio of these chambers to the aorta is used to assess the effect of shunts upon the heart, especially the arterial duct. The normal left atrial to aortic root ratio is 0.84–1.39 in preterm babies and 0.95–1.38 at term (10th and 90th centiles). Ratios of more than 1.4:1 or 1.5:1 suggest volume loading (see Chapter 7).

Recent data in hypotensive newborns suggests that a LVEDD:Ao ratio of more than 2.0:1 (>90th centile) makes further volume loading of the neonatal ventricle unlikely to produce a sustained increase in cardiac output.[6]

Doppler assessment of systolic function

Ventricular output Stroke volume and cardiac output can be calculated from the product of the integral of the ascending aortic Doppler velocity–time curve (also known as stroke distance) and the cross-sectional area of the aorta derived from its diameter. This is covered in detail in Chapter 5. However, it is worth noting now that

serial changes in the mean velocity or the stroke distance correlate directly to change in stroke volume.* For serial study it is not necessary to measure the aortic root diameter.[12,13]

Systolic time intervals The *shape* of the aortic Doppler velocity–time curve also yields information about ventricular function, though the shape is also affected by changes in afterload (e.g. due to left-to-right ductal shunting) and preload. If function is normal, the isovolumetric ('pre-ejection') phase is short, the rate of pressure rise is rapid, and the period from the onset of flow to maximum velocity ('time to peak velocity') is short. If ventricular function is reduced, these phases are both prolonged.

In the neonatal heart, the heart rate is so fast that measurement of acceleration time is prone to error, making it less clinically useful. The analysis is used little in clinical practice. Furthermore, mitral regurgitation (a common accompaniment to poor ventricular function) shortens the time to peak velocity, confusing the picture further.

Assessing right ventricular function

M-mode echocardiography

The right ventricle is more complex in shape than the left and is 'wrapped' around the left ventricle. This complex anatomy makes quantitative evaluation by M-mode difficult at any age and not very useful in the neonate because it is not possible to get a reliable 'slice' through the ventricle that represents overall function. Furthermore the ventricular septum is dominated by the left ventricle, so fractional shortening of the diameter of the right ventricle means little.

Despite these drawbacks, a dilated outflow tract may be seen (in the standard parasternal long-axis view) in pathological right ventricular dilatation, and the right ventricular chamber will appear larger than the left. In adults and children, dilatation is described as mild (enlarged but RV<LV), moderate (RV=LV) and severe (RV>LV). However, the right ventricle is dominant at birth and is greatly

---

*Stroke volume has also been measured at the mitral orifice in adults assuming the annulus to be circular and using the long-axis parasternal view. The transmitral flow is then estimated using pulsed Doppler at the mitral leaflets from an apical four-chamber view (Fig. 2.2.6). Left ventricular output can be calculated in a way analogous that described for the aorta, but this method has yet to be validated in the newborn.

enlarged compared with later life. This can be very striking – especially in the first few hours of life.

The motion of the interventricular septum as seen in the parasternal long-axis view or with M-mode echocardiography is influenced by right ventricular pressure or volume overload. Normally the septum moves as if it were part of the left ventricle, i.e. towards the centre of the ventricle and towards the left ventricular posterior wall. However, as the right ventricle becomes volume loaded, the motion becomes flatter until the septal motion reverses and becomes 'paradoxical'. This indicates right ventricular volume overload. It is seen with atrial septal defects and pulmonary incompetence, but also in severe PPHN. It is also important as it renders indices of left ventricular systolic function based upon M-mode measurements useless (see Fig. 4.5).

☞ *Practical Point*
- **Marked RV dominance leads to marked inaccuracy in all of the calculations of LV function from M-mode measurements including FS and Vcf.**

Cross-sectional echocardiography

Useful subjective assessment of right ventricular systolic function can be done with experience from apical, subcostal and parasternal short-axis views. In asphyxia with PPHN, the right ventricle appears grossly enlarged and stiff, and the high end-

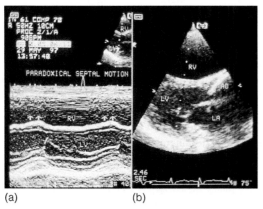

(a)　　　　　　　(b)

Fig. 4.5 Paradoxical septal motion (in a patient with severe tricuspid valve regurgitation). (a) The arrows indicate that the interventricular septum paradoxically moves away from the LV posterior wall during systole.
(b) The parasternal view shows the large RV cavity.

diastolic pressure reduces diastolic inflow so the right atrium becomes distended (see Chapter 10.2).

Doppler assessment of systolic function

As with ascending aortic Doppler and the left ventricle, it is possible to obtain serial assessment of change in right ventricular stroke volume by serial assessment of the pulmonary arterial flow velocity–time integral (stroke distance), most usefully obtained with pulsed Doppler at the pulmonary valve as discussed in Chapters 3, 5 and 9.2.

The isovolumic (pre-ejection) phase is measurably prolonged with RV dysfunction, and it is prolonged further by a high pulmonary vascular resistance.[14] This is discussed in more detail in Chapter 6.

☞ *Practical Point*
- **The clinically most useful assessment of RV systolic function is made by subjective review of cross-sectional images.**

DIASTOLIC FUNCTION

Background

Recent years have seen an enormous increase in interest in adult cardiology in the role of diastole in ventricular performance, particularly in ischaemic heart disease, ventricular hypertrophy, cardiomyopathies and pericardial disease. Now that diabetic cardiomyopathy and dexamethasone-induced cardiac hypertrophy[15] are recognized in the neonate, the assessment of diastolic function should be an important subject for research. Hypertrophic cardiomyopathy is characterized by supernormal systolic function and grossly impaired diastolic relaxation. This reduces cardiac output by limiting ventricular filling, and results in atrial dilatation. However, relatively few studies of diastolic function have been carried out in neonates.[16–18] We can be sure that diastolic dysfunction is common in pathological states though; profound right-to-left atrial shunting in some hypoxaemic infants is testimony to that.

Defining diastole

Ventricular diastole is defined as the interval between closure of the outlet (aortic or pulmonary) valve to closure of the inlet valve. Initially, the ventricular pressure falls rapidly during the isovolumic relaxation phase. When ventricular pressure falls below atrial pressure, the mitral or tricuspid valve opens and blood flows into the ventricle. Assuming that the inlet valve is normal, the rate and pattern of flow (which can be seen with pulsed Doppler studies) depends upon the pressure gradient across it. This is determined by several factors:

1. the rate of ventricular relaxation
2. the end-diastolic pressure in the ventricle
3. venous filling of the atrium
4. atrial contraction.

The ventricle fills passively at first until the pressures equalize and flow slows or ceases for a short time (diastasis). Atrial systole then boosts flow into the ventricle.

Doppler inflow studies

Normative data exist for the inflow patterns across the mitral and tricuspid valves; these are discussed in Chapter 2.2. Flow pattern is influenced by ventricular relaxation. However, there is a wide range of normal findings and tachycardia often causes the E and A waves to merge.

Left ventricular filling

Doppler recordings of left ventricular filling velocities correspond with those measured by other techniques. Pulsed wave Doppler is used from the apical four-chamber view (Chapter 2.2, Figs 2.2.5 and 2.2.6). In the normal patient, rapid, passive flow of blood following mitral opening produces an E velocity wave. This is followed by a variable period of minimal flow before the A wave due to atrial contraction. Quantitative measurements can be made from the Doppler velocity curve:

1. maximum velocities – the E and A velocities and their ratio
2. acceleration and deceleration times – time from onset to peak velocity
3. time intervals – duration of the components of diastole
4. velocity–time integrals – for volumetric analysis.

At high heart rates the period of diastasis is shortened, producing an A wave closely after an E wave. The two usually merge in the neonate with a high heart rate. In normal children E filling is

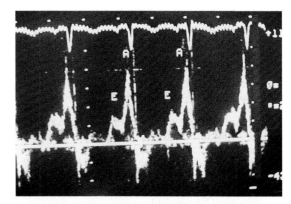

Fig. 4.6 Abnormal inflow through the mitral valve: the A wave is much higher than the E wave. This example was taken from an infant after closure of the arterial duct with indomethacin; the dramatic reduction in LV cavity size seemed to result in this transient abnormality of diastolic relaxation of the LV.

greater than A; 80% of filling occurs early in diastole. With age the atrial component becomes more important with equalization of velocities at about 60 years of age. Before birth, the fetal mitral A wave is dominant or at least equal to the E wave.[19] Postnatally, the mean normal ratio in the premature neonate is 1.0:1, and 1.1:1 at term.[17,18] Interpretation is therefore difficult owing to the wide range of normality, but a ratio of <0.6:1 in preterm and <0.7:1 in term babies may suggest a diastolic filling abnormality (see Fig. 4.6).

REFERENCES

1. Gill AB, Weindling AM. Echocardiographic assessment of cardiac function in shocked very low birthweight infants. *Archives of Disease in Childhood* 1993;68:17–21.
2. Halliday HL, McClure G, McCreid M. Transient tachypnoea of the newborn: two distinct entities? *Archives of Disease in Childhood* 1981;56:322–325.
3. Skinner JR, Boys RJ, Hunter S, Hey EN. Pulmonary and systemic arterial pressure in hyaline membrane disease. *Archives of Disease in Childhood* 1992;67:366–373.
4. Skinner JR, Hunter S, Hey EN. Haemodynamic features at presentation in persistent pulmonary hypertension of the newborn and outcome. *Archives of Disease in Childhood* 1996;74:26–32.
5. Evans N, Kluckow M. Early determinants of right and left ventricular output in ventilated preterm infants. *Archives of Disease in Childhood* 1996;74(2):F88–F94.
6. Wyllie JP, Hunter S, Hey EN. *Towards logical treatment of hypotension*. Presentation to the Neonatal Society. Newcastle upon Tyne, July 1996.
7. Sahn DJ, DeMaria A, Kisslo J, Weyman A. Recommendations regarding quantitation in m-mode echocardiography: results of a survey of

echocardiographic measurements. *Circulation* 1978;6:1072–1083.

8. American Society of Echocardiography Committee on Standards, Subcommittee on Quantitation of Two-Dimensional Echocardiograms. Recommendations for quantitation of the left ventricle by two-dimensional echocardiography. *Journal of the American Society of Echocardiography* 1989;2:361–367.

9. Lee LA, Kimball TR, Daniels SR, Khoury P, Meyer RA. Left ventricular mechanics in the preterm infant and their effect on the measurement of cardiac performance. *Journal of Pediatrics* 1992;120(1):114–119.

10. Karliner JW, Gault J, Eckberg D, Mullins C, Ross J. Mean velocity of fiber shortening – a simplified measure of left ventricular contractility in man. *Circulation* 1971; 44:323.

11. Sahn DJ, Terry R, O'Rourke R, Leopold G, Friedman WF. A new technique for the non-invasive diagnosis of cyanotic congenital heart disease. *Circulation* 1973;48 (suppl IV):224.

12. Sahn DJ, Deely WJ, Hagan AD, Friedman WF. Echocardiographic assessment of left ventricular performance in normal newborns. *Circulation* 1974;XLIX:232–236.

13. Hudson I, Houston A, Aitchison T, Holland B, Turner T. Reproducibility of measurements of cardiac output in newborn infants by Doppler ultrasound. *Archives of Disease in Childhood* 1990;65:15–19.

14. Skinner JR, Boys RJ, Heads A, Hey EN, Hunter S. Estimation of pulmonary artery pressure in the newborn: study of the repeatability of four Doppler echocardiographic techniques. *Pediatric Cardiology* 1996;17:360–369.

15. Evans N. Cardiovascular effects of dexamethasone in the preterm infant. *Archives of Disease in Childhood* 1994;70(1):F25–F30.

16. Trang T, Tibballs J, Mercier J, Beafils F. Optimization of oxygen transport in mechanically ventilated newborns using oximetry and pulsed Doppler-derived output. *Critical Care Medicine* 1988;16:1094–1097.

17. Johnson GL, Moffett CB, Noonan JA. Doppler echocardiographic studies of diastolic ventricular filling patterns in premature infants. *American Heart Journal* 1988;116:1172–1174.

18. Riggs TW, Rodriguez R, Snider AR. Doppler evaluation of right and left diastolic function in normal neonates. *Journal of the American College of Cardiology* 1989;13:700–705.

19. Allan LD. Normal fetal cardiac anatomy – Doppler echocardiography. In: Allan LD (ed.) *Manual of Foetal Echocardiography*, pp 56–73. Lancaster, England: MTP Press, 1986.

CHAPTER 5

Cardiac output

Dale C Alverson

INTRODUCTION

Cardiac output is one of the major determinants of systemic blood flow, which, in turn, provides oxygen delivery throughout the body[1]:

O$_2$ delivery = cardiac output (CO) × arterial oxygen content

Cardiac output monitoring should therefore be useful and important in the newborn intensive care unit, providing additional data to ensure adequate systemic oxygen delivery in order to preserve organ function and viability and prevent tissue damage and death.[2] It is common practice to monitor blood pressure in the critically ill or preterm neonate, but this is only an indirect indicator of blood flow or cardiac output since it is also dependent upon systemic vascular resistance (SVR). Thus:

Mean arterial pressure = CO × SVR

Changes in blood pressure over time may reflect changes in either cardiac output, vascular resistance or a combination of the two. Isolated values are even more difficult to interpret. The more critical variable is cardiac output since it is a major determinate of overall oxygen delivery. However, its measurement has been difficult in the past because of the small size and clinical instability of the patients and the invasiveness of most methods. Echocardiography provides a suitable non-invasive method.

This chapter focuses on measurement of left ventricular output (LVO). It is also possible to measure right ventricular output; this technique is incompletely evaluated in the neonate but is discussed briefly at the end of this chapter.

The technique to assess LVO involves measuring the mean velocity of blood flow in the ascending aorta using either pulsed or continuous wave (CW) Doppler, and determining the diameter of the aortic root using cross-sectional or M-mode echocardiography. It is important to remember that this method is actually measuring LVO rather than total or effective systemic cardiac output; in the presence of left-to-right ductal shunting, for example, more blood is flowing through the ascending aorta than is reaching the descending aorta beyond the duct. With a closed duct, however, LVO equals systemic cardiac output. This important issue is addressed again later.

To calculate LVO from the velocity and diameter measurements, two equally suitable equations can be used; both are shown below. In both cases AoCSA represents ascending aortic cross-sectional area. The two equations give exactly the same end result.

$$\text{LVO (ml/min)} = \text{VAo (cm/s)} \times 60 \text{ s/min} \times \text{AoCSA (cm}^2) \qquad (1)$$

where VAo is the = temporal and spatial mean ascending aortic flow velocity.[3]

$$\text{LVO (ml/min)} = \text{AoSD (cm)} \times \text{heart rate (bpm)} \times \text{AoCSA (cm}^2) \qquad (2)$$

where AoSD is the aortic stroke distance* (also 'FVI', flow velocity integral).

It is usual in neonatology to represent ventricular output as an index in relation to body weight, i.e. x ml/kg/min. (In cardiology cardiac output is usually related to body surface area (litres/min/m^2).)

METHODS AND INSTRUMENTATION

There are a variety of approaches to obtain Doppler-derived cardiac output measurements. The choice of approach depends upon available equipment, technical expertise, the size of the infant and personal preference.

To obtain Doppler signals one may use:

1. non-imaging or duplex (simultaneous Doppler and imaging) techniques (Fig. 5.1);
2. pulsed or CW Doppler (Figs 5.2, 5.3);
3. suprasternal, apical or subcostal approaches (Fig. 5.1).

In determining the cross-sectional area of the aorta one can:

1. make the measurement at the LVOT or at or above the aortic valve (Fig. 5.4);
2. use cross-sectional or M-mode imaging (Fig. 5.5).

All have been used in reported literature. The most important factors are to keep repeatability error as low as possible, and consistently use the same method.

AoSD equals the area under the velocity curve. Conceptually, it represents the distance a single red cell would travel up the ascending aorta in systole. When this distance is multiplied by the cross-sectional area (AoSD × AoCSA), a volume is obtained; the left ventricular stroke volume. Multiplying by heart rate gives the LVO per minute.

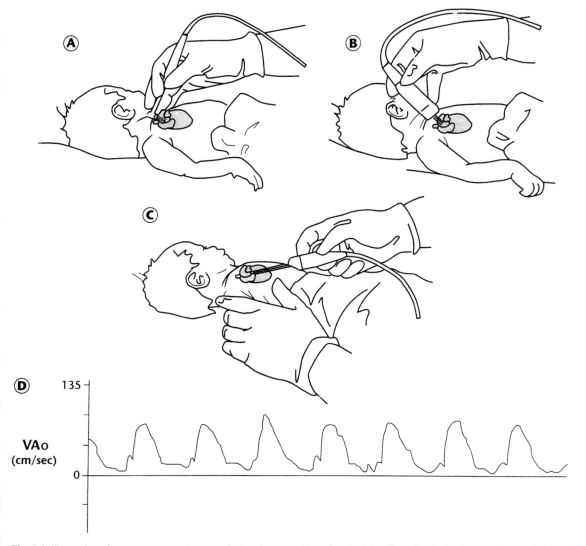

Fig. 5.1 Illustration of some common ultrasound transducer positions for obtaining Doppler-derived ascending aortic blood flow velocity signals.

(a) Suprasternal approach using a 'hammer-head' non-imaging Doppler transducer with the ultrasound beam directed down the ascending aorta towards the aortic valve.

(b) Suprasternal approach using a 'duplex' imaging and Doppler transducer allowing image verification of Doppler sample volume location and the angle of insonance (see also Fig. 5.2).

(c) Subcostal approach using a 'duplex' imaging and Doppler transducer with the ultrasound beam directed into the LVO tract and ascending aorta with image verification of Doppler sample volume location and angle of insonance.

(d) Typical phasic ascending aortic blood flow velocity signals which can be obtained using any of these approaches.

This section discusses some of these approaches. It concentrates only on assessment of LVO.

Beginning the procedure

It is always wise to begin by performing a routine echocardiogram (as well as clinical examination) as described earlier in this book, with a settled, quiet infant. Do not assume that there is a normal heart. Particular attention should be paid to the aortic valve, to assure the absence of stenosis and to ascertain whether or not the arterial duct is open. During this study the diameter of the aorta can be measured, before going on to the Doppler measurements.

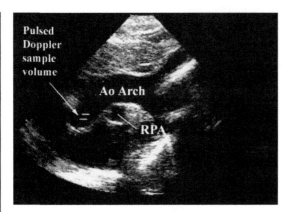

Fig. 5.2 Ultrasound image from a 'duplex' transducer using a suprasternal approach showing the Doppler sample volume in the ascending aorta above the aortic valve. RPA, right pulmonary artery.

☞ *Practical Point*
- **Always confirm normal cardiac anatomy prior to the assessment of cardiac output, and in particular exclude aortic valve disease and assess ductal patency.**

Non-imaging suprasternal

At our institution we prefer a 'blind' suprasternal approach to obtain ascending aortic Doppler velocity signals and use a pulsed wave Doppler probe without simultaneous 'duplexed' ultrasound images of the sampled region.[4] Blood flow velocity signals are obtained using a 5 or 3.5 MHz, range-gated, pulsed Doppler velocimeter and a 'hammer-head' shaped suprasternal transducer. This type of equipment is less expensive than combined Doppler and imaging 'duplex' systems but perhaps requires more technical skill in order to obtain reliable and reproducible measurements.

The hand-held transducer is placed on a layer of airless contact gel in the suprasternal notch with the infant in a supine position and the ultrasound beam is directed towards the ascending aorta (Fig. 5.1). By correct anatomical orientation, careful movement of the transducer, and use of the range gate to determine appropriate depth of sampling (usually 1.5–3.5 cm in newborns, dependent on their size), the operator searches 'blindly' for the highest characteristic aortic velocity signals. The operator both listens to the signals and watches the trace. The characteristic signals should indicate that the sample volume is in the ascending aorta just above the valve leaflets at an angle of insonance less than

15°. Aortic blood flow velocity signals have a characteristic high-pitched, clean, homogeneous sound. Displayed on screen, there is a rapid systolic upstroke followed by an initial rapid downstroke and variable degrees of positive and negative velocities during diastole close to the baseline (Figs 5.1 and 5.3). Excessive positive or negative velocities far from the baseline during diastole usually indicate inappropriate placement of the sample volume. The flow profile should be of a laminar type, i.e. non-turbulent, with most of the blood at any one time travelling at roughly the same speed. This is shown by 'hollow' rather than 'filled' signals on the spectral display. Even mild aortic stenosis renders the technique invalid, as does placing the sampling towards the side of the aorta where viscous friction reduces the local velocity.

The system software can often measure the temporal mean velocity automatically, rather than

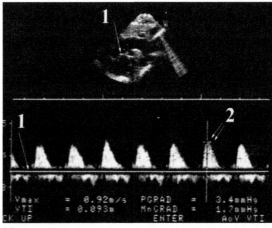

(a)

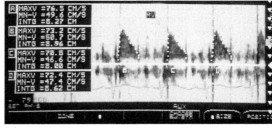

(b)

Fig. 5.3 (a) Ultrasound image showing the direction of the CW Doppler beam in the ascending aorta using a suprasternal approach and the ascending aortic blood flow velocity signals. (1) represents the zero baseline and (2) the maximum peak velocity.
(b) Doppler flow in the ascending aorta from a blind CW pencil probe. MAXV and MN-V, maximum and mean velocity; INTG, flow velocity integral (or stroke distance).

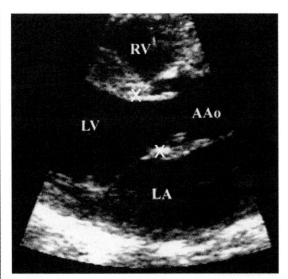

Fig. 5.4 Ultrasound long-axis cardiac image showing the ascending aorta (AAo) and aortic valve in region where ascending aortic diameter measurements can be taken. The crosses indicate the aortic valve annulus, at the hinge points of the aortic valve.

having to trace over the waveform by hand. The analogue velocity signals can be characterized most accurately by using a zero crossing counter (ZCC) or from the maximum or mode of the velocity spectral dispersion envelope displayed over time (Fig. 5.6).[5]

To calculate volume of flow, measurement of the ascending aortic diameter is required. We prefer to measure the diameter where we expect the Doppler sample region to be, i.e. just above the aortic valve leaflets. M-mode or cross-sectional echocardiography can be used (Fig. 5.5). Some authors have found that M-mode measurements are more repeatable than cross-sectional measurements. This may in part be due to the relatively high definition to wall edges given by M-mode. However, with good images, cross-sectional echocardiography can also be used. Cross-sectional area (AoCSA) is derived from diameter (d) thus:

$$AoCSA = p\,(d^2/4)$$

Duplex: apical and suprasternal

Duplex ultrasound scanners which combine and integrate Doppler with cross-sectional imaging are now available in many institutions. They allow more accurate visual placement of the Doppler ultrasound beam in the area of interest, as well as assuring a small angle of insonance or (if the angle

is greater than 20°) direct measurement of that angle in order to calculate the true velocity using the Doppler equation (see Chapter 2.1). Many machines can do this correction automatically.

LVO measurements can be obtained using either a suprasternal or apical approach to view the ascending aorta. Figure 5.5 shows a long-axis view obtained from the apical approach; the sample volume can be moved along the left ventricular outflow tract or into the aorta (Fig. 5.1).[6] Values obtained from the apical position tend to be slightly lower than those obtained from the suprasternal position, so it is important to use only one approach in serial study of the same patient.

CW doppler

Pulsed wave Doppler has the advantage that the sample volume can be placed at various depths, potentially allowing the operator to avoid superfluous or undesired signals from other flow

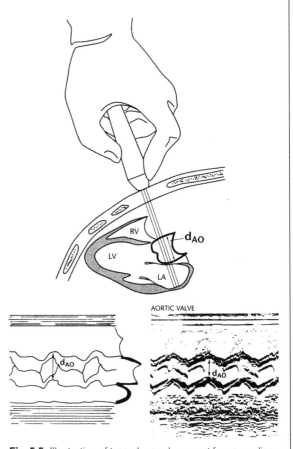

Fig. 5.5 Illustration of transducer placement for ascending aorta diameter (d_{Ao}) measurement and M-mode tracings from which d_{Ao} measurement can be made.

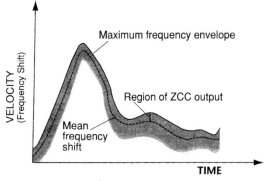

VELOCITY (Frequency Shift)

Maximum frequency envelope

Region of ZCC output

Mean frequency shift

TIME

Doppler spectral display

Fig. 5.6 Illustration of a spectral display of an aortic blood flow velocity signal over time and the region of the signal representing the maximum frequency envelope versus region of zero crossing counter (ZCC) output versus mean frequency shift. Any of these regions can be used to characterize the temporal velocity signal for subsequent integration (area under the curve) and determination of the temporal mean velocity and ultimate volumetric flow calculations. The method used would normally show minimal differences in the ascending aorta and result in similar temporal mean velocity measurements. However, if there is significant spectral dispersion, characterization of the velocity signal using these different methods could differ significantly and affect temporal mean velocity determination.

streams elsewhere along the path of the ultrasound beam. However, CW Doppler has also been used successfully in neonates[7,8] with very acceptable results for repeatability. The absolute values are also similar to those obtained with pulsed wave Doppler.

One reason for the success of this method may be the very fact that accurate depth positioning is not necessary. Provided the beam passing down the ascending aorta is in line with the ascending aorta, it will continue down through the aortic valve and into the LVOT. The highest velocity anywhere along the beam will be represented as the peak velocity in the velocity profile.

The preferred technique is to insonate from the suprasternal notch using a 'blind' (non-imaging) small pencil probe, similar to the pulsed Doppler probes (see Fig. 2.3.1). Interpretation of the signals is rather different, however (Fig. 5.3b). The aim is that the Doppler beam should pass through the aortic valve, such that opening and closing valve 'clicks' should be present on the spectral trace at the onset and end of systolic flow (seen best on Fig. 5.3b). The upstroke should be smooth, and there should be

little flow away (downward) from the probe during systole. If the beam is tilted too far posteriorly it insonates the aortic arch, so that flow is across the beam and both upward and downward flow is detected during systole. Further posterior tilt leads to detection of flow into the descending aorta, away from the probe, leading to a downwards only deflection on the trace. If the probe tilts too far anteriorly, the signal becomes weak until it is lost altogether. Confusion can also be caused by a higher upward velocity arising from the innominate artery to the right of the midline. This is avoided by taking care to keep the probe in the mid-suprasternal notch, and to have valve clicks simultaneously on the trace.

Limitations

There are physical and technical limitations to obtaining Doppler-derived measurements of cardiac output. As with any ultrasound method, interspersed free air interferes with transmission and reception of the ultrasound signal and the area of interest. Thus a pneumothorax (commonly) and pneumomediastinum, pnuemopericardium or even subcutaneous emphysema (rarely) may preclude Doppler-derived measurement of cardiac output. Since accurate determination of blood flow velocity is best achieved in a stream of laminar flow, turbulent flow with a high velocity, wide spectral spread and varying directions of flow also precludes accurate measurements of spatial mean velocity representing the entire flow stream. Thus the technique is unreliable in patients with aortic valve stenosis or regurgitation. Excessive movement of the infant may make consistent vascular insonation difficult; patients can only be studied while quiet.

VALIDATION OF THE METHOD

We compared Doppler-derived values with measurements obtained using the Fick principle in 33 paediatric patients (age 3 days to 17 years) during cardiac catheterization.[3] There was close correlation between the two methods. Linear regression analysis of values ranging from 403 to 5540 ml/min revealed a correlation coefficient of 0.98 with a slope of 1.07 and a y-intercept of –4.5 ml (Fig. 5.7). Other investigators have also shown similar strong correlation between Doppler-derived values and those obtained using invasive methods

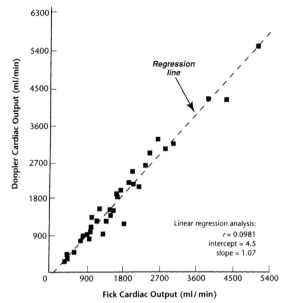

Fig. 5.7 Graphical linear regression comparison of Doppler-derived and Fick-derived left ventricular cardiac output measurements in 33 paediatric cardiac catheterization patients revealing close correlation of the two methods.

in the paediatric age group.[9] The accuracy has been validated in vitro using flow phantoms and a pulsatile pump where absolute flow can be measured directly.[5]

We have evaluated reproducibility of the pulsed Doppler velocity measurement among four investigators in 10 healthy term newborns between 8 and 24 hours of age.[10] The coefficient of variation between operators (interoperator variability) was only 2.5%. The coefficient of variation for intraoperator measurements was 11.7% for single measurements and 6.6% for the average of the three repeated measures by a single operator. On the basis of that variability study, the corresponding 95% confidence interval for the true cardiac output measurement would be ±33.7 ml/min/kg where the average cardiac output was 226 ml/min/kg in the 10 infants studied. As an example, where a single operator has averaged three measurements on two separate occasions, the absolute change would have to be 33.7 ml/min/kg in order to be considered statistically significant at $p < 0.05$, or 47.7 ml/min/kg if the averaged measurements were done by two different operators on the two separate occasions. This level of reproducibility compares favourably with that reported for Fick, thermodilution, as well as echo Doppler methods in adults.[11–14]

- **The largest measurement error comes from measurement of aortic root diameter. In serial measurements, the diameter may be assumed to remain the same, and one single cross-sectional area measurement may be used.**

NORMAL VALUES

Prior to echo Doppler there were few data on cardiac output in neonates and infants owing to the invasiveness of other techniques. It was therefore necessary to establish normal values for echo Doppler[15] to compare with values obtained in critically ill infants. We studied a total of eight preterm (29–36 weeks) and 14 term newborns in the first week of life; all were healthy, stable, the appropriate weight for gestational age and had a closed arterial duct. The range was 158 to 325 ml/min/kg. The preterm infants averaged 221 ± 56 ml/min/kg and the term infants averaged 236 ± 47 ml/min/kg. These findings are similar to values reported using thermodilution or Fick methods where mean systemic blood flow averaged 232 ml/min/kg between 2 and 28 hours of age.[16] Walther *et al.* reported a more extensive study of Doppler-derived cardiac outputs in newborns over a wide range of gestational ages and weights.[17] Their results were similar to ours in term infants but they reported gradually increasing values per kilogram with diminishing gestational age and weight. It is important for each institution to establish its own 'normal' values because of technical and observer variables.

In longitudinal studies in 31 healthy infants over the first year of life[18] mean ascending aortic blood flow velocity remained relatively constant, averaging 20.5 ± 3.4 (SD) cm/s. However, changes in calculated aortic cross-sectional area over time correlated strongly with corresponding changes in weight or body surface area. Therefore, changes in calculated absolute cardiac output correlated strongly with increases in weight gain and increases in body surface area over the first year. Cardiac output corrected for body weight or body surface area also remained relatively constant over the first year. Averaging by weight, values were 204 ± 45 ml/min/kg with a range of 180 to 226 ml/min/kg with a slight trend downward. By body surface area mean values were 3.48 l/min/m² ranging from 3.06

to 3.76 l/min/m² with a slight trend upward over the first year.

INFLUENCE OF DUCTAL SHUNTING

The Doppler methods so far described involve measurement of left ventricular outflow or preductal ascending aortic blood flow velocity. Since patency of the arterial duct is common in newborns, particularly in the premature neonate, it is important to recognize the influence of left-to-right ductal shunting on left ventricular cardiac output and on overall systemic blood flow – the blood flow variable of greatest importance in determining systemic oxygen transport. Assuming there are no intracardiac shunts causing recirculation through the pulmonary vascular bed, LVO is equal to pulmonary blood flow (Qp). Qp is, in turn, the combination of systemic blood flow (Qs) returning to the right heart from the systemic circulation and any left-to-right ductal blood flow (Qpda). This all returns to the left heart. That is (see Fig. 5.8):

$$LVO = Qp = Qs + Qpda$$

The left-to-right ductal shunt does not participate in overall systemic blood flow and thus is not a contributor to systemic oxygen transport. This is the concept of the **ductal steal**. In the presence of a left-to-right ductal shunt, echo-Doppler-derived LVO cannot be used as a reliable reflection of systemic blood flow and oxygen delivery. It is important therefore to determine whether a left-to-right ductal shunt exists. If such a shunt exists, any changes seen in LVO could reflect changes in systemic blood flow, ductal shunting or a combination of the two.

The effect of ductal shunting on LVO and other indicators of systemic blood flow have been studied using Doppler techniques.[19,20] In the newborn the LVO will increase in response to increasing preload from increased pulmonary venous return secondary to the left-to-right ductal shunting. Ascending aortic blood flow and LVO are usually elevated in infants despite evidence of ductal steal causing diminished systemic blood flow and reducing systemic blood pressure. When the duct closes, LVO falls to normal levels as systemic blood pressure rises towards normal. If a large left-to-right ductal shunt persists, there is a continued coronary arterial steal which may impair left ventricular function[21] and diminish the ability to compensate for the increased pulmonary venous return. Thus, LVO will

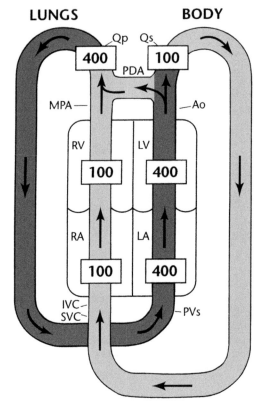

Fig. 5.8 Illustration of the effect of left-to-right patent ductus arteriosus (PDA) shunting on LVO and relationship to ascending aortic flow and systemic flow (Qs). Pulmonary flow (Qp) = LVO = ascending aortic flow = PDA shunt flow + Qs.

eventually decrease and even fall below normal, with worsening congestive heart failure and seriously impaired systemic blood flow. This can be called a **malignant** duct and, if not corrected, is associated with high mortality, particularly in the extremely premature neonate. Inotropic support, such as with digitalis, may increase myocardial oxygen demand even further in the face of decreasing oxygen delivery. This haemodynamic situation is best treated by **closure** of the duct.

The influence of the duct on systemic blood flow can be monitored in a variety of ways using other ultrasound techniques; these are covered in Chapter 7.

CLINICAL APPLICATIONS

It has now been possible to observe the impact of a variety of clinical conditions and therapies on cardiac output in the newborn.[2]

In cases of haemodynamic instability, myocardial dysfunction or shock, echo Doppler cardiac output measurements can determine the effectiveness of inotropes and assist in adjusting or weaning off therapy. Cardiac output determination is a more sensitive reflection of the cardiovascular haemodynamics than blood pressure alone.[22] Blood pressure may remain within normal limits while cardiac output is significantly impaired because systemic vascular resistance increases owing to the α-adrenergic effects of certain inotropes or an intrinsic adrenergic response. Blood pressure may not fall until the body's natural compensatory mechanisms finally fail. Serious falls in cardiac output (and thus tissue oxygen delivery) may be detected earlier and early intervention may prevent such circulatory collapse. We have observed a strong association between persistently low LVO in the first 24 hours of life, low cortisol levels and a significantly higher mortality in preterm infants with respiratory distress syndrome (RDS) treated with surfactant despite inotropic therapy and normal blood pressure.

Cardiac output may be impaired during conventional mechanical or high-frequency ventilatory support, particularly with higher positive end-expiratory pressure (PEEP) or high mean airway pressure (Paw). Measuring cardiac output by echo Doppler can therefore assist in determining the optimal PEEP or Paw needed to obtain the best level of overall oxygenation and systemic oxygen transport. We found no deleterious effects of high-frequency jet ventilation on cardiac output in neonates with pulmonary interstitial emphysema as compared with conventional mechanical ventilation.

Other studies have shown a markedly low Doppler-derived cardiac output (116 ± 15 ml/min/kg) in the presence of supraventricular tachycardia (SVT) in the neonate with a rapid, significant and dramatic improvement to normal levels (207 ± 15 ml/min/kg) after conversion to normal sinus rhythm. These data are consistent with fetal hydrops and neonatal congestive heart failure in association with SVT and indicate the importance of early conversion to sinus rhythm. We found a statistically significant rise in cardiac output after partial exchange transfusions for polycythaemic hyperviscosity associated with an 80% improvement in laser Doppler measures of peripheral skin blood flow.

When oxygen consumption is measured along with cardiac output, systemic oxygen extraction or oxygen utilization can be calculated defining the relationship between oxygen supply and demand.[23,24] A high level of oxygen extraction may indicate the need to improve systemic oxygen transport (e.g. by blood transfusion) or diminish oxygen demand.[25]

DETERMINING RIGHT VENTRICULAR OUTPUT

The same principles can be used to determine output from the right ventricle (RVO). First, diameter of the pulmonary artery is determined from cross-sectional imaging and then pulmonary artery stroke distance is determined from pulsed wave Doppler (Fig. 5.9). The diameter of the pulmonary artery is probably best determined from the hinge points of the pulmonary valve seen in the standard parasternal short-axis view. Some authors prefer a parasternal long-axis view of the pulmonary valve and artery[26]; this is obtained by tilting the scanning probe towards the left shoulder from the standard parasternal long-axis view. The reproducibility of measurement of valve diameter is not established, and may be prone to more error than measurement of aortic root diameter. This is because the pulmonary valves and pulmonary arterial walls are parallel to the ultrasound beams and are therefore defined by the lateral resolution of the ultrasound imaging. Lateral resolution is usually poorer than axial resolution (see Chapter 1.1). M-mode echocardiography cannot be used because the pulmonary arterial walls are parallel to the ultrasound waves rather than perpendicular to them. Furthermore, because the pulmonary arterial walls are more elastic, expanding during systole, the exact timing of measurement during systole may be more critical.

The pulsed Doppler sample is placed at the tips of the pulmonary valve and the area under the Doppler flow curve is assessed in the same way as ascending aortic flow, to calculate pulmonary artery stroke distance (PASD), also called the pulmonary artery flow velocity integral. CW Doppler should probably not be used here because the velocity can be artificially increased by the detection of increased velocity through the branch pulmonary arteries and descending aorta as they are insonated beyond the pulmonary artery.

RVO is then calculated thus:

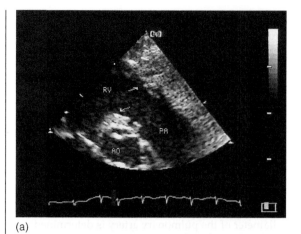

(a)

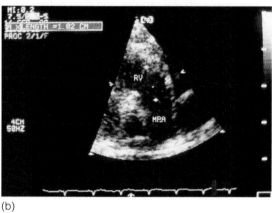

(b)

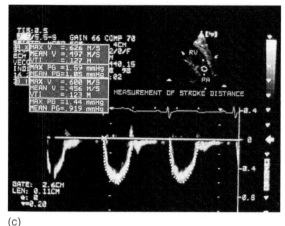

(c)

Fig. 5.9 Measurement of RVO. (a) Tilted parasternal long-axis view to show the hinge points of the pulmonary valve (arrowed) where diameter can be measured.
(b) Better alignment with direction of flow prior to placing pulsed Doppler sample at the pulmonary valve. The valve measures 1.02 cm in diameter.
(c) Using on-line software, the Doppler trace is manually followed with a tracker ball. The stroke distance (here shown as 'VTI', velocity time integral, among all the other unwanted measurements) is 12.7 cm and 12.3 cm in two beats.

RV stroke volume (ml) = PASD (cm) × PACSA (cm²)

where PACSA is pulmonary artery cross-sectional area, and PASD is pulmonary artery stroke distance (or pulmonary artery flow velocity integral). Then

RV output (ml/min/kg) = RV stroke volume (ml) × heart rate (bpm)

Interpretation of values

It should be remembered that turbulence from pulmonary stenosis invalidates the technique, and turbulence in the pulmonary artery from left-to-right ductal flow can disturb the flow pattern, making accurate determination of stroke distance very difficult.

RVO should equal LVO when there is no shunting across the duct or across the oval foramen, and studies have shown a correlation between the values under these circumstances. LVO output is raised by pure left-to-right ductal shunting, but RVO is not; indeed, it may be reduced if there is so

much ductal steal that effective systemic cardiac output is reduced, thereby reducing systemic venous return. However, RVO is also affected by interatrial shunting across the often patent oval foramen. The interrelationship between atrial and ductal shunting and the effect of these on both ventricular outputs is discussed in Chapter 3.

Low values (<150 ml/kg/min) are found in low output states, particularly in hypoxaemic infants, and high values are a feature of a large left-to-right atrial shunt.

☞ *Practical Point*
- As with LVO, serial changes in RVO can be made by using a single measurement of pulmonary artery diameter, or by reporting pulmonary stroke distance alone; this avoids repeatability error in the measurement of pulmonary artery diameter.

FUTURE INNOVATIONS

Present systems are expensive and require technical expertise and operator time which currently preclude their wide utilization. Future technological improvements may allow more practical integration of echo Doppler cardiac output measurements, intermittently or continuously, into routine monitoring in neonatal intensive care units. Doppler cardiac output monitoring could someday be included along with heart rate, respiratory rate, ECG, blood pressure, and transcutaneous blood gas monitoring capability at the bedside.

REFERENCES

1. Alverson DC. Neonatal cardiac output measurement using pulsed Doppler ultrasound. In: *Noninvasive Neonatal Diagnosis. Clinics in Perinatology* 1985;12:101–127.

2. Alverson DC. Pulsed Doppler assessment of ascending aortic flow velocity in newborns and infants: clinical application. *Echocardiography* 1988;5:1–22.

3. Alverson DC, Eldridge MW, Dillon T *et al*. Noninvasive pulsed Doppler determination of cardiac output in neonates and children. *Journal of Pediatrics* 1982;101:46–50.

4. Alverson DC. Noninvasive measurement of cardiac output in the newborn. *Journal of Perinatology* 1984;4:16–20.

5. Voyles WF, Altobelli SA, Fisher DC, Greene ER. A comparison of digital and analog methods of Doppler spectral analysis for quantifying flow. *Ultrasound in Medicine and Biology* 1985;11:727–734.

6. Mandelbaum-Isken VH, Linderkamp O. Cardiac output by pulsed Doppler in neonates using the apical window. *Pediatric Cardiology* 1991;12:13–16.

7. Hatle L. Assessment of aortic blood flow velocities with continuous wave Doppler ultrasound in the neonate and young child. *Journal of the American College of Cardiology* 1985;5:113S–119S.

8. Hudson I, Houston A, Aitchison T, Holland B, Turner T. Reproducibility of measurements of cardiac output in newborn infants by Doppler ultrasound. *Archives of Disease in Childhood* 1990;65:15–19.

9. Goldberg SJ, Sahn DJ, Allen HD *et al*. Evaluation of pulmonary and systemic blood flow by two dimensional Doppler echocardiography using fast Fourier transform spectral analysis. *American Journal of Cardiology* 1982;50:1394–1400.

10. Claflin KS, Alverson DC, Pathak D, Angelus P, Backstrom C, Werner S. Cardiac output determination in the newborn: reproducibility of the pulsed Doppler velocity measurement. *Journal of Ultrasound Medicine* 1988;7:311–315.

11. Nishimura RA, Callahan MJ, Schaff HV *et al*. Noninvasive measurement of cardiac output by continuous-wave Doppler echocardiography: initial experience and review of the literature. *Mayo Clinic Proceedings* 1984;59:484–489.

12. Gardin JM, Dabestani A, Matin K *et al*. Reproducibility of Doppler aortic blood flow measurements: studies on intraobserver, interobserver and day-to-day variability in normal subjects. *American Journal of Cardiology* 1984;54:1092–1098.

13. Holmgren A, Pernow B. The reproducibility of cardiac output determination by the direct Fick method during muscular work. *Scandinavian Journal of Clinical and Laboratory Investigation* 1960;12:224.

14. Stetz CW, Miller RG, Kelly GE *et al*. Reliability of the thermodilution method in determination of cardiac output in clinical practice. *American Review of Respiratory Disease* 1982;126:1101–1104.

15. Alverson DC, Eldridge MW, Johnson JD *et al*. Noninvasive measurement of cardiac output in healthy preterm and term newborn infants. *American Journal of Perinatology* 1984;1:148–151.

16. Burnard ED, Granang A, Gray RE. Cardiac output in the newborn infant. *Clinical Science* 1966;31:121–133.

17. Walther FJ, Siassi B, Ramadan NA *et al*. Pulsed Doppler determinations of cardiac output in neonates: normal standards for clinical use. *Pediatrics* 1985;76:829–833.

18. Alverson DC, Aldrich M, Angelus P *et al*. Longitudinal trends in left ventricular cardiac output in healthy infants over the first year of life. *Journal of Ultrasound Medicine* 1987;6:519–524.

19. Alverson DC, Eldridge MW, Johnson JD *et al*. Effect of patent arterial duct on left ventricular output in premature infants. *Journal of Pediatrics* 1983;102:754–757.

20. Alverson DC, Eldridge MW, Aldrich M *et al*. Effect of patent arterial duct on lower extremity blood flow velocity patterns in preterm infants. *American Journal of Perinatology* 1984;1:216–222.

21. Way GL, Pierce JR, Wolfe RR *et al*. ST depression suggesting subendocardial ischemia in neonates with respiratory distress syndrome and patent arterial duct. *Journal of Pediatrics* 1979;95:609–611.

22. Kluckow M, Evans N. Relationship between blood pressure and cardiac output in preterm infants requiring mechanical ventilation. *Journal of Pediatrics* 1996;129:506–512.

23. Lister G, Moreau G, Moss M. Effects of alterations in of oxygen transport in the neonate. *Seminars in Perinatology* 1984;7:192–204.

24. Alverson DC. The physiologic impact of anemia in the neonate. *Clinics in Perinatology* 1995;22:609–625.

25. Alverson DC, Isken VH, Cohen RS. The effect of booster blood transfusions on oxygen utilization in infants with bronchopulmonary dysplasia. *Journal of Pediatrics* 1988;113:722–726.

26. Evans N, Iyer P. Assessment of ductus arteriosus shunt in preterm infants supported by mechanical ventilation: effects of interatrial shunting. *Journal of Pediatrics* 1994;125:778–785.

CHAPTER 6

Pulmonary arterial pressure

Jon Skinner

INTRODUCTION

Some 30 years ago there was tremendous interest in the aetiology of neonatal respiratory failure in the preterm infant. Direct cardiac catheterization revealed that pulmonary arterial (PA) pressure was elevated in most babies with hyaline membrane disease (HMD). 'Pulmonary ischaemia' was considered to be the primary underlying pathology. Though surfactant deficiency is accepted now as the major aetiological factor, recent studies using Doppler echocardiographic techniques confirm that PA pressure is indeed elevated during the course of the disease, even when blood gas status is satisfactory.

There has followed a resurgence of interest in PA pressure measurement. Recent studies suggest that PA pressure falls more slowly as HMD resolves in patients who subsequently develop bronchopulmonary dysplasia (BPD).[1] Doppler echocardiographic techniques have also been used to assess PA pressure in babies with persistent hypoxia and it has been claimed that they can be used to predict the patients who will benefit from pulmonary vasodilator therapy.[2]

Such studies may lead to changes in clinical management by altering treatment protocols and by using echocardiography in minute-to-minute bedside management. For the neonatologist to make balanced decisions from such information, the limitations of the techniques (which are many) need to be understood, even if the clinician never actually performs echocardiography.

This chapter gives a brief summary and background of each method and then a step-by-step practical guide as to how to make the measurements. Then follows a review of the advantages and limitations of each method and some clinical implications and research findings.

METHODS TO ASSESS PA PRESSURE

Broadly speaking, there are three methods. They respectively involve measurement of:

1. peak velocity of tricuspid valve regurgitation
2. velocity of flow throught the arterial duct
3. right ventricular systolic time intervals.

The way these measurements are made can be summarized briefly as follows:

1. Peak velocity of tricuspid regurgitation (TR). Most preterm infants have some TR in the first

days of life.[3,4] From the peak velocity, measured with continuous wave (CW) Doppler ultrasound (m/s), a peak right ventricle to right atrial pressure drop (mmHg) is determined by applying the modified Bernoulli equation[5,6] (see Chapters 2.1 and 2.3).

2. Velocity of flow through the arterial duct. The speed of flow through the arterial duct and the pattern of flow during the cardiac cycle reflect the balance of aortic and pulmonary arterial pressures. These can be recorded with Doppler ultrasound. The flow can be categorized into patterns associated with pure right-to-left, intermediate or pure left-to-right, and velocity of flow can be measured. Some authors have applied the modified Bernoulli equation to the velocities (m/s) to derive a pressure difference (mmHg) between aorta and pulmonary artery.[7–9]

3. Right ventricular systolic time intervals. There are a number of different time intervals that can be measured during the cardiac cycle. Those measured at the pulmonary valve during systole either with M-mode or Doppler echocardiography are the systolic right ventricular time intervals. These change in a manner which is related to pulmonary arterial pressure. They are less reliable than the first two methods, and conceptually difficult to understand, but they are easy to measure. They are unreliable in the presence of many congenital heart diseases (unlike measurement of TR and ductal flow) but remain important because many babies have neither TR nor a patent duct.

Each method has advantages and disadvantages; these are summarized towards the end of the chapter. None is perfect and all rely on the expertise of the operator.

In this chapter it is assumed that structural cardiac abnormalities have already been excluded. The ultrasound machine should be linked to an ECG.

MEASUREMENT OF PEAK VELOCITY OF TR

Theoretical background (see Fig. 6.1)

The peak velocity of TR, measured with Doppler ultrasound, is converted into a pressure drop by application of the modified Bernoulli equation, $p = 4 v^2$, p is the pressure drop (mmHg) and v is the velocity of blood (ms/s). This equation was

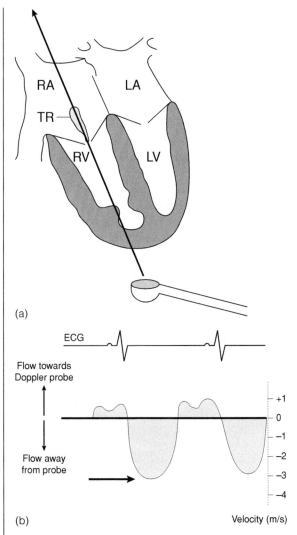

(a)

(b)   Velocity (m/s)

Fig. 6.1 Estimation of systolic pulmonary arterial pressure from peak velocity of tricuspid regurgitation. (a) The beam of CW Doppler ultrasound passes through the jet of TR. (b) The Doppler waveform, showing peak velocity (v) of TR

introduced earlier in Chapters 2.1 and 2.3. The drop in pressure from the right ventricle (RV) to the right atrium (RA) in systole can be assessed as follows:

RV pressure − RA pressure = 4 × (TR jet velocity)^2

Systolic pulmonary arterial pressure approximates to right ventricular systolic pressure if there is no pulmonary stenosis. Hence systolic PA pressure is equal to the drop in pressure in systole between RV and RA plus the RA pressure. If RA pressure is measured invasively, then this can be added to give an approximate systolic PA pressure. In spontaneously breathing newborn infants RA

pressure is very low, approximating to zero, so that RA pressure can effectively be ignored, and the RV–RA pressure drop assumed to approximate to systolic PA pressure.[10] In ventilated babies, particularly those with right ventricular failure, such as following perinatal asphyxia, RA pressure is usually higher, between 5 and 10 mmHg. An allowance for RA pressure in these babies is sensible, and 5 or 10 mmHg can be added to the RV–RA pressure drop.[9,10]

In practice, the changes in RV–RA pressure drop are so much greater than RA pressure that the RA pressure is relatively unimportant, particularly in serial measurement, and can be disregarded in most circumstances.

How to do it

The aim is to measure the highest recordable velocity of a regurgitant jet through the tricuspid valve.

A

The first step is to see if there is any regurgitation. This is easiest using cross-sectional echocardiography with colour Doppler. An apical or subcostal four-chamber view is obtained and the colour mapping area is superimposed over the tricuspid valve and right atrium. Regurgitation is seen as a jet squirting away from the scanning head, from the right ventricle into the right atrium (see Figs 2.3.6 and 2.3.7). If apical or subcostal views are difficult, a good view of the tricuspid valve can be obtained from a parasternal position by angling the scanning plane to the subject's right from a standard long-axis view (see Fig. 1.4.5d; the scanning head points away from the left shoulder). If colour Doppler is not available, pulsed Doppler interrogation just above the tricuspid valve in the right atrium will reveal a high-velocity, aliasing jet in diastole (Fig. 2.3.6a).

B

Similar interrogation of the mitral valve is necessary to exclude mitral regurgitation (which is relatively uncommon). Doppler signals of mitral and tricuspid regurgitation are very similar in the newborn, and often of similar velocity, so one must be sure that a regurgitant signal arises from the tricuspid and not the mitral valve (see below, *D*). This is especially important if a non-imaging pencil probe is used to measure the peak velocity.

c

Measurement of peak TR velocity is made with CW Doppler because the velocities being measured are usually too high for pulsed wave Doppler, and would cause aliasing. If the ultrasound machine has an in-line CW Doppler facility, this can then be superimposed onto the colour jet. By small angulations of the probe, the CW line seen on the screen is brought into line with the colour jet.

If there is only a non-imaging pencil probe, the probe is first positioned at the lower left sternal edge and directed towards the tricuspid valve. This takes practice and tuition. Start with the Doppler beam pointing roughly towards the spine (i.e. slightly medially) with a cranial tilt of 30–45° (see Fig. 6.2). The Doppler low-frequency filtering is set high or maximal, and gain settings usually need to be high. A regurgitant jet is first heard before it is seen on the Doppler tracing, and is a relatively

high-pitched hiss or whoosh coming out of one of the stereo speakers on either side of the machine during systole. Small, subtle movements of the probe aim to increase the intensity of the sound and the Doppler trace on the screen.

The Doppler tracing reveals low-velocity diastolic flow above the zero line (away from the probe), representing diastolic inflow into the RV, followed by a higher velocity downward deflection of tricuspid regurgitation (see Figs. 6.1b and 6.2c). The peak velocity is measured only when there is a clear envelope throughout systole; the highest velocity on screen is recorded. This process is repeated from at least two other positions to ensure that the highest velocity is recorded (this is essential with in-line CW as well as with the pencil probe; see Chapter 2.3). Higher up the left parasternal edge at about the second or third intercostal space, the beam is directed somewhat caudally towards the

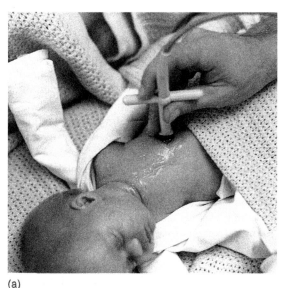

(a)

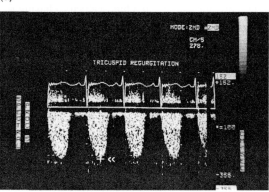

(c)

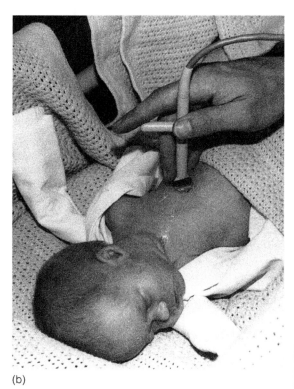

(b)

Fig. 6.2 Measurement of peak velocity of TR using a blind (non-imaging) CW Doppler pencil probe. (a) The TR jet is usually easiest to find at the lower left sternal edge. (b) Subtle movement is needed to optimize the Doppler envelope. Here the probe is moved a little towards the apex and directed medially. (c) The arrows highlight the peak velocity of 2.78 m/s.

tricuspid valve; from the apical position it is directed roughly towards the right scapula; and from the subcostal position the beam is initially directed towards the left of the spine between the scapulae.

The highest recordable velocity is noted, because it is assumed that at that time the Doppler beam and regurgitant jet are in alignment. *Failure to align correctly will result in underestimation of the RV–RA pressure drop.*

D

If there is no mitral regurgitation (MR) the measurement is complete. If MR is present there may be confusion as to which signal is being

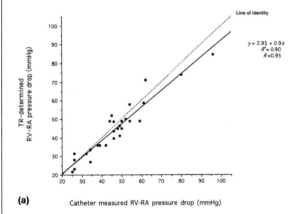

(a)

Catheter measured RV-RA pressure drop (mmHg)

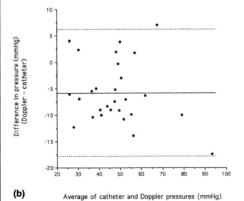

(b)

Average of catheter and Doppler pressures (mmHg)

Fig. 6.3 A comparison of Doppler-derived peak RV–RA pressure drop with that derived from cardiac catheterization in infants. (a) Correlation coefficient of 0.95. (b) Bland–Altman plot demonstrates that the Doppler-derived pressure drop underestimates peak RV pressure by an average of 7 mmHg – roughly equivalent to the expected right atrial pressure. (Dashed lines represent two standard deviations above and below mean pressure difference.)

recorded; this velocity will also be high velocity and pansystolic. MR is uncommon in association with HMD whereas TR is the norm in the first three or four days; however, babies with myocardial ischaemia and/or PPHN may well have both MR and TR. It is important to be sure which velocity is being measured, and there are a number of ways they can be differentiated.

When simultaneous imaging is possible it is usually easy to be sure the CW beam is not passing through the MR jet by studying the colour Doppler jets on screen. It is also possible to distinguish mitral and tricuspid regurgitant (TR) signals using the pencil probe alone, but this requires experience and practice (see Figures 6.1–6.3).

1. The first point is that two separate jets are found in different positions. From the lower left sternal edge or the apex, the signal of TR is more medial, and disappears as the beam is angled slowly laterally, and after about a 30°C movement, the signal of MR appears.
2. TR is usually easiest to obtain from the left parasternal or subcostal positions, and MR from the apex.
3. The measured peak velocities are usually different from the same scanning position. The peak velocity of MR is related to the left ventricle to left atrial pressure difference during systole in a similar manner to TR and the RV–RA pressure drop. If systemic arterial pressure is higher than PA pressure then the MR jet will be higher than the TR jet.

☞ *Practical Point*
● **To differentiate mitral from tricuspid regurgitation when using non-imaging probe:**
1. **TR is more medial when insonating from the apex.**
2. **TR is usually easiest to obtain from low left parasternum, and MR from apex.**
3. **Peak velocities are usually different from the same insonation point.**
4. **Application of the modified Bernoulli equation to the MR jet gives the left ventricle to left atrial pressure difference, which approximates to systemic arterial blood pressure.**
5. **Diastolic inflow characteristics (E and A waves) are often different – check first with pulsed wave Doppler.**

4. Finally, the diastolic inflow pattern, recorded previously with pulsed Doppler, may be different (the E:A ratio is typically higher; see Chapter 2.2), although this is not always the case in the newborn.

PATTERN AND VELOCITY OF DUCTAL FLOW

Theoretical background

The direction and speed of flow through the arterial duct depend upon the balance of pressures between the aorta and the pulmonary artery.

Using Doppler ultrasound it is possible to record both the direction and the speed of flow in the arterial duct throughout the cardiac cycle. The duct therefore provides a useful insight into the relationship of these two pressures that can be critical in the sick newborn baby.

Pattern of flow through the cardiac cycle.

Simultaneous Doppler and cardiac catheterization studies have shown that the pattern of flow through the duct alters in a recognizable way as the balance of aortic and pulmonary arterial pressures change (see Fig. 6.4–6.6).

Pure right-to-left ductal flow indicates that pulmonary arterial pressure is higher than aortic pressure throughout the cardiac cycle. This never occurs in healthy babies during postnatal life. It can occur with failure of the transitional circulation or in hypoxaemic babies with severe respiratory failure. When pure right-to-left ductal flow is seen it is especially important to be sure that there is not structural heart disease such as aortic coarctation or anomalous pulmonary venous drainage (see Chapters 9.1 and 9.2).

When aortic and pulmonary arterial pressures are approximately equal, then flow is bidirectional; right-to-left flow occurs during systole and left-to-right during diastole. Right-to-left flow occurs earlier in the cardiac cycle because the pulmonary arterial pressure wave reaches the arterial duct before the aortic pressure wave, the pulmonary valve being closer to the duct than the aortic valve.

Healthy newborn babies have bidirectional flow in the first few hours of life. This changes to pure left-to-right by 12 hours of age because aortic pressure is then higher than pulmonary arterial pressure throughout the cardiac cycle. Initially the left-to-right velocity is low during systole (less than 1 m/s) and higher in diastole. PA pressure

continues to fall and at the same time systemic arterial pressure rises such that the velocity of left-to-right flow gradually increases until the duct closes. Prior to closure the left-to-right velocity is high throughout the cardiac cycle and is typically highest at end systole/early diastole (usually 2–3 m/s).

Deriving aortopulmonary pressure difference from ductal velocity and the Bernoulli equation

Several authors have derived the pressure drop across the duct by applying the modified Bernoulli equation to the measured velocities. These calculated pressure drops were then compared with simultaneously directly measured pressure differences at cardiac catheterization.[7,8] This idea for deriving pressure drop is attractive to neonatologists because ductal patency is the norm during the critical phases of neonatal respiratory failure,[4,11] and aortic pressure is often measured invasively. PA pressure could be derived easily by subtracting the pressure drop across the duct from

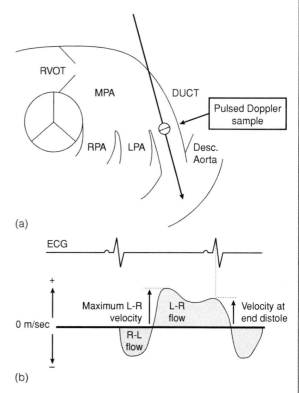

(a)

(b)

Fig. 6.4 Measurement of velocity of flow through the arterial duct. (a) 'Ductal view' from high left parasternal position, with beam of pulsed Doppler ultrasound passing through the arterial duct. (b) Doppler tracing showing bidirectional ductal flow.

Ductal flow patterns		
		Pulmonary: Aortic systolic pressure ratio
ECG		
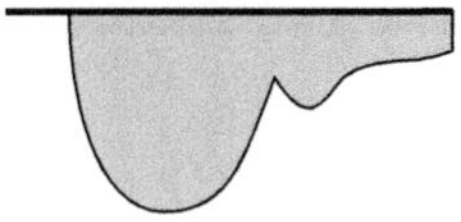	1. Pure right-to-left. Not seen in healthy infants. Occurs in severe PPHN, rare in HMD.	> 1.0:1
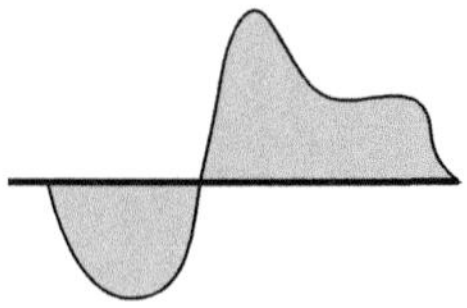	2. Bidirectional. Common in healthy infants <12 hours old.	0.8:1-1.3:1
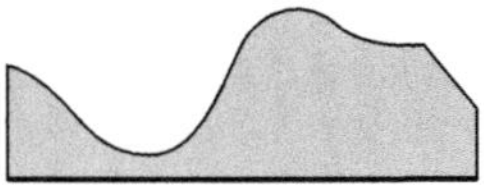	3. Left-to-right, low systole higher diastole. Transitional between 2. and 4. Common in healthy infants <36 hours old.	0.70:1-0.95:1
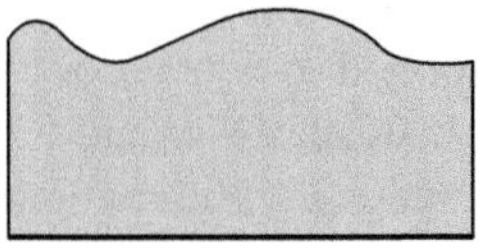	4. Left-to-right, high throughout. Common in healthy infants prior to ductal closure (up to four days of age).	<0.75:1
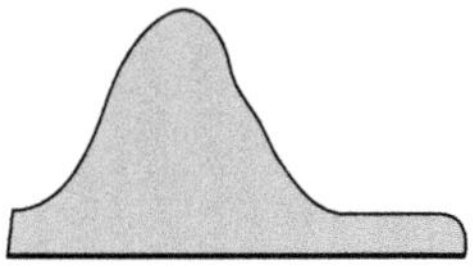	5. Left-to-right, high systole, low end diastole. Not seen in healthy infants. Characteristic of large L-R ductal shunt.	0.5:1-0.9:1
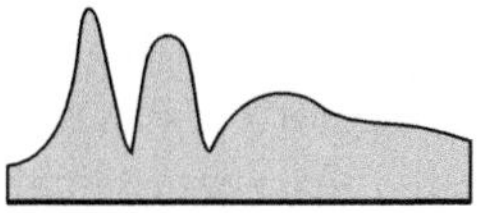	6. Left-to-right, complex low velocity. Not seen in healthy infants. Often occurs with large duct and systemic hypotension.	0.7:1-1.1:1

Fig. 6.5 Diagram to illustrate the relationship of the pattern of ductal flow to the pulmonary:aortic systolic pressure ratio (derived from TR jet and aortic pressure) in newborns.

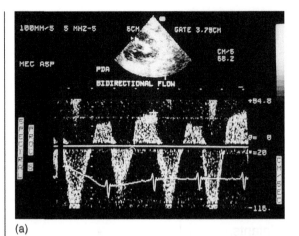

(a)

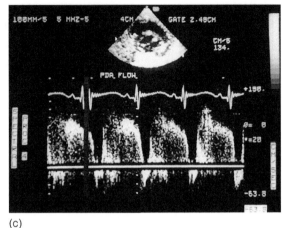

(c)

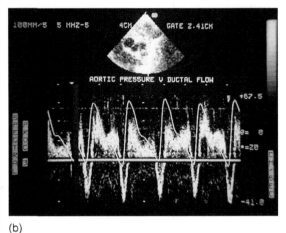

(b)

Fig. 6.6 Examples of bidirectional ductal flow. (a) The right-to-left (downward) phase is as long as the left-to-right phase in this infant with PPHN. (b) The right-to-left phase is much shorter in this infant; the pulmonary:systemic pressure ratio is lower. The simultaneous aortic pressure trace illustrates how the ductal flow is dictated by pressure differential across it. (c) The right-to-left phase is very short, and the peak left-to-right velocity is 1.34 m/s compared with 0.68 m/s in (a)).

aortic pressure. However, results of validatory studies, most of which were performed in children beyond the first month of age, have been inconsistent.

It is not known how accurate the method is in the preterm. Underestimation of the pressure drop may arise from failure to align properly with the jet. Alignment may at times be impossible; the jet seen with colour Doppler often swings across the pulmonary artery during the cardiac cycle. Constriction of the duct makes it very small prior to closure and this may lead to viscous friction. This can result in reduced velocity at a given pressure such that applying the modified Bernoulli equation again results in an underestimation of the true pressure drop. Overestimation of the pressure drop is also described, and is harder to explain. The varying shape of the duct may be to blame. It is our impression that large pressure differences in either direction are underestimated using this method, but further work is required.

We would suggest that the modified Bernoulli equation should not be applied to ductal flow velocities in the preterm. Instead, we would recommend using serial analysis within patients over time observing changes in pattern of flow and/or velocity of flow (in m/s) without applying the Bernoulli equation.

How to do it

Visualize the duct

With practice, the arterial duct becomes quite easy to visualize, particularly in the preterm with HMD (see Chapter 7), and this is made even easier with colour Doppler. The starting point is the high left parasternal edge; the 'three-legged' view of the duct appears when a standard short-axis parasternal cut (Chapter 1.4) is modified by sliding up the chest by one intercostal space and applying slight anticlockwise rotation and a little caudal tilt (see Figs 1.1.10 and 7.4–7.6).

Record the pattern of flow

The pattern of flow throughout the cardiac cycle is first recorded with pulsed wave Doppler ultrasound, by placing the sampling gate at the pulmonary end of the duct.

Bidirectional flow The velocity of left-to-right flow can be recorded from the pulmonary end of the duct. When there is right-to-left flow, the peak velocity of this component increases as the pulsed Doppler sample is moved by the operator towards the aortic end of the duct. The velocity of the right-to-left component is best measured towards the aortic end of the duct. It may be useful to measure the duration of right-to-left and left-to-right flow during the cardiac cycle and express it in ratio form (see Figs 6.4 and 6.6); the right-to-left phase shortens as PA pressure falls.

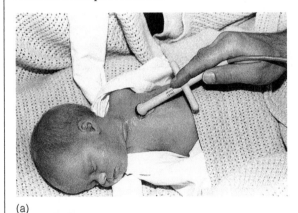

(a)

(b)

Fig. 6.7 Measurement of left-to-right ductal flow with a blind continuous wave Doppler pencil probe. (a) It is positioned in the second left intercostal space and pointed posteriorly and slightly towards the clavicle. (b) The Doppler trace shows a peak left-to-right velocity (A) of 2.32 m/s translating to a pressure drop between the aorta and pulmonary artery of 21.5 mmHg at this point.

Pure left-to-right flow Low velocities can be recorded in the same way with pulsed wave Doppler. High velocities causing aliasing must be measured with CW Doppler. The CW cursor is positioned guided by the colour flow map. Care is taken to record the highest left-to-right velocity; the direction of the colour jet cannot be relied on alone to ensure optimal alignment.

If only a non-imaging pencil probe is available, this is first positioned at the mid-to-upper left sternal edge and directed posteriorly (Fig. 6.7). Slow cranial angulation will detect the left-to-right flow seen as upward flow, above the zero line, on the Doppler trace. Continuous left-to-right flow has a characteristic high-pitched 'machinery murmur' sound, similar to that heard with a stethoscope. The Doppler low-frequency filtering and gain settings are usually best in the middle ranges, but this depends on the speed of the jet and size of the duct.

Small, subtle movements of the probe (typically towards the left sternoclavicular junction) may increase the intensity of the sound and the Doppler trace on screen.

The left-to-right peak velocity is measured when there is a clear envelope throughout the cardiac cycle; the highest velocity on screen is recorded which is typically in late systole/early diastole.

Pure right-to-left flow The right-to-left velocity can usually be measured with the pulsed wave Doppler as above. However, it has been shown that if the modified Bernoulli equation is applied to the measured velocity, the derived pressure drop in this direction is usually inaccurate. Peak right-to-left velocity should not be measured with the non-imaging pencil probe alone because many structures (branch pulmonary arteries and descending aorta) can also produce velocities away from the probe, making it difficult to know which velocity is being measured. CW Doppler should

☞ *Practical Points*

● **Measuring velocity of flow in the arterial duct:**
1. **Do not rely only on the colour Doppler jet to align with flow – instead always seek the highest velocity.**
2. **Do not use a non-imaging probe to measure right-to-left velocity.**
3. **Record values in m/s rather than deriving pressure drop.**

only be used in conjunction with imaging (i.e. 'in line') to measure right-to-left ductal velocity.

RIGHT VENTRICULAR SYSTOLIC TIME INTERVALS

Theoretical background

The timing and duration of right ventricular systolic events change with increased PA pressure. The classical changes of pulmonary hypertension are summarized in Figure 6.8. The period between closure of the tricuspid valve and opening of the pulmonary valve (the 'right ventricular pre-ejection period') is prolonged, and the flow profile in the pulmonary artery is altered from a smooth round shape to a triangular shape with an early peak velocity. There is then early, rapid deceleration of pulmonary blood flow, followed by a brief

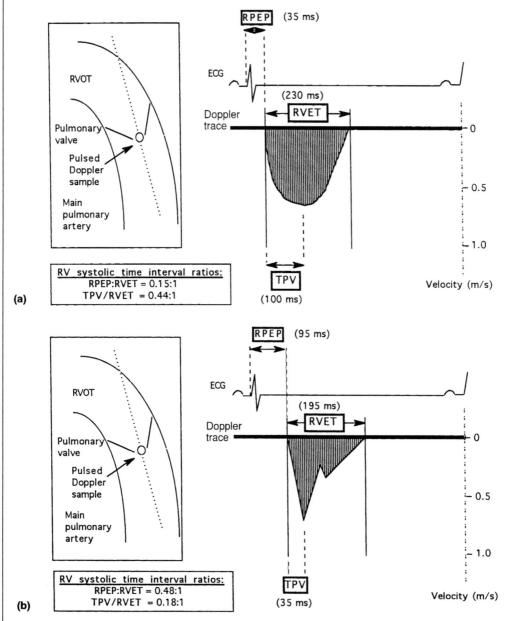

Fig. 6.8 Measurement of right ventricular systolic time intervals using pulsed wave Doppler at the pulmonary valve. (a) Term infant with *low* PA pressure. (b) Term infant with *high* PA pressure.

secondary rise, giving a classical 'notched' appearance to the flow velocity profile at the pulmonary valve. This is reflected in mid-systolic partial closure of the valve (seen best using M-mode echocardiography).

The pre-ejection period was investigated in the 1970s by M-mode echocardiography,[12-15] and the PA flow profile (measuring the 'time to peak velocity') in the 1980s with Doppler.[16] It is, however, important to recognize that these systolic time intervals are not closely or reliably related to invasively measured PA pressure. This is particularly true in congenital heart disease, where the presence of intracardiac shunts changes haemodynamics dramatically. For this reason they are not used in congenital heart disease. However, they are experiencing a revival in neonatology where subjects typically have a structurally normal heart.

Abbreviations

This area has been plagued with abbreviations, which make the subject difficult to digest. For brevity and to aid comprehension, only three time intervals will be discussed here. Sorry, but you need to learn and understand them!

- **RPEP** right ventricular pre-ejection period
- **TPV** time to peak velocity of pulmonary blood flow*
- **RVET** right ventricular ejection time.

RPEP is directly related to pulmonary arterial pressure and TPV is inversely related to PA pressure. Both are directly related to heart rate, so to allow for this both RPEP and TPV are usually expressed as a ratio of RVET (RPEP/RVET and TPV/RVET, respectively).

Physiology of systolic time intervals and pulmonary hypertension

In essence, as pulmonary arterial pressure increases, RPEP/RVET rises and TPV/RVET falls (see Fig 6.9). However, an understanding of the underlying physiology gives insight into the limitations of these ratios.

TPV is sometimes known as the acceleration time, 'AcT'. Some authors have further corrected for the influence of heart rate by using regression equations or dividing the time interval or interval ratio by the square root of the cardiac cycle length (the R–R interval); this is denoted by a small 'c', e.g. 'TPVc' or 'TPV/RVETc'.

Prolongation of RPEP

RPEP approximates to the time during which the right ventricle undergoes isovolumic contraction, i.e. the time between closure of the tricuspid valve

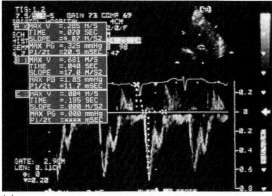

(a)

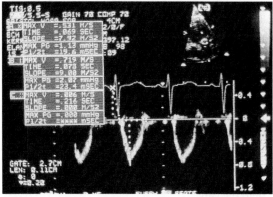

(b)

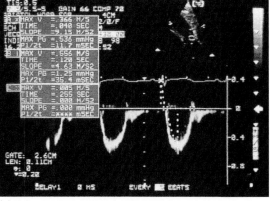

(c)

Fig. 6.9 Example of the change in flow pattern at the pulmonary valve in a term infant over the first day of life (a) At 3 hours, RPEP (A) is 70 ms, TPV (B) is 40 ms, RVET (C) is 185 ms. (b) At 6 hours, RPEP (A) is 69 ms, TPV (B) is 78 ms, RVET (C) is 216 ms. (c) At 18 hours, RPEP (A) is 40 ms, TPV (B) is 120 ms, RVET (C) is 255 ms.

at end diastole and opening of the pulmonary valve. This period is prolonged in pulmonary hypertension because the right ventricle has to generate a higher pressure before the pulmonary valve will open.

Other factors also prolong RPEP, namely right ventricular dysfunction, right ventricular volume overload and right bundle branch block.

Shortening of TPV

A rapid increase in right ventricular pressure during the pre-ejection period results in rapid acceleration of flow in the pulmonary artery when the pulmonary valve opens. Early deceleration of flow probably results from reduced capacitance and high impedance of the pulmonary vasculature, and possibly also from an early reflection of the pulsatile wave from stiff peripheral vessels. The time between onset of flow to peak flow (TPV) is thus shortened. This is analogous to the systemic circulation and pressure profiles seen in essential hypertension.

A mid-systolic notch in the flow profile is present in severe pulmonary hypertertension (see Fig. 6.9a). This is also seen as sharp retrograde movement of the pulmonary valve on M-mode. This notch has, however, been noted in idiopathic main pulmonary artery dilatation without pulmonary hypertension. It may therefore be a secondary phenomenon due to dilatation of the main pulmonary artery, producing eddy currents within the artery that reflect back onto the valve.

Other factors that may alter TPV are unclear as yet. TPV may be shortened by tricuspid regurgitation because it is known that the TPV at the aortic valve is shortened by mitral regurgitation. TPV or RVET can be difficult to measure in the presence of significant left-to-right ductal shunting because turbulence at the valve disturbs the Doppler signals. The effect of right ventricular dysfunction is not known. Values for TPV/RVET are also affected by gestational age and/or body size; TPV/RVET is higher at a given PA pressure in term babies[18] than in preterm babies. (Values for RPEP/RVET are comparable between babies of different size.)

How to do it

RPEP,* TPV and RVET can all be measured at the same Doppler ultrasound examination; the procedure is simple.

Obtain a standard short-axis parasternal view (see Chapter 1.3). Slide along the short axis away

from the left shoulder so that the pulmonary valve is directly below the transducer, and the ultrasound beam is in line with the main pulmonary artery. The pulsed Doppler sample is placed at the pulmonary valve, with a small sample volume. Align with flow as far as possible, although this is may not be critical for these time measurements (unlike measurements of velocity). The sample gate must be in the middle of the valve.

Another way to view the pulmonary valve is to tilt the scanning plane over towards the left shoulder from a standard long-axis view (a long-axis view of the pulmonary artery). Many find this view preferable to the short-axis view.

The pulmonary valve must be seen in its maximal width to ensure that the sample is not positioned eccentrically. Any movement away from this position can cause large errors. TPV is always longer in the right ventricular outflow tract than at the valve, and it is shorter beyond the valve in the main pulmonary artery.[19] If the sample is to one side of the valve or artery, the effect is also to shorten TPV.

A clear onset and cessation of flow should be seen and a clean Doppler envelope recorded. RPEP is measured from the Q-wave on the ECG to the

---

☞ *Practical Point*
- **Measurement of right ventricular systolic time intervals:**
1. **Do not use in the presence of large intracardiac shunts.**
2. **Positioning of the pulsed Doppler sample is critical in measurement of TPV (see text).**
3. **Measure four cardiac cycles at each measurement.**
4. **Reproducibility tends to be poor, therefore repeat measurements at least once; re-apply probe and re-measure.**
5. **Do not directly compare TPV/RVET values between babies of greatly different size (see text).**

RPEP approximates to the time during which the right ventricle undergoes isovolumic contraction, between closure of the tricuspid valve at end diastole and opening of the pulmonary valve. Both of these events can be recorded with M-mode. However, in practice, RPEP is measured from the Q-wave of the ECG (rather than from closure of the tricuspid valve) to the onset of flow at the pulmonary valve. This method is described here. The earlier method using M-mode was described by Riggs et al.[12]

onset of flow through the pulmonary valve. TPV is measured from the onset of flow to the peak velocity, and RVET from the onset to the end of forward flow.

Most authors record between three and five beats and average the values to allow for variation due to respiration. Because the potential for observer error is high, it is wise to remove the probe, restart and repeat the measurements to make sure they are consistent.

LIMITATIONS AND REPEATABILITY OF THE METHODS AND REFERENCE TO CLINICAL STUDIES

A comparison of the different techniques is summarized in Table 6.1.

Measurement of TR

For

In skilled hands this is undoubtedly the most reliable method for determining systolic PA pressure; this is reflected in its regular use in clinical paediatric cardiology. It is also a highly repeatable technique (repeatability index (95% confidence limits for repeatability) <10%). A change in velocity of 0.3–0.4 m/s usually represents genuine clinical change in PA pressure and there is a large potential for change; the range found in the preterm is 1.8–4 m/s.

Against

It is often time-consuming to achieve good signals, and TR is not present in most babies with BPD. During HMD the incidence of measurable TR falls from about 95% in the first 36 hours to about 50% at 7–10 days.[4] Surprisingly, it is also absent in about one third of hypoxaemic term babies.[20]

Ductal flow velocities

For

These are easier to acquire than TR velocities and can be very helpful in clinical practice. An example of how the patterns and flow velocities can change during oxygen therapy is shown in Figure 6.13. The method is very sensitive to small changes in pulmonary or systemic arterial pressure; it is easy to observe the change from right-to-left or bidirectional flow to left-to-right flow with improvement in oxygenation or ventilation in hypoxaemic infants. It is, after all, the relationship of PA pressure to aortic pressure that is of most clinical interest rather than any absolute measurements of PA pressure. Normal values for healthy newborns and those with HMD have been published.[4]

With care, the repeatability is acceptable (repeatability index of about 35%) because of the large degree of change that can occur. We have found that in a clinically stable baby left-to-right velocity changes of the order of 0.6–0.9 m/s can be

Table 6.1 Features of four Doppler echocardiographic methods of PA pressure estimation in the newborn

Method	Repeatability[21]	Relation to systolic PA pressure	Complicating factors	Strongest points	Weakest points
TR (m/s)	Very good	Direct relationship. Accurate.	Assumption of right atrial pressure.	Accurate. Repeatable.	Not feasible to measure in many babies. Technically demanding.
Ductal velocity (m/s)	Reasonable	Inverse relationship.	Affected by systemic pressure and ductal constriction.	Usually easy to measure. Large range of values.[b] Reflects balance of Ao and PA pressures.	Need patent duct. Uncertain whether modified Bernoulli equation can be applied.
TPV/RVET ratio	Poor	Inverse relationship. Accuracy unpredictable.	Not all known; heart rate, gestation, ?RV function.	Usually easy to measure.	Poor repeatability. Many complicating factors. Narrow range of values.[b]
PEP/RVET ratio	Poor[a]	Direct relationship. Accuracy unpredictable; better in restricted groups with closed duct.	Ventricular dysfunction.	Usually easy to measure. Link to RV dysfunction can be an advantage.	Poor repeatability. Narrow range of values.[b]

[a] May be better with M-mode rather than Doppler.
[b] The expected range of values in the neonatal population.

detected reliably and indicate genuine haemodynamic change; the range seen in the newborn is 0.0–3.5 m/s.[21]

Against

It can be difficult to align accurately with the jet, leading to underestimation of the pressure difference. Furthermore, deriving PA pressure by applying the modified Bernoulli equation to the velocity and subtracting this from systolic aortic pressure is of uncertain accuracy and of even less certain clinical value. As with TR measurements, ductal patency gradually becomes less frequent with time during severe HMD (90% plus in the first three days to less than 40% at one week[4,11]), and is uncommon in BPD. Even in hypoxaemic term infants about a quarter have a closed duct.[20]

Right ventricular systolic time intervals

For

These are easy to measure and can be acquired in almost every baby, and therefore provide the only methods by which every subject can be studied. They have been useful in cross-sectional studies of newborns in health and disease, and have potential to provide 'predictive' indices for later development of BPD in babies with HMD.

The fact that RPEP prolongs with right ventricular failure may paradoxically be an advantage; even though 'true' PA pressure values derived from regression equations will be inaccurate in a baby with RV failure, RPEP will shorten as *either* RV function improves or PAP falls. Early studies found a close link between RPEP/RVET and severity in HMD, whereas other methods have not shown this, suggesting that RV dysfunction is a common and significant problem in HMD. This ratio has recently found less favour than the TPV/RVET ratio but may well be superior in many respects, and can easily be measured at the same examination.

Against

Repeatability can be a problem. We have not been able to achieve reliably better than 30% repeatability index for either method, and this may be significantly worse in inexperienced hands. TPV/RVET for example has, in our hands, a repeatability coefficient of 0.10:1, which is large when the range of values in the neonate is about

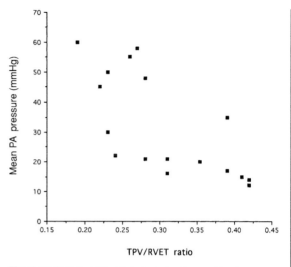

Fig. 6.10 Relationship of mean pulmonary artery pressure measured at cardiac catheterisation in children by Kosturakis *et al.*[16] versus TPV:RVET ratio. There is a wide spread of values around the correlation.

0.32:1 (0.18:1 to 0.50:1). It is worth noting that there was a wide spread of values around the correlation of TPV:RVET ratio with PA pressure in the initial study by Kosturakis *et al.*[16] (see Fig. 6.10).

FURTHER DISCUSSION

Both RPEP/RVET and TPV/RVET are subject to a variety of other complex haemodynamic variables. TPV/RVET is still subject to change with heart rate; some authors have further 'corrected' for heart rate by dividing the ratio by the square root of the R–R interval. The problems with systolic time intervals are reflected in the numerous publications which have sought to improve correlation with PA pressure with various mathematical manoeuvres. One study comparing seven different Doppler echocardiographic techniques in children found that when TPV was measured in the RVOT the relationship to PAP was closer than when positioned at the pulmonary valve.[6] This has not yet found favour in neonatology, perhaps because of problems with accurate positioning of the sample in such small hearts.

Our own studies found that the TPV/RVET ratio was particularly unreliable in PPHN when babies with suprasystemic PA pressure may have normal TPV/RVET ratios.[20]

Both RPEP/RVET and TPV/RVET ratios may find their best clinical use in babies with BPD, in whom other measures of PA pressure are often impossible, but even then they must be interpreted cautiously.

Halliday *et al.* (1980) reported that after four weeks of age the RPEP/RVET ratio rises above 0.35:1 in babies with BPD during episodes of hypoxia.[13] Another group found that a value below 0.30:1 in infants with BPD indicated a subsequent favourable outcome.[22] These values are quite different from the first days of life; for example, a much higher RPEP/RVET value of 0.55:1 indicated infants with PPHN who would subsequently respond to tolazoline.[14] However, when RPEP/RVET ratios were compared with direct measurement in six infants with BPD, three of the values were found to be significantly misleading: one baby had a value of 0.25:1 with a systolic PA pressure of 58 mmHg, and another had a ratio of 0.30:1 with a PA pressure of 55 mmHg while breathing 100% oxygen.[23]

The RPEP/RVET ratio seems to be unaffected by varying body size, and our studies suggest a closer relationship to systolic PA pressure reasonably in healthy babies with a closed duct (see Fig. 6.11).

The TPV/RVET ratio has not been compared with direct measurement in the preterm or in babies with BPD. However, provided it is used in comparisons of babies of similar gestation and body weight, there is some evidence that it may prove to be of value. At four weeks of age healthy preterm infants (born at an average of 27 weeks' gestation) have a TPV/RVETc ratio above 0.45:1, whereas in babies with BPD it is lower.[1] Further studies are underway to see if this ratio can also predict outcome.

These systolic time intervals clearly have a role in research, and may ultimately have a clinical role in neonatology. However, their unpredictability dictates that they should not be used in clinical decision making in paediatric cardiology; several studies have now demonstrated that they fail to predict PA pressure reliably in infants and children with intracardiac shunts.[17]

RESEARCH AND CLINICAL APPLICATIONS

There have been so many publications with these techniques that it is beyond the scope of this book to discuss them all. Some have already been discussed above and others are referred to in Chapter 9.2 in the assessment of the hypoxaemic infant.

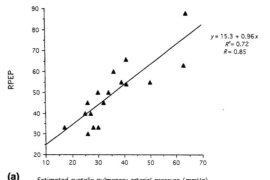

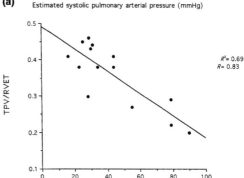

(a) Estimated systolic pulmonary arterial pressure (mmHg)

(b) Estimated systolic pulmonary arterial pressure (mmHg)

Fig. 6.11 (a) RPEP versus systolic PA pressure derived from peak velocity of tricuspid regurgitation in babies <33 weeks with a closed duct. (b) TPV/RVET versus systolic PA pressure derived from peak velocity of tricuspid regurgitation in term babies with a closed duct.

Reference values for each measurement are summarized below.

Direct measurement

Values for directly measured systolic PA pressure are available from healthy term infants who underwent cardiac catheterization.[24] These are presented first in Table 6.2 as a useful point of comparison.

Table 6.2 Systolic pulmonary and systemic arterial pressure determined by cardiac catheterization in healthy term infants

	Age group		
	0–12 h N = 20	13–36 h N = 25	37–72 h N = 6
Systolic PA pressure (mmHg)	53 (40–76)	48 (32–68)	39 (32–46)
Systolic Ao pressure (mmHg)	64 (50–78)	70 (46–84)	66 (62–88)
PA:Ao ratio	0.89 (0.51–1.09)	0.72 (0.51–0.84)	0.55 (0.26–0.74)

Values are median and (range).

Using peak velocity of tricuspid regurgitation

Values for systolic PA pressure in healthy term and preterm babies have been derived from tricuspid regurgitation and the modified Bernoulli equation.[3] The results presented in Tables 6.3 and 6.4 make no allowance for RA pressure and have therefore been termed (more correctly) the RV–RA pressure drop.

Table 6.3 Healthy term infants: TR velocity and calculated RV–RA pressure drop

	Age group		
	0–12 h N = 7	13–36 h N = 8	37–72 h N = 7
TR velocity (m/s)	3.5 (3.3–4.1)	3.0 (2.9–4.0)	2.7 (2.6–3.2)
RV–RA drop (mmHg)	55 (44–66)	37 (34–64)	30 (28–41)

Values are median and (range).

In a longitudinal study of systolic PA pressure in HMD using TR,[4] derived values showed that the PA:Ao pressure ratio remained elevated during the course of the disease (see Fig. 6.12). No clear link to disease severity could be established. Larger and more mature babies (>32 weeks' gestation) tended to have a higher PA:Ao pressure ratio on the second and third days, coinciding with the most severe

Table 6.4 Healthy preterm infants (28–36 weeks'): TR velocity and calculated RV–RA pressure drop[3]

	Age group		
	0–12 h N = 8	13–36 h N = 7	37–72 h N = 5
TR velocity (m/s)	3.2 (2.9–3.5)	2.6 (2.4–2.8)	2.4 (2.2–2.9)
RV–RA drop (mmHg)	41 (34–49)	27 (23–31)	23 (20–33)

Values are median and (range).

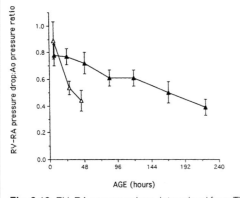

Fig. 6.12 RV–RA pressure drop determined from TR and the modified Bernoulli equation, expressed as a ratio of aortic pressure in healthy preterms (△) and those with HMD (▲).

phase of their disease, whereas the ratio fell quicker in the very low birth weight babies. Systemic arterial pressure also rose slower over the first three days than in healthy babies.

Measurement of ductal flow velocity

Values during health are presented in Table 6.5. Velocity across the duct is much lower during HMD, and this partly reflects the lower systemic arterial pressure.[4] In healthy babies bidirectional flow is very unusual after 12 hours of age, but is present in the majority with HMD until beyond the second day. After 72 hours pure left-to-right flow is most common, other than in those with systemic hypotension or persistent hypoxaemia. Studies during surfactant therapy currently suggest an earlier increase in left-to-right velocity during recovery from HMD, possibly related to more rapid resolution of the disease.

Table 6.5 Peak velocity of L–R ductal flow (m/s) in healthy newborns[4]

	Age group		
	0–12 h	13–36 h	37–72 h
Term	1.0 (1.0–1.9)	2.1 (1.4–2.8)	2.7
Preterm (28–36 weeks)	1.4 (0.4–1.4)	2.4 (1.9–2.7)	2.4

Values are median and (10th and 90th centiles).

Peak L–R ductal flow velocity during HMD[4] was similar at 0–12 hours (1.3 m/s), but then was much lower than in the healthy infants: 1.2 m/s at 13–36 hours, 1.3 m/s at 37–72 hours and 1.6 m/s at 72–96 hours. Values as high as those seen in healthy newborns after 12 hours were not usually seen until after the fifth day. In babies with PPHN qualifying for extracorporeal membrane oxidation (ECMO), peak L–R velocity remains less than 1 m/s, and usually less than 0.5 m/s, even after 12 hours of age.[25] In minute to minute changes of haemodynamics secondary to changes in ventilation or blood gas status, changes in ductal blood flow velocity are often the most obvious of all Doppler measurements (see Fig. 6.13).

RPEP/RVET ratio

There is considerable disagreement between studies about normal values (see Table 6.6), but most agree that a RPEP/RVET ratio >0.50:1 after 12 hours of age is abnormal, and is typical for babies with HMD in the first 12–24 hours, PPHN, or for hypoxaemic babies with BPD. A ratio >0.6:1 after 72 hours is very uncommon in HMD but is consistent with

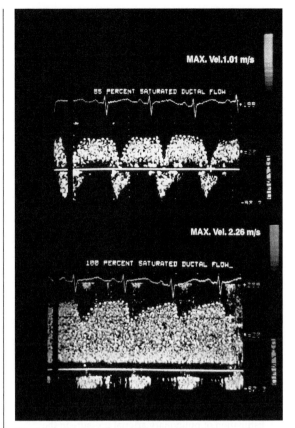

Fig. 6.13 Change in ductal flow pattern during a rise in arterial oxygen saturation from 85% to 100% due to change in ambient oxygen. The peak left-to-right velocity increases markedly from 1 m/s to 2.3 m/s, and the lowest velocity from zero to almost 2 m/s.

right ventricular failure or severe PPHN. The ratio increases with hypoxia in babies with BPD; it has been suggested that the ratio should be kept below 0.35:1 after four weeks of age to prevent the development of cor pulmonale.[13] Another group found that babies with BPD did better ultimately if the ratio was less than 0.30:1 at four weeks.[22]

This ratio is more closely related to disease severity in HMD than other estimates of PA pressure.[15] This may be due to its relationship also

Table 6.6 RPEP/RVET values in healthy newborns

	Age group			
	0–12 h	13–36 h	37–72 h	>72 h
RPEP/RVET[12,26,27] healthy term	0.39–0.51[a]	0.32	0.28–0.34[a]	
RPEP/RVET[15] healthy preterm	0.33	0.28	0.27	0.28

Mean values are presented.
[a] This is a range of *mean* values from three different studies.

to RV dysfunction; babies with severe HMD probably have combined pulmonary hypertension and RV dysfunction, both of which prolong RPEP.

We found a close relationship of RPEP/RVET and RPEP alone to systolic PA pressure determined from TR in preterm babies with a closed duct[18] (see Fig. 6.11). This correlation ($r = 0.85$ for RPEP and 0.86 for RPEP/RVET) was very much weaker, indeed virtually zero, if the duct was patent; this was possibly due to the more marked elevation of diastolic and mean PA pressure in babies with a patent duct.

TPV/RVET ratio

The TPV/RVET values shown in Table 6.7 are taken from a study which compared TPV/RVET values in term and preterm infants. The authors suggested that because TPV/RVET rose somewhat more slowly in the preterm group, pulmonary arterial pressure may fall more slowly in the preterm. A similar study[3] using TR and ductal flow patterns found no difference in the rate of fall in PA pressure between term and preterm babies. The discussion continues!

Table 6.7 TPV/RVET ratio in healthy newborns

	Age group			
	1–6 h	25–36 h	37–72 h	73–96 h
TPV/RVET[28] healthy term[a]	0.23 ± 0.04	0.36 ± 0.04		0.38 ± 0.02
TPV (ms)[27] healthy term	47 ± 11	82 ± 14		
TPV/RVET[18] healthy preterm	0.20 ± 0.04	0.29 ± 0.05		0.35 ± 0.05

[a] When the pulsed Doppler sample was placed in the RVOT[26] of term infants, mean value at 1–12 h was 0.37, and at >72 h was 0.56.

In HMD, TPV/RVET values are on average lower, consistent with the elevation of PA pressure seen in this population. Whether this ratio can be relied upon in the presence of an arterial duct or ventricular dysfunction is not known. Values in term or preterm babies with PPHN bear little relationship to PA pressure determined by other means.[20]

In contrast, the TPV/RVET ratio correlated quite closely ($r = 0.83$) with PA pressure derived from TR in healthy term babies with a closed duct[18] (see Fig. 6.11). The value of this ratio and its derivative TPV/RVETc (TPV/RVET is divided by the square root of the R–R interval) in predicting the development of chronic lung disease is under investigation; a ratio <0.46:1 at 7 days predicted chronic lung disease with a specificity of 94% and sensitivity of 55% among 73 very low birth weight infants.[22]

REFERENCES

1. Gill AB, Weindling AM. Raised pulmonary artery pressure in very low birthweight infants requiring supplemental oxygen at 36 weeks after conception. *Archives of Disease in Childhood* 1995;72:F20–22.
2. Johnson GL, Cunningham MD, Desai NS, Cottrill CM, Noonan JA. Echocardiography in hypoxemic neonatal pulmonary disease. *Journal of Pediatrics* 1980;96:716–720.
3. Skinner JR, Boys RJ, Hunter S, Hey EN. Non-invasive determination of pulmonary arterial pressure in healthy neonates. *Archives of Disease in Childhood* 1991;66:386–390.
4. Skinner JR, Boys RJ, Hunter S, Hey EN. Pulmonary and systemic arterial pressure in hyaline membrane disease. *Archives of Disease in Childhood* 1992;67:366–373.
5. Skinner JR, Stuart AGS, O'Sullivan J, Heads A, Boys RJ, Hunter S. Validation of right heart pressure determination by Doppler in infants with tricuspid regurgitation. *Archives of Disease in Childhood* 1993;69:216–220.
6. Stevenson GS. Comparison of several non-invasive methods for estimation of pulmonary artery pressure. *Journal of the American Society of Echocardiography* 1989;2:157–171.
7. Houston AB, Lim MK, Doig WB *et al*. Doppler flow characteristics in the assessment of pulmonary artery pressure in ductus arteriosus. *British Heart Journal* 1989;62:284–290.
8. Musewe NN, Smallhorn JF, Benson LN, Burrows PE, Freedom RM. Validation of Doppler-derived pulmonary arterial pressure in patients with ductus arteriosus under different hemodynamic states. *Circulation* 1987;76:1081–1091.
9. Musewe NN, Poppe D, Smallhorn JF *et al*. Doppler echocardiographic measurement of pulmonary artery pressure from ductal Doppler velocities in the newborn. *Journal of the American College of Cardiology* 1990;15:446–456.
10. Skinner JR, Milligan DWA, Hunter S, Hey EN. Central venous pressure in the ventilated neonate. *Archives of Disease in Childhood* 1992;67:374–377.
11. Evans NJ, Archer LNJ. Doppler assessment of pulmonary artery pressure and extrapulmonary shunting in the acute phase of hyaline membrane disease. *Archives of Disease in Childhood* 1991;66:6–11.
12. Riggs T, Hirschfeld S, Borkat G, Knoke J, Liebman J. Assessment of the pulmonary vascular bed by echocardiographic right ventricular systolic time intervals. *Circulation* 1977;5:939–947.
13. Halliday HL, Dumpit FM, Brady JP. Effects of inspired oxygen on echocardiographic assessment of pulmonary vascular resistance and myocardial contractility in bronchopulmonary dysplasia. *Pediatrics* 1980;65:536–540.
14. Riggs T, Hirschfeld S, Fanaroff A, Liebman J, Fletcher

B, Meyer R. Persistence of fetal circulation syndrome: An echocardiographic study. *Journal of Pediatrics* 1977;91:626–631.
15. Halliday H, Hirschfeld S, Riggs T, Liebman J, Fanaroff A, Bormuth C. Respiratory distress syndrome: echocardiographic assessment of cardiovascular function and pulmonary vascular resistance. *Pediatrics* 1977;60:444–449.
16. Kosturakis D, Goldberg SJ, Allen HD, Loeber C. Doppler echocardiographic prediction of pulmonary arterial hypertension in congenital heart disease. *American Journal of Cardiology* 1984;53:1110–1115.
17. Vogel M, Weil J, Stern H, Buhlmeyer K. Responsiveness of raised pulmonary vascular resistance to oxygen assessed by pulsed Doppler echocardiography. *British Heart Journal* 1991;66:277–280.
18. Skinner JR. Relationship of right ventricular systolic time intervals to systolic pulmonary arterial pressure determined from tricuspid regurgitation. In: Skinner JR, MD thesis *Non-invasive determination of pulmonary arterial pressure in the newborn*, ch 15, pp 251–294. University of Leicester, UK, 1993.
19. Panidis JP, Ross J, Mintz GS. Effect of sampling site on assessment of pulmonary artery blood flow by Doppler echocardiography. *American Journal of Cardiology* 1986;58:1145–1147.
20. Skinner JR, Hunter S, Hey EN. Haemodynamic features at presentation in persistent pulmonary hypertension of the newborn and outcome. *Archives of Disease in Childhood* 1996;74:F26–32.
21. Skinner JR, Boys RJ, Heads A, Hey EN, Hunter S. Estimation of pulmonary arterial pressure in the newborn: a study of the repeatability of four Doppler echocardiographic techniques. *Pediatric Cardiology* 1996;17:360–369.
22. Fouron JC, Le Guennec JC, Villemant D, Bard H, Perreault G, Davignon A. Value of echocardiography in assessing the outcome of bronchopulmonary dysplasia of the newborn. *Pediatrics* 1980;65:529–535.
23. Newth CJL, Gow RM, Rowe RD. The assessment of pulmonary arterial pressure in bronchopulmonary dysplasia by cardiac catheterisation and M-mode echocardiography. *Pediatric Pulmonology* 1985;1:59–63.
24. Emmanouilides GC, Moss AJ, Duffie ER, Adams FH. Pulmonary arterial pressure changes in human newborn infants from birth to 3 days of age. *Journal of Pediatrics* 1964;65:327–333.
25. Walther FJ, Benders MJ, Leighton JO. Early changes in the neonatal circulatory transition. *Journal of Pediatrics* 1993;123:625–632.
26. Shiraishi H, Yaganisawa M. Pulsed Doppler echocardiographic evaluation of neonatal circulatory changes. *British Heart Journal* 1987;57:161–167.
27. Takenaka K, Waffarn F, Dabestani A, Gardin JM, Henry WL. A pulsed Doppler echocardiographic study of the postnatal changes in pulmonary artery and ascending aortic flow in normal term newborns. *American Heart Journal* 1987;113:759–766.
28. Evans NJ, Archer LNJ. Postnatal circulatory adaptation in healthy term and preterm neonates. *Archives of Disease in Childhood* 1990;65:24–26.

CHAPTER 7

Ductal shunting

Jon Skinner

INTRODUCTION

This chapter deals specifically with the assessment of left-to-right ductal shunting during neonatal respiratory failure.

There have been hundreds of publications on ductal shunting over the last two decades. From their clinical practice, neonatologists are very much aware of the importance of assessing ductal shunting and wish to learn echocardiography to be able to assess ductal shunting without always consulting the paediatric cardiologist. It is something that a neonatologist may reasonably expect to be able to learn to do, provided that advice is sought from a paediatric cardiologist when appropriate. We are convinced that echocardiography should always be done prior to therapeutic ductal closure to confirm the diagnosis.

Some centres routinely screen their very low birth weight (VLBW) babies at a fixed age (sometimes combining the examination with cranial ultrasound). This practice places too great a burden on the busy paediatric cardiologist. There is thus a need for someone in the neonatal team to do the echocardiography, and to understand how the findings should be interpreted.

There are important caveats, however. Echocardiography should not replace clinical acumen, but add to it. Always feel for full pulses in the feet in an infant about to undergo therapeutic ductal closure, so that when left-to-right ductal shunting is detected by Doppler ultrasound, the clinician is reassured that there is no coincidental aortic coarctation. Aortic coarctation can be a difficult echocardiographic diagnosis to make and closing the duct is usually detrimental in its presence. One hundred percent arterial oxygenation should be achieved at least once to eliminate cyanotic congenital heart disease. Left-to-right ductal shunting may occur in pulmonary atresia, for example, and closing the duct would be disastrous. It is not only through sophisticated echocardiographic knowledge that congenital heart disease that is duct-dependent is ruled out, but also through common sense, clinical acumen and straight-forward echocardiography.

This chapter sets out a logical and practical approach to assessing ductal shunting with echocardiography, and discusses the advantages and limitations of different measurement techniques at each stage. Echocardiographic monitoring during therapy is discussed, as well as some important research findings with clinical implications.

HOW TO DO IT

The procedure is summarized as follows.

1. Clarify the aims of the examination.
2. Clinical examination should include feeling for full foot pulses and being certain that cyanotic heart disease is not suspected.
3. A routine echocardiogram is performed (as described in Chapter 8), sequentially identifying chambers, and looking for left-sided chamber dilatation.
4. In the short-axis parasternal view, the main pulmonary artery is scanned with pulsed or colour Doppler, looking for turbulent flow.
5. The duct is imaged with cross-sectional and colour Doppler echocardiography to determine its size.
6. The direction and pattern of ductal flow is determined with pulsed and/or continuous wave (CW) Doppler.
7. The size of the shunt is graded into small, moderate or large using a variety of techniques.

Clarifying the aims of the examination

'Is the duct significant?'

The echocardiographer is commonly asked 'Is the duct clinically significant?', a question which the echocardiographer cannot answer. A good echocardiogram will reveal whether ductal shunting is present or not and whether it is small, medium or large. It can also reveal some circulatory side-effects such as reduced diastolic flow in the systemic arteries. It is remarkable how stretched the left atrium and ventricle appear in some babies very early in the course of their respiratory failure due to left-to-right ductal shunting. Such a finding does not necessarily mean that the duct needs to be closed. Nor does it mean that fluid deprivation will be helpful. These are complex and difficult questions; they depend on the relative likelihood of spontaneous ductal closure, which itself is multifactorial, and the potential side-effects of treatment. Every neonatologist has his or her own views on these points!

One should therefore be careful in one's own mind to avoid dictating treatment by saying whether a shunt is 'significant' or not. Because of the confusion that this word can cause, it is probably best also to avoid the popular term 'haemodynamically significant duct'. The echocardiographer should instead set out to determine the approximate size (and direction) of the shunt, describe it as small, medium or large, and ascertain the circulatory effects that it is having. This information can then be added to the whole clinical picture so that an informed decision can be made.

Clinical examination

A careful clinical examination should include feeling for full foot pulses and being certain that cyanotic heart disease is not suspected.

It is obviously important to ensure that there is no congenital heart disease that will deteriorate with pharmacologically induced ductal closure. This can be done successfully with careful clinical examination in combination with echocardiography. Demonstrating no gradient between right arm and leg blood pressures is also reassuring. However, mild aortic coarctation can become more severe with indomethacin (probably because of ductal-like tissue at the aortic isthmus). It is good clinical practice, therefore, to keep a careful check on foot pulses during a course of indomethacin or other anti-prostaglandin medication.

Routine echocardiogram

A routine echocardiogram is performed, sequentially identifying chambers, and looking for left-sided chamber dilatation.

The importance of a logical approach to each scan is discussed in Chapter 8. Repeating this routine series of images ensures that the examiner becomes used to what is normal, and thereby rapidly identifies what is abnormal. In particular, the examiner must be sure that the aortic and pulmonary valves are opening normally, and that the velocities beyond them are normal.

Classical cross-sectional echocardiographic features of a large left-to-right ductal shunt

The most striking feature is left atrial and left ventricular enlargement. This is seen in a number of views, particularly the four-chamber and long-axis views. The left ventricle becomes globular and the interatrial septum bows to the right (see Fig. 7.1). Pulsed Doppler interrogation of the interatrial flow reveals entirely, or almost entirely, left-to-right flow.

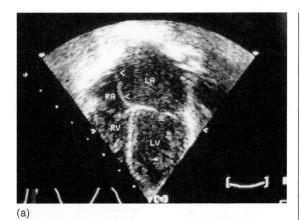
(a)

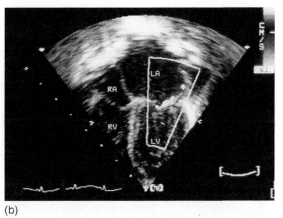
(b)

Fig. 7.1 (a) Apical four-chamber view showing dilated left atrium (LA) and left ventricle (LV). The arrows indicate the atrial septum bulging to the right. (b) Same view with colour Doppler demonstrating mild mitral regurgitation. This is common with this degree of volume loading.

The degree of left atrial enlargement depends not only on the size of the ductal shunt, but also on the size of the oval foramen. If the oval foramen is large and stretched, the left atrium can decompress through it into the right atrium. Left-to-right atrial shunt velocity will be correspondingly lower, because the pressure difference between left and right atria is lower, and the right ventricle will become relatively dilated (see Chapter 3). If the oval foramen is small, the velocity through it can be greater than 2 m/s, indicating marked elevation of left atrial pressure. (Applying the modified Bernoulli equation to this, 2 m/s suggests a 16 mmHg pressure difference between LA and RA.) The left atrial and ventricular cavities in this circumstance are typically very much enlarged.

LV function appears hyperdynamic. A volume-

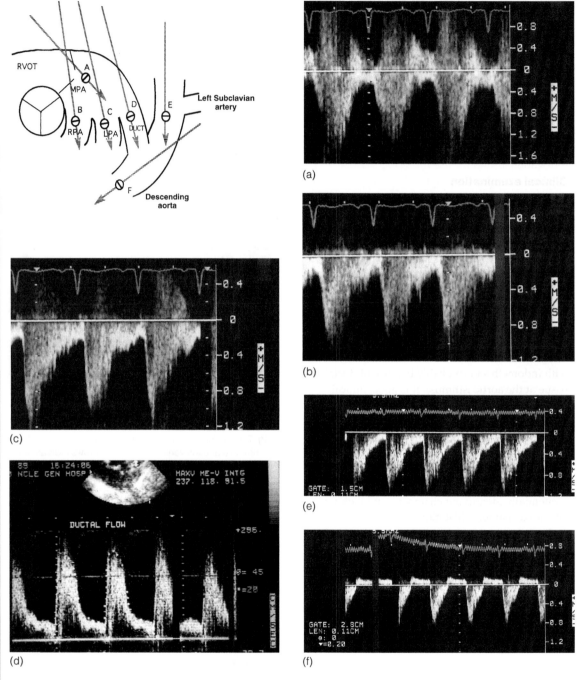

Fig. 7.2 Pulsed Doppler samples in various positions in the presence of a large left-to-right ductal shunt. Parts (a) to (f) correspond to the sample positions indicated in the line diagram. ⊖, pulsed Doppler sample. (a) In the main pulmonary artery instead of pure forward (downward) flow restricted to systole there is chaotic flow throughout the cardiac cycle. (b) In the right pulmonary artery forward flow continues throughout diastole, as in (c), in the left pulmonary artery. (d) In the duct there is pure left-to-right flow which is quite smooth ('hollow' spectral display) because of little ductal constriction, and the velocity is low at end diastole. (e) In the arch of the aorta forward flow continues through diastole. (f) In the descending aorta there is retrograde diastolic flow.

loaded left ventricle with some depression of systolic function may therefore appear normal to the naked eye, and even have a normal (or only slightly reduced) shortening fraction (this measurement is described in Chapter 4). In one study, 29% of preterms had a LV shortening fraction in the normal range prior to ductal ligation; in the remainder it was greater.[1]

Trivial mitral regurgitation is common, seen either with colour Doppler or pulsed Doppler interrogation just above the valve (Fig. 7.1b).

It should be remembered that there are other potential causes of LA and LV enlargement. Left atrial enlargement can occur with moderate or severe mitral regurgitation. This is uncommon and may indicate other pathology such as myocardial or papillary muscle insufficiency, or congenital heart disease such as common arterial trunk or coarctation. If LV function is depressed, both LV and LA will dilate.

Search for turbulence

In the short-axis view, turbulence in the main pulmonary artery is looked for with pulsed wave or colour Doppler.

In the standard short-axis parasternal view, the pulsed Doppler sample volume is placed in the main pulmonary artery, just beyond the pulmonary valve. The trace may be irregular due to the retrograde flow from the duct into the pulmonary artery (see Fig. 7.2). There should, however, be clear forward flow through the pulmonary valve.

Fig. 7.3 A small duct in a healthy term infant at 4 hours. (a) A bright colour Doppler jet, narrow it its narrowest point (towards the bottom of the flare). (b) Pulsed Doppler sample in the duct shows aliasing high velocity.

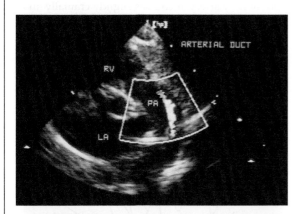

(a)

(b)

Be sure that the pulmonary valve opens and that forward flow is registered as a downward (negative) signal on the Doppler trace. (In pulmonary atresia, there can similarly be turbulence in the main pulmonary artery from ductal flow, and apparent forward flow just beyond the valve as the blood circulates around the pulmonary artery.) Move the sample further down into the pulmonary artery. Typically the signal becomes more disorganized as a result of the turbulence. With smaller shunts, the turbulence may be only locatable on the anterior side of the main pulmonary artery (to the right of the screen).

Colour Doppler makes localization and visualization of the duct much easier. Typically a bright flare is seen along the anterior portion of the main pulmonary artery (see Fig. 7.3). Moving the imaging probe will localize the origin of the jet to the arterial duct, near the origin of the left pulmonary artery.

Determination of duct size

The duct is imaged with cross-sectional and colour Doppler echocardiography to determine its size.

Ductal patency is easily confirmed by combining cross-sectional and Doppler modalities. Turbulence in the main pulmonary artery can occasionally arise from aortopulmonary collateral arteries in babies with chronic lung disease,[2] or more rarely from aortopulmonary window or coronary artery fistulas. Thus it is important to image the duct.

Imaging

The anatomy of the duct is seen in Figure 7.4. It typically arises from the main pulmonary artery near the origin of the left pulmonary artery, with a course slightly to the left of that of the main pulmonary artery. It courses slightly cranially and posteriorly to join with the descending aorta opposite to, and just beyond, the origin of the left

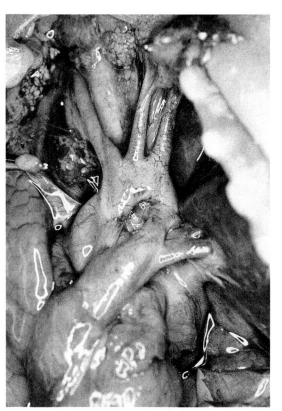

(a)

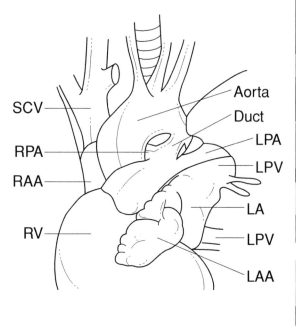

(b)

Fig. 7.4 Anatomical photograph (a) and corresponding drawing (b) showing the course of the arterial duct. SCV, superior caval vein; RAA, right atrial appendage; LPV, left pulmonary vein. (Photo kindly supplied by Dr. Michael Ashworth, Bristol Children's Hospital, UK)

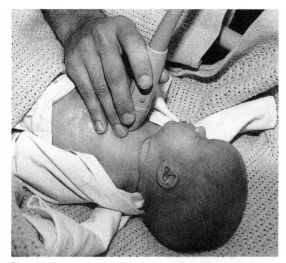

Fig. 7.5 Photograph of the ultrasound position to obtain a view of the arterial duct (see also Fig. 1.4.10).

subclavian artery, which comes off laterally from the arch of the aorta.

The duct may be visualized by sliding up the chest from the standard short-axis view with some anticlockwise rotation (Fig. 7.5; see also Fig. 1.4.10). The 'three-legged stool' appearance is seen (see Fig. 7.6a), with the right and left pulmonary arteries forming the right and middle legs and the duct being the third leg. By starting with a clear view of the aortic arch from the suprasternal notch, and slowly moving back towards the three-legged view, it is usually possible to obtain a view of the duct in its entirety and beyond down the descending aorta (Fig. 7.6b). At birth the duct has no constriction and is as wide as the descending aorta, just as in the fetus. Ductal constriction typically begins at the pulmonary end or in the middle of the duct.[3]

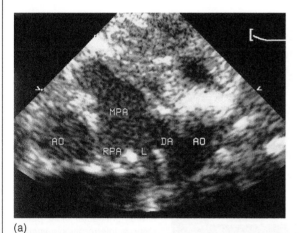

(a)

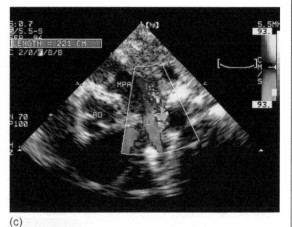

(c)

Fig. 7.6 Cross-sectional views of a large arterial duct. (a) The so-called 'three-legged stool' view: RPA, LPA and the duct form the three legs. (b) The probe is slightly higher up the chest; left: a complete view of the duct from MPA into descending aorta; right: colour Doppler is deep orange, suggesting non-turbulent and relatively low-velocity left-to-right flow. (c) Measurement of the ductal internal diameter at the narrowest point of the colour Doppler in the duct.

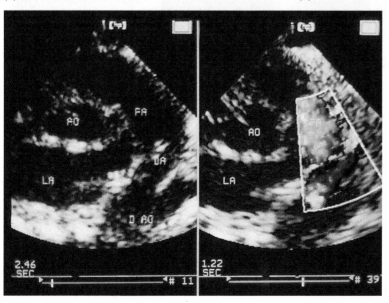

(b)

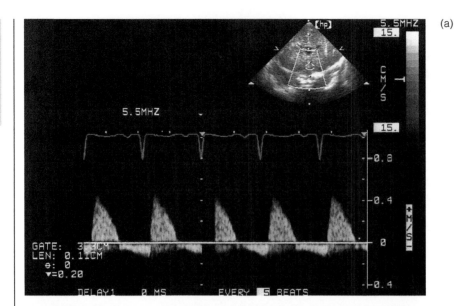

(a)

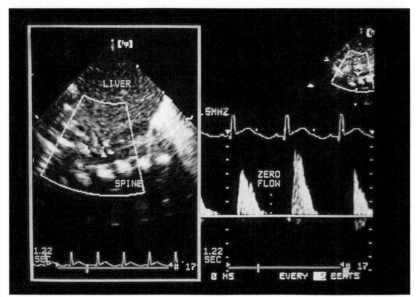

(b)

Fig. 7.7 In an infant with a large left-to-right ductal shunt, pulsed Doppler interrogation reveals further evidence of ductal steal with absence of the normal forward flow in diastole in (a) a cerebral artery and (b) a mesenteric artery.

Pulsed Doppler ultrasound

When the sample is placed at the pulmonary end of the duct, continuous left-to-right flow is detected (see Fig. 7.2). At the origin of the left pulmonary artery there is high velocity forward flow in diastole as blood continues to pour from the aorta into the pulmonary arteries during diastole.

CW Doppler ultrasound

The non-imaging pencil probe is placed at the mid to upper left sternal edge and directed posteriorly. Fine adjustments bring a continuous upward deflection on the Doppler trace (see Fig. 6.7). This technique is

very sensitive in experienced hands – a tiny duct can be missed using just the other methods.

Colour Doppler ultrasound

The bright flare of colour in the main pulmonary artery makes the detection of a patent duct very easy (see Fig. 7.6). The size of this flare when a ductal view is obtained is also helpful in grading the size of the duct and the size of the shunt (see below).

How large is the duct?

Measuring the internal diameter of the duct can be difficult even when clear images are obtained.

Accurate measurement of the narrowest part of the duct is unreliable – the edge of the area of constriction, often a 'shelf', is often difficult to see. Sometimes the duct may appear to be large although it is actually closed by a narrow ridge.

Measuring the width of the colour Doppler jet within the duct can be useful. A recent study in preterms less than 1500 g suggests that a minimal colour map diameter of greater than 1.4 mm[4] was necessary before a large left-to-right ductal shunt could occur (see Fig. 7.6c). While this can be a useful guide, one should not overestimate its reliability. Colour Doppler gain, filter and map controls must be the same with each sequential examination; a narrow jet can easily be made artificially into a fat one! This technique has been applied to sizing ASDs and VSDs, but it remains controversial. Irregularly shaped orifices have different measurements in different planes and the variability of colour Doppler maps and gain settings causes inaccuracies.

It is probably reasonable to try to judge the internal size of the duct as closed, small, moderate (mild constriction) or large (no evidence of constriction), but attempts at measuring diameter with colour Doppler are legitimate if done regularly and care is taken to standardize machinery settings. Remember that the size of the shunt depends not only on the size of the duct, but on the balance of resistances on each side of it. There is a huge duct at birth, but very little left-to-right shunt!

Direction and pattern of ductal flow

The direction and pattern of flow through the duct is determined with pulsed and/or CW Doppler.

The measurement techniques have been discussed in Chapter 6. Large left-to-right shunts characteristically have continuous left-to-right flow, but instead of continuous high-velocity flow, as in healthy babies before the duct finally closes, the higher velocity is in late systole, and the velocity at end diastole is very low (less than 1 m/s, and less than half the peak velocity in systole), or even zero. An example is shown in Figure 7.2d. This flow pattern indicates that the aortic and pulmonary arterial pressures are roughly equal at end diastole; this is never seen in normal healthy infants.

Bidirectional flow (right-to-left in systole, left-to-right in diastole) or right-to-left flow indicates that there is elevated pulmonary vascular resistance; anti-prostaglandins should be avoided in this situation.

Grading shunt size

The size of the shunt is graded into small, moderate or large using a variety of techniques.

Those new to echocardiography will be surprised at how unsophisticated and subjective measurement of left-to-right ductal shunt size is. There are, sadly, good reasons for this.

- Volume of flow through the duct cannot be quantified directly with Doppler ultrasound (like ascending aortic flow – see Chapter 5) because of inaccuracy in measurement of ductal diameter, and because there is turbulent rather than laminar flow.
- Theoretically one could measure right and left ventricular outputs and calculate the difference; left ventricular output should be twice as high with a 2:1 ductal shunt. This is, however, complicated by the coexistence of an interatrial shunt of variable size (see Chapter 3), and by difficulty in getting good flow signals in the pulmonary artery when there is turbulence due to the flow from the duct.

We are left with semiquantitative techniques that can, at best, differentiate ductal shunts into small, moderate and large after establishing that there is a patent duct. These involve:

1. assessment of left atrial and left ventricular size;
2. assessment of ductal size;
3. 'quantifying' colour flow in the main pulmonary artery; and
4. pulsed Doppler evaluation of abnormal diastolic flow in systemic arteries and branch pulmonary arteries.

Useful additional techniques are:

5. the analysis of ductal flow pattern; and
6. assessment of left ventricular output.

It is not necessary to perform all of these at each examination! However, each method has its uses, and needs to be understood. Using a combination of techniques improves sensitivity and specificity of the examination, and much can be done in a short time with practice.

Left atrial and ventricular size

One of the most popular techniques is to measure the width of the left atrium or left ventricle in diastole in relationship to the width of the aorta. Using the aorta as a constant like this allows comparison between babies of different size. The 'LA:Ao ratio' was first described in 1974 by Silverman *et al.*[5] Using M-mode echocardiography they found that 10 preterm infants requiring ductal ligation had a mean LA:Ao ratio of 1.38:1 (all were above 1.15:1) compared with a mean of 0.86:1 in controls with a closed duct.

How to do it Once a good long-axis view is obtained from the third or fourth intercostal space at the left sternal border, the M-mode cursor is dropped through the aortic cusps into the left atrium (see Chapter 1.5).

By convention, the measurements are made from leading edge to leading edge (i.e. the front of the aorta to the front of the posterior wall of the aorta, and from the front of the posterior wall of the aorta to the front of the back wall of the left atrium). Left atrial maximal diameter is measured at the point of maximal forward excursion of the aorta – see Fig. 7.8).

Limitations and repeatability Hundreds of studies have used this technique since Silverman's paper, and it is still popular in clinical practice. The repeatability of the technique, with care, can be very good. Alone it has poor specificity and sensitivity because other factors such as LV dysfunction can enlarge the left atrium and different fluid regimes also affect it. The left atrium is not only smaller in dehydrated babies, but also in those with a large interatrial communication as discussed above. However, in combination with the newer methods, which at the very least can prove ductal patency, it

remains very useful. We, and many others,[6,7] have found that a ratio of >1.4:1 is specific enough to indicate at least a moderate shunt, but this figure varies between echocardiographers and between institutions. For reasons that are not fully understood, this ratio is not reliable in the first 24 hours of life. Having an easily measurable 'number' such as this allows at least semiobjective monitoring of the effect of therapy, and comparison between different centres.

Similarly the left ventricular end-diastolic dimension (LVEDD):Ao ratio has been used; values over 2.1:1 are usually found with large shunts.[6]

In clinical practice, subjective assessment of LA and LV volume loading from four-chamber views is just as useful.

Assessment of ductal size (Fig. 7.6c)

If a duct is narrower than 1.4 mm in preterms under 1500 g a large shunt is unlikely to be present.[4] Using this method in healthy term infants, minimum internal diameter of the duct was 4.2 ± 0.6 mm at 2 hours of age and 2.3 ± 0.5 mm at 12 hours.[8]

Quantifying ductal shunt size by assessing colour Doppler flow in the main pulmonary artery

Obtaining a colour Doppler 'flare' in the main pulmonary artery has already been described. The size of the flare, and the distance it travels in the main pulmonary artery, depends on how much blood is going through the duct. A tiny shunt is seen as a narrow jet which does not reach the pulmonary valve; a moderate shunt produces a jet which is wider, passes

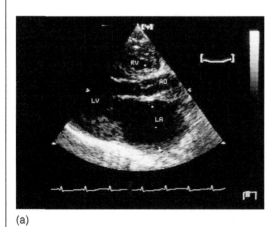

(a)

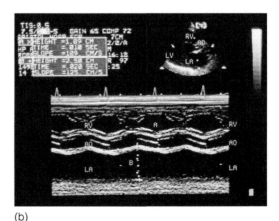

(b)

Fig. 7.8 (a) Parasternal long-axis view showing gross dilatation of the left atrium and ventricle. (b) The left atrial:aortic root ratio is 2.50 cm:1.09 cm, i.e. 2.3:1.

well into the pulmonary artery but not quite to the pulmonary valve; and a large shunt has a jet which is very wide and reaches the pulmonary valve and swirls back down into the artery.

Limitations and repeatability Quantification of blood flow with colour Doppler ultrasound is inaccurate. Many authors have attempted to quantify valvular regurgitation by outlining the area of retrograde flow. Unfortunately because so much depends on the machine and the colour map, filters and gain settings, this type of measurement has not found regular use. Instead, regurgitation is usually classified into mild, moderate and severe. It needs to be remembered also that the distance a jet travels relates to its *speed* as much as its *volume*. A relatively small duct with high aortopulmonary pressure difference can be expected to produce a jet which reaches a long way into the pulmonary artery.

Nevertheless, most paediatric echocardiographers do find such semiquantitative information useful in clinical practice. Provided care is taken to ensure gain settings are not too high, colour Doppler ultrasound can be a valuable subjective way to assess ductal shunting.

Pulsed Doppler evaluation of abnormal diastolic flow in systemic and branch pulmonary arteries
Diastolic aortic pressure is low with a large left-to-right ductal shunt owing to the phenomenon known as 'ductal steal'. Blood passing down the descending aorta during systole goes backwards up the arterial duct and into the pulmonary arteries during diastole. This results in relative underperfusion of all of the systemic arteries, including those supplying the cerebral hemispheres and the gut.

How to do it Pulsed Doppler ultrasound is particularly useful in observing this phenomenon as the sampling gate can be placed in any artery. Classical findings with a large ductal shunt are shown in Figure 7.2.

The procedure is simply to align as closely as possible with flow in the branch pulmonary arteries parasternally and the arch and descending aorta from the suprasternal notch. Similar interrogation can be made in the mesenteric arteries from the subcostal position, and also in cerebral arteries from the fontanelles. Absent or retrograde diastolic cerebral blood flow is said to be present at all times in babies requiring ductal ligation,[9] and rare in babies without a duct. Similar findings in brachial and femoral arteries are less specific; they commonly occur in babies with a closed duct.[9]

As the Doppler sample is moved around, retrograde diastolic flow is seen in the descending aorta, gut and cerebral arteries, whereas abnormally high antegrade diastolic flow is seen in both branch pulmonary arteries (particularly the left) as the continuous stream of blood from the aorta pours into them via the duct. Low-velocity antegrade diastolic flow is also seen in the arch of the aorta, (above or proximal to the duct) as blood returning from the head and neck arteries passes down the aorta and into the duct during diastole.

Such findings certainly tempt the investigator to use the term 'haemodynamically significant' for such a ductal shunt. There have been attempts to quantify these changes and correlate them with either cardiac catheter findings or other echocardiographic features. Some results are summarized in Table 7.1.

Limitations and repeatability These findings are useful and increase the specificity of the examination in terms of selecting the left-to-right ductal shunts with the most profound circulatory effects.

Table 7.1 Doppler echocardiographic studies relating arterial flow velocities to quantity of ductal shunting

Position of sample gate	Feature quantified	No duct	Small	Moderate	Large
Centre of MPA[10] (maximum velocity)	Antegrade diastolic flow	0	0–20 cm/s	>20 cm/s	
Origin of LPA[11a] (mean velocity)	Antegrade diastolic flow	–	>30 cm/s	30–50 cm/s	>50 cm/s
Descending Ao[12b] (as percentage of forward flow)	Retrograde diastolic flow	10%	<30%	30–50%	>50%

MPA, main pulmonary artery; LPA, left pulmonary artery.
[a]This study demonstrated a linear relationship between mean antegrade flow velocity during diastole determined by pulsed Doppler ultrasound in the left pulmonary artery and left-to-right shunt ratio during cardiac catheterization in 26 patients aged from 1 day to 3.5 years.
[b]This study demonstrated a linear relationship between the ratio of the retrograde flow velocity integral to antegrade flow velocity integral and the size of left-to-right ductal shunt assessed by radionuclide angiography in children from 2 weeks to 9 years. The investigators used CW Doppler ultrasound.

Like the other measurements, however, they are not truly quantitative, and in addition they have not been subjected to rigorous tests of repeatability.

Abnormal retrograde diastolic flow in the descending aorta and in the aortic arch is seen with severe aortic incompetence and aortopulmonary window. Neither of these conditions deteriorates with indomethacin treatment, and the former should be easily detectable with colour Doppler echocardiography. Aortopulmonary window is extremely rare but is not an easy echocardiographic diagnosis and will also cause turbulence in the main pulmonary artery and left-sided chamber dilatation. It should, of course, be excluded, along with other intracardiac left-to-right shunts, if cardiac failure persists after ductal closure.

Ductal flow pattern

While much is known of the relationship of ductal flow patterns to pulmonary arterial pressure (PA pressure; see Chapter 6), relatively little is known about how the flow patterns change with quantity of flow through the duct.

It has been shown that the classical pattern of flow with a large shunt in the preterm infant is high in systole and very low in diastole[13] (see Fig. 7.2d and compare with the other flow patterns in Chapter 6). The ratio of systolic:end diastolic velocities is usually greater than 2:1, often as high as 5:1. The velocity at

end diastole is less than 1 m/s, and is frequently almost zero, indicating that the pulmonary and aortic pressures are balanced at end diastole. This is consistent with low diastolic aortic pressure and elevated diastolic PA pressure. This pattern is not seen in healthy infants.

As the duct constricts during treatment or spontaneous closure, the velocity throughout the cardiac cycle rises, most noticeably at end diastole, indicating that the aortic to PA pressure gradient is increasing (see Fig. 7.9). The ratio of systolic to diastolic velocities decreases. Interestingly, if there is a murmur present, this usually disappears even though the velocity across the duct carries on increasing.

Measurement of left ventricular output

The method for measuring left ventricular output has been described earlier in Chapter 5. Stroke volume increases markedly with left-to-right ductal shunting (much more so than heart rate[14,15]). An increase of 60% has been shown to predict the development of symptomatic ductal shunting.[16]

A possible use for this method is to evaluate shunt size. We found that an aortic stroke distance of greater than 12 cm in babies at less than 32 weeks' gestation is as specific as an LA:Ao ratio greater than 1.4:1 in detecting babies who have, or will subsequently develop, signs and symptoms of

---

☞ *Practical Point*

- In summary, echocardiographic features of a left-to-right ductal shunt are:
1. Bowing of the interatrial septum to the right with enlarged left atrium and left ventricle – four-chamber views.
2. Left atrium enlarged; LA:Ao ratio >1.4:1 – long-axis view.
3. Colour Doppler – continuous flare in the main pulmonary artery from arterial duct.
4. Pulsed wave Doppler – Turbulent flow in the main pulmonary artery, continuous antegrade flow in diastole in left pulmonary artery and arch of aorta, retrograde diastolic flow in descending aorta, cerebral and gut blood vessels.
5. CW Doppler – continuous left-to-right (upward) flow in main pulmonary artery, with higher velocity in systole and low velocity at end diastole.
6. Raised left ventricular stroke volume.

Suggested grading of L–R ductal shunts into small, medium or large:

	Small	Medium	Large
LA:Ao ratio	<1.4:1	1.4:1–1.6:1	>1.6:1
Ductal diameter (colour)	<1.5 mm	1.5–2.0 mm	>2.0 mm
Diastolic flow in descending Ao	Antegrade	0% to <30% of forward flow	>30% of forward flow

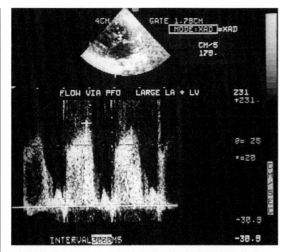

Fig. 7.9 Pulsed Doppler at the small oval foramen shows high velocity (1.8 m/s) due to left atrial hypertension.

a large shunt. This is consistent with other reports.[17]

The problem with the method is that some large ducts may coexist with left ventricular dysfunction. These babies will be unable to respond by increasing stroke volume. They would potentially not be detected by this method, and are probably the babies at greatest risk of developing circulatory failure (this 'malignant ductus' is referred to in Chapter 5).

MONITORING EFFECT OF THERAPY

In essence, all of the above features should gradually revert to normal as the duct constricts. There are a few useful tips, however.

When the duct is closed therapeutically, the left atrium may take time to reduce in size, and can sometimes even enlarge. As the left ventricle is off-loaded of excess volume it becomes relatively thick-walled and stiff, and diastolic relaxation is impaired due to sudden reduction in cavity size. This often

causes transient disturbance of diastolic filling. During mitral inflow the E wave disappears and there is a prominent A wave (see Chapter 2.2). When this happens, the left atrium may be very distended, even if the duct is completely closed. Mitral regurgitation can also occur. There may still be overt cardiac failure with pulmonary congestion and further indomethacin would not be helpful. Left atrial size should not be used alone to monitor progress during treatment.

During constriction ductal velocities increase markedly, and aortic stroke distance reduces. Table 7.2 shows mean results from 11 babies during ductal constriction during a course of indomethacin therapy, and Figure 7.10 shows serial change in left-to-right ductal velocity in these 11 babies.

Note that LV output has fallen on average by about one third, and that almost all of this fall is due

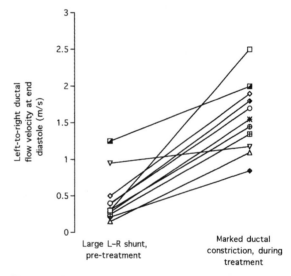

Fig. 7.10 Graph showing increased end-diastolic left-to-right ductal flow velocity during ductal constriction secondary to indomethacin treatment.

Table 7.2 Mean haemodynamic measurements from 11 preterm infants (23–30 weeks' gestation, birth weight 615–1625 g) during ductal constriction (prior to eventual closure) during indomethacin treatment

	Pre-constriction	During indomethacin treatment	Average change	Significance[a]
LA:Ao ratio	1.59:1	1.28:1	−19%	<0.0001
LV output (ml/kg/min)	521	352	−32%	<0.0001
Heart rate	161	154	−4%	<0.05
LV stroke volume index (ml/kg)	3.3	2.3	−29%	<0.0001
Systolic blood pressure (mmHg)	49	56	+14%	<0.05
Maximal L–R ductal flow velocity (m/s)	1.8	2.6	+44%	<0.01
Ductal flow velocity at end diastole (m/s)	0.5	1.4	+157%	<0.001

[a]Paired *t* test.

to a fall in stroke volume rather than heart rate. Note also the significant rise in systolic systemic arterial pressure, and the increase in ductal flow velocities, the largest percentage change being in the velocity at end diastole. The ratio of maximal left-to-right flow velocity (mid–late systole) to velocity at end diastole changed from a mean of 3.6:1 to 1.9 :1.

CLINICAL RESEARCH

Clinical research has recently challenged some long-held beliefs. For instance: (1) prolonged ductal patency is a feature of prematurity per se; (2) the preterm neonate is only able to elevate left ventricular output through increase in heart rate and not stroke volume; (3) a large left-to-right ductal shunt is usually clinically obvious; and (4) clinically 'silent' ductal shunting is unimportant.

Ductal patency and prematurity

Echocardiographic studies confirm that prolonged ductal patency is a feature of respiratory failure in the preterm neonate. However, healthy preterms, down to 28 weeks' gestation, do not have prolonged ductal patency. The results of two studies[18,19] are summarized in Figure 7.11. Timing of ductal closure was by cross-sectional echocardiography with either colour Doppler or pulsed and CW Doppler. Ducts were closed in term and preterm infants by the end of the fourth day.

Healthy preterm infants below 28 weeks' gestation without increased oxygen requirements

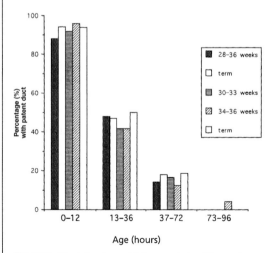

Fig. 7.11 Ductal patency histogram in healthy preterms (28–36 weeks) over the first five days, from studies of Reller et al. (1988)[18] and Skinner et al. (1991)[19] (see text).

are uncommon, and there are no data about ductal closure in this group. However, it seems that prematurity per se (down to 28 weeks' gestation) does not result in prolonged ductal patency.

Regulation of cardiac output in the preterm neonate – stroke volume or heart rate?

Research in newborn lambs has shown that cardiac output is dependent on heart rate during the early neonatal period.[20] This information has subsequently been applied incorrectly to the preterm infant with left-to-right ductal shunting.

Using the Doppler echocardiographic technique described in Chapter 5 to assess left ventricular output it is now obvious that the major response of the left ventricle to the increased demand from left-to-right ductal shunting in the preterm infant is a doubling of stroke volume.[14–17] Heart rate changes much less – in the order of 20% – and not always in the same direction.

The earlier animal work is not necessarily at variance with these new findings because the studies in animals were done with stable preload and afterload and a closed arterial duct. With a large duct and low pulmonary vascular resistance, there is increased preload due to the increased pulmonary venous return, and reduced afterload due to the low pulmonary vascular resistance. The left ventricle can thus stretch and, in accordance with Starling's law, eject its contents effectively.

Heart rate is thus an unreliable clinical guide with which to monitor ductal shunting, whereas echocardiographic monitoring of LV output can be very useful. Furthermore (as discussed above), if there are echocardiographic features of a large shunt but LV output is not elevated, this may be a sign that the LV cannot cope and the systemic circulation is in danger of collapse.

Are clinical signs of left-to-right ductal shunting reliable?

Those not yet accustomed to echocardiography in the preterm may still believe that clinical signs are reliable in detecting large ductal shunts. Unfortunately this is not the case, even with experienced clinicians.

McGrath et al. in 1978 first described the 'silent ductus'.[21] Using aortography they showed that a large left-to-right ductal shunt could be present in infants with respiratory distress but without a murmur or other clinical signs. Clinicians were sceptical of these findings, but when clinical examination has been directly compared with echocardiography[10] it was found that clinical examination was both insensitive (as low as 37%) and non-specific, with a positive predictive power as low as 60%. In another study[9] a murmur was absent in at least 20% of cases with a large shunt, although hyperactive precordium was a more sensitive feature. Contrary to popular belief, pulse pressure, another classical clinical sign, is also frequently normal with a large ductal shunt, particularly in babies less than 1000 g but also in some larger babies. This is because systolic systemic arterial pressure falls as much as diastolic pressure with a large shunt.[22]

Clinical signs of a large shunt appear on average 72 hours later than echocardiographic signs.[16,23]

Clinical examination cannot therefore be relied upon to detect or rule out a large left-to-right ductal shunt.

Is clinically 'silent' ductal shunting unimportant?

After the 'silent ductus' was first recognized, there followed a number of studies randomizing preterms with HMD into early ductal closure or not. Results were disappointing, showing little or no difference in mortality or morbidity. This led to the view that silent shunting was unimportant, and that reliance on clinical signs was satisfactory in detecting patients for treatment.[24] This would suggest that echocardiographic screening is unnecessary.

The studies did not, however, differentiate babies on the basis of whether or not they had a ductal shunt. Therefore many babies received indomethacin or surgical ligation when it was not clinically needed. The real question, which still remains unanswered, is whether early closure of the large but silent duct (only) reduces morbidity.

There is considerable evidence that silent shunting is detrimental to clinical well-being. In a study of 20 infants with severe HMD,[23] we followed ductal shunting echocardiographically while the clinicians, who were unaware of the results of the echocardiography, performed daily clinical cardiovascular examination. After recovery from the severe phase of HMD, three babies post extubation suffered cardiorespiratory collapse within the next 24 hours requiring re-ventilation and resuscitation. All three were felt to have had a septic episode or necrotizing enterocolitis (NEC), and were treated as

such. Neonatologists may recognize this as not a too unfamiliar scenario. A mean of 24 hours later obvious clinical signs of ductal shunting appeared for the first time, and after repeat echocardiography indomethacin was given and all three were successfully extubated. None had blood film or eventual bacteriological evidence of sepsis and all got better with ductal closure.

The sting in the tail is that all three of these babies had a large ductal shunt on echocardiography for an average of three days prior to the collapse; LA:Ao ratios were >1.6:1 and LV output was markedly elevated in all until specific treatment to close the duct (indomethacin) was given. (An example of one baby's course is given in Fig. 7.12.) The attending physicians believed that the duct had 'opened up' secondary to stress, but the echocardiography proved otherwise. It seems likely that the ductal shunt was directly responsible for the deterioration in all three of these babies.

There is a lot of other evidence that silent shunting has potentially harmful effects. It worsens pulmonary compliance, reduces cerebral, gut and renal blood flow, reduces effective systemic cardiac output[25] along with both systolic and diastolic systemic arterial pressure, and places a huge demand on the left ventricle, increasing net energy expenditure just to maintain the circulatory status quo. All of these render the infant vulnerable to any additional circulatory disturbance.

Indomethacin causes such major circulatory disturbances (including dramatic reduction in gut and cerebral blood flow and possibly coronary arterial constriction) that it would not be surprising if these changes counterbalanced the benefits of ductal closure itself. Ibuprofen is thought to have fewer side-effects and in a recent randomized trial in VLBW babies[26] it was given at three hours of age and markedly reduced the number of preterm infants with a subsequent symptomatic ductal shunt, and almost halved the time on ventilation and length of hospitalization.

Further, larger control trials are required, selecting babies with large silent shunts only and randomizing them into treatment or non-treatment groups, using such a drug with less severe side-effects.

In the mean time, neonatal echocardiographers will continue to find it hard to believe that silent ductal shunting is not important.

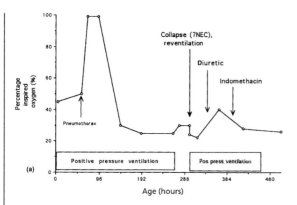

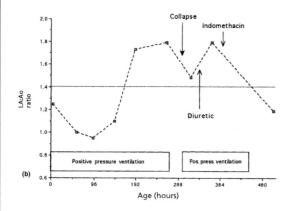

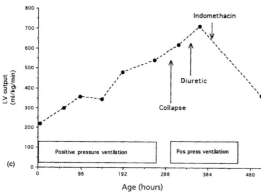

Fig. 7.12 Development of left-to-right ductal shunting in a preterm infant (27 weeks, 895 g) with HMD. (a) Time course of respiratory disease. Extubation at day 11 from intermittent mandatory ventilation (IMV) and 23% inspired oxygen is followed a day later by collapse, resuscitation and re-ventilation. The first clinical signs of a patent duct appear 48 hours later (see text). Attending clinicians felt he had 'opened his duct' at this stage. Indomethacin closes the duct and he is extubated uneventfully. (b) The LA:Ao ratio had been high for 3–4 days before the collapse, despite the absence of clinical signs (the duct had never constricted since birth). (c) Left ventricular output rises throughout, mediated by a three-fold increase in stroke volume and little change in heart rate.

REFERENCES

1. Baylen B, Meyer RA, Korfhagen J, Benzing G, Bubb ME, Kaplan S. Left ventricular performance in the critically ill premature infant with patent ductus arteriosus and pulmonary disease. *Circulation* 1977;55:182–188.
2. Skinner JR, Silove ED. Aorto-pulmonary collateral arteries mimicking symptomatic ductal shunting in a preterm infant. *British Heart Journal* 1995;74:93–94.
3. Smallhorn JF, Gow R, Olley PM *et al*. Combined noninvasive assessment of the ductus arteriosus in the preterm infant before and after Indomethacin treatment. *American Journal of Cardiology* 1984;54:1300–1304.
4. Kluckow M, Evans N. Early echocardiographic prediction of symptomatic patent ductus arteriosus in preterm infants undergoing mechanical ventilation. *Journal of Pediatrics* 1995;127:774–779.
5. Silverman NH, Lewis AL, Heyman MA, Rudolph AM. Echocardiographic assessment of ductus arteriosus shunt in premature infants. *Circulation* 1974;50:821–825.
6. Johnson GL, Breart GL, Gewitz MH *et al*. Echocardiographic characteristics of premature infants with patent ductus arteriosus. *Pediatrics* 1983;72:864–871.
7. Evans N. Diagnosis of patent ductus arteriosus in the preterm newborn. *Archives of Disease in Childhood* 1993;68:58–61.
8. Harada K, Shiota T, Takahashi Y, Tamura M, Toyono M, Takada G. Doppler echocardiographic evaluation of left ventricular output and left ventricular diastolic filling changes in the first day of life. *Pediatric Research* 1994:35:506–509.
9. Kupfershmid C, Lang D, Pohlandt F. Sensitivity, specificity and predictive value of clinical findings, m-mode echocardiography and continuous-wave Doppler sonography in the diagnosis of symptomatic patent ductus arteriosus in preterm infants. *European Journal of Pediatrics* 1988;147:279–282.
10. Hirsimaki H, Kero P, Wanne O. Doppler ultrasound and clinical evaluation in detection and grading of patent ductus arteriosus in neonates. *Critical Care Medicine* 1990;18:490–493.
11. Hiraishi S, Horiguchi Y, Misawa H *et al*. Nonivasive Doppler echocardiographic evaluation of shunt flow haemodynamics of the ductus arteriosus. *Circulation* 1987;75:1146–1153.
12. Serwer GA, Armstrong BE, Anderson PAW. Continuous wave Doppler ultrasonographic quantitation of patent ductus arteriosus flow. *Journal of Pediatrics* 1982;100:297–299.
13. Skinner JR, Hunter S, Hey EN. A new method to assess ductal shunting. *Paediatric Reviews and Communications* 1991;6:58–59 (Abstr).
14. Alverson D, Eldridge M, Johnson J *et al*. Effect of patent ductus arteriosus on left ventricular output in premature infants. *Journal of Pediatrics* 1983;102:754–757.
15. Skinner JR, Hunter S, Hey EN. Regulation of cardiac output in the premature neonate: stroke volume or heart rate? *Pediatric Cardiology* 1991;12(4):258 (Abstr).

16. Walther F, Kim D, Ebrahimi M, Siassi B. Pulsed Doppler measurement of left ventricular output as early predictor of symptomatic patent ductus arteriosus in very preterm infants. *Biology of the Neonate* 1989;56:121–128.

17. Lindner W, Seidel M, Versmold H, Dohlemann C, Riegel K. Stroke volume and left ventricular output in preterm infants with patent ductus arteriosus. *Paediatric Research* 1990;27:278–281.

18. Reller MD, Ziegler ML, Rice MJ, Solin RC, McDonald RW. Duration of ductal shunting in healthy preterm infants: An echocardiographic color flow Doppler study. *Journal of Pediatrics* 1988;112:441–446.

19. Skinner JR, Boys RJ, Hunter S, Hey EN. Non-invasive determination of pulmonary arterial pressure in healthy neonates. *Archives of Disease in Childhood* 1991;66:386–390.

20. Rudolph AM. Circulatory changes during the perinatal period. *Pediatric Cardiology* 1993;4(Suppl 2):17–20.

21. McGrath RL, McGuinness GA, Way GL, Wolfe RR, Nora JJ, Simons MA. The silent ductus arteriosus. *Journal of Pediatrics* 1978;93:110–113.

22. Evans N, Moorcraft J. Effect of patency of the ductus arteriosus on blood pressure in very preterm infants. *Archives of Disease in Childhood* 1992;67:1169–1173.

23. Skinner JR, Hunter S, Hey EN. Cardiorespiratory collapse and the silent ductus. *Klinische Padiatrie* 1991;203:52 (Abstr).

24. Archer LNJ, Glass EJ, Godman MJ. The silent ductus arteriosus in idiopathic respiratory distress syndrome. *Acta Paediatrica Scandinavia* 1984;73:652–656.

25. Evans N, Kluckow M. Early determinants of right and left ventricular output in ventilated preterm infants. *Archives of Disease in Childhood* 1996;74:F88–F94.

26. Varvarigou A, Bardin CL, Beharry K, Chemtob S, Papegeorgio A, Aranda JV. Early Ibuprofen administration to prevent patent ductus arteriosus in premature newborn infants. *Journal of the American Medical Association* 1996;275:539–544.

Putting it into Practice

CHAPTER 8

A logical approach to cardiac scanning

Stewart Hunter

INTRODUCTION

For whatever reason a scan is being done, it is important for the operator to consider that congenital heart disease may be present, and should be excluded. This can be done by always following a set examination sequence and positively identifying cardiac structures and their position from venous inflow to arterial outflow. Once an abnormality is identified, or if normality is in doubt, expert cardiological opinion should be sought.

This chapter highlights important practical differences between adult and neonatal echocardiography (for those more used to scanning adults or older children), describes a simplified and modern way to classify congenital heart disease, and suggests a scanning routine to be used for every examination. Examples of some abnormalities are given.

SPECIAL FEATURES OF NEONATAL ECHOCARDIOGRAPHY

The neonatologist has much greater flexibility of approach when scanning the heart than does the adult cardiologist. The subcostal and suprasternal approaches give clinically invaluable anatomical information in a much higher percentage of patients in infancy than at any other time of life. The heart is also relatively larger compared to the thoracic cavity and more of it is apposed to the chest wall, such that it can be scanned parasternally from the second to the fifth intercostal space compared with only the fourth and fifth spaces in older patients. It is therefore possible, for example, to construct a family of sequential views in the anatomical short axis (see Fig. 1.4.6). Imaging is usually particularly easy during HMD, since the poorly aerated lungs provide little barrier to ultrasound, but becomes more difficult in the infant with chronic lung disease and hyperinflated lungs.

Because of the potential complexity of the relationships between the cardiac structures, all possible echo windows are utilized – some views being better for some lesions than others. For example, from the apical window the interatrial septum lies along the interrogating scan beam and is so thin that it frequently appears to be absent when it is in fact intact (Fig. 8.1a). In comparison, the interatrial septum viewed subcostally is scanned en face and absence of echoes from the central part

of the septum reliably diagnoses an atrial septal defect (Fig. 8.1b).

Orientation of the image on screen

All kinds of clinical imaging have conventions for orienting the images. Some, such as computerized axial tomography (CAT) scans, follow the bizarre pathological habit of considering anatomical sections as if the observer were lying under the section looking upwards! Echocardiographers who deal only with adults and acquired heart disease tend to orient their cross-sectional scans with the sharp end upwards. This results in the ventricles lying above the atria and the great arteries hanging below the

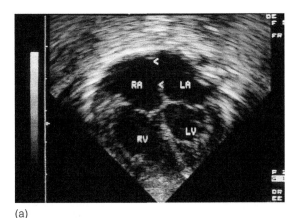

(a)

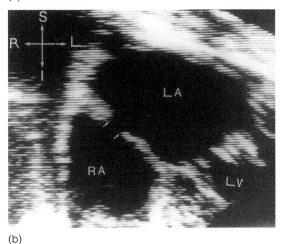

(b)

Fig. 8.1 (a) Apical four-chamber view showing the two ventricles and the two atria. The area arrowed appears to be a defect in the interatrial septum. This was in fact an artifact and the septum was intact.
(b) Paracoronal subcostal view showing left and right atria. There is a small central atrial septal defect, the outlines of which are defined with certainty because the ultrasound beam is hitting the interatrial septum at right angles.

ventricles. Congenital heart disease is complex enough without this added iatrogenic inconvenience.

Neonatal echocardiographers should orient their cardiac imaging in an anatomically correct way. 'The right side of the scan should contain left-sided cardiac structures and vice versa, as if viewing a chest X-ray for example. The atria and great arteries should be shown above the ventricles. This is all easily achieved in modern echo machines at the flick of a switch and most transducers have a mark on their side to match with the screen marker to ensure that the laterality of the scan is correct.

Systematic approach

It is important when scanning the cardiovascular system of infants to have a systematic approach. We always start with the subcostal views (Fig. 8.2). This offers a variety of views including four-chambered

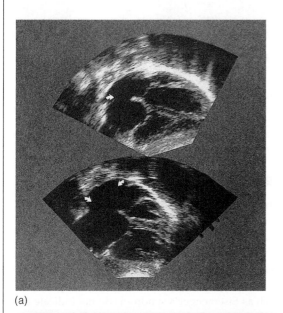

(a)

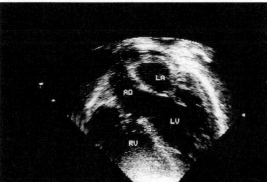

(b)

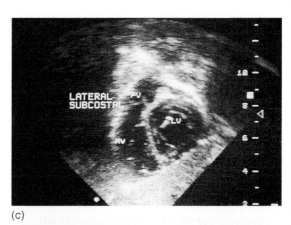

(c)

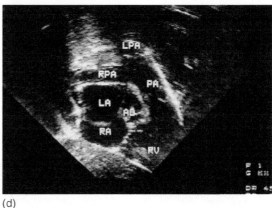

(d)

Fig. 8.2 (a) Subcostal four-chambered view showing the atria situated above the ventricles and slightly to the right side. There is a large interatrial septal defect and three of the four pulmonary veins are seen arrowed. Within the smooth-walled left ventricle the mitral valve inserts onto the free wall. Within the right ventricle the tricuspid valve inserts onto the septum. The attachment of the mitral ring is further away from the apex than that of the tricuspid ring.
(b) Apical four-chamber, plus aortic root view showing in addition a large subaortic VSD. AO, ascending aorta.
(c) A sagittal view subcostally of a normal heart showing a short-axis cut across the left ventricle and the equivalent cut through the right ventricle and main pulmonary artery. This is equivalent to a lateral angiogram. PV, pulmonary valve.
(d) A subcostal view equivalent to a right anterior oblique angiogram with the anterior part of the heart to the right and the posterior to the left. The whole of the right heart is seen and part of the interatrial septum and aortic root. AO, aorta; PA, pulmonary artery.

views, short-axis views and two oblique views which are equivalent to lateral and right anterior oblique angiography. These subcostal views allow the operator to assess the great veins and their atrial attachments, pulmonary venous drainage, the integrity of the interatrial septum, the atrioventricular junction, the inlet and trabecular ventricular septum and both outlets up to the bifurcation of the pulmonary arteries or the ascending aorta. The right ventricle may appear smaller in the subcostal four-chamber view, and the relative size of the two ventricles and their inlets is then best assessed from the apical four-chamber view.

Long-axis parasternal views delineate the outlets of the heart, the ventricular arterial connections, left atrial size and left ventriculo-function (Fig. 8.3). The previously mentioned family of parasternal short-axis views runs from low ventricular level to the ascending aorta and gives important diagnostic information about wall thickness, cavity dimension, ventricular function, coronary artery anatomy and the arterial duct (Fig. 1.4.6a–d). Finally the suprasternal approach merges in the infant with the high left parasternal view and delineates the arch and its branches better than at any other time of life (Fig. 8.4).

☞ *Practical Point*

- **A logical sequence of scanning approaches is subcostal, followed by apical, parasternal long-axis and short-axis, ductal and suprasternal arch views.**

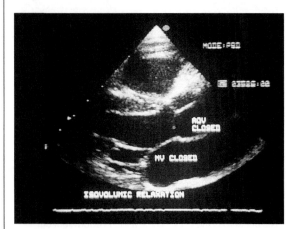

Fig. 8.3 A long-axis parasternal view showing the aorta to the right, left atrium posteriorly and the left ventricle to the left. The structures are shown in isovolumic relaxation with both aortic and mitral valves closed.

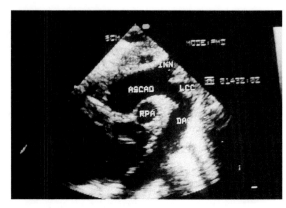

Fig. 8.4 A suprasternal scan in the plane of the arch of aorta. It shows the ascending aorta from the left side of the picture proceeding backwards before giving off the innominate and left common carotid arteries. The origin of the left subclavian is not well seen. The descending aorta is shown on the right of the picture descending inferiorly. ASCAO, ascending aorta; INN, innominate artery; LCC, left common carotid artery; DAO, descending aorta.

SEQUENTIAL CHAMBER LOCALIZATION

The underlying principle

An essential and helpful part of new cardiac anatomical nomenclature is 'sequential chamber localization'[2] Congenital heart disease often appears very complex to the non-cardiac eye. In part this is because of previously confusing names. Eponyms such as Eisemenger's syndrome do not indicate the underlying pathology. It may be a little long winded to say 'a VSD with pulmonary vascular disease', but at least everybody knows what you are talking about.

Latin is a dead language, beautiful in its own right and interesting, but 'Greek' to the average doctor or lay person! Even Latin words that you think you understand may mislead you. 'Solitus' doesn't mean solitary, for instance, but 'usual'. 'Inversus' doesn't mean mirror imaged, it means 'upside down'. It therefore makes a lot of sense to eschew Latin when naming parts of the body.

Paediatric cardiologists have for years used terms which infer underlying embryological bases for some of the malformations of the heart. 'Primitive ventricle' and 'endocardial cushion defect' have been used to describe congenital cardiac lesions as if these were truly the result of persistence of embryological structures – which they are not. Such terms are fortunately less frequent today and should be dropped from clinical use.

Instead congenital heart disease is characterized descriptively using anatomical and physiological terms in a sequential fashion. If you wish to build a safe house, you first consolidate the foundation before proceeding to the subsequent floors. Similarly, when you start to examine an infant with congenital heart disease, start at the venous inflow and the atria and work appropriately until you finish up at the great arteries.

Putting it into practice and establishing normality

An ideal sequence of scanning views and positions is described below with classical normal features to be *positively* identified. Notes on relevant aspects of congenital heart disease follow each section.

Transverse subcostal view

The liver and inferior vena cava (IVC) lie on the right of the spine (see Fig. 1.4.3), and the IVC drains into the right-sided atrium. The pulsatile aorta lies to the left and in front of the spine (see Fig. 8.5).

Notes The position and morphology of the atria are particularly important in complex cases. There are several alternatives. The atria may be morphologically normal and usually arranged – right atrium to the right, left atrium to the left; they

may be mirror imaged – right atrium to the left and left atrium to the right; or isomeric – two left atria or two right atria. The echocardiogram is unfortunately not reliable in deciding on the atrial arrangement, although some clues are obtained from the transverse subcostal view of the abdominal vessel (Fig. 8.5). If the atrium that receives the caval veins is on the right, then it is most likely to be an anatomical right atrium. Similarly if the atrium that is posterior receives the pulmonary veins, then it is most likely to be a left atrium. These are not totally reliable criteria. The appearances of the atrial appendages are the only totally reliable guide to differentiating and identifying the atria, but they are not well seen by transthoracic or subcostal echo.

Fortunately in clinical practice there is a simple alternative – the plain chest X-ray. The atria and lung always go together, thus a short bronchus on the right on the chest X-ray suggests a three-lobed right lung on that side with early branching, and a right atrium on the right. On the left, the bronchus is normally longer and bifurcates to supply a two-lobed lung (i.e. the morphological left atrium lies in the left). Mirror imaging of the lungs will give a long bronchus on the right and a short one on the left. Two long bronchi means two left lungs and two short bronchi means two right lungs – left atrial isomerism and right atrial isomerism, respectively (Fig. 8.6).

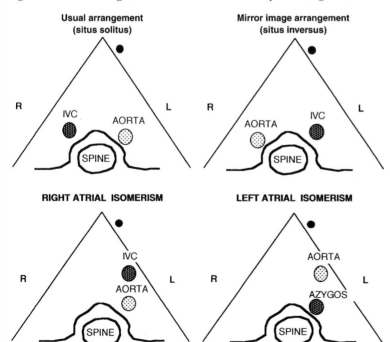

Fig. 8.5 Diagram of transverse section across the abdomen in the normal situation (situs solitus), and common abnormalities of situs.

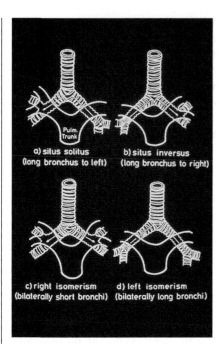

Fig. 8.6 Possible variations in bronchial and therefore pulmonary and atrial arrangements. (a) Usual arrangement with the atria and lungs on their proper sides. (b) Mirror imaging of normal with the right atrium and right lung on the left side and vice versa. The two isomeric options are shown in the lower diagrams (c,d).

Subcostal view of the atria and atrioventricular junctions

The superior vena cava (SVC) is seen to join the right atrium and the pulmonary veins drain into the left atrium. The atrial septum is intact, usually with a visible oval foramen, and is central, bowing to the left in infants with reduced pulmonary blood flow (such as persistent pulmonary hypertension of the newborn (PPHN) or anomalous pulmonary venous drainage), or to the right in infants with increased pulmonary blood flow (such as with a left-to-right ductal shunt). The atrioventricular valves lead to the ventricles which are on the patient's left.

Notes Whether the heart is in the right or left chest is obviously important, but mirror imaging of the heart's position is really quite rare in comparison with other congenital malformations. An isolated right heart is more likely to have congenital cardiac malformations than if a right-sided heart is part of overall mirror imaging of all organs (situs inversus). In the latter the incidence of congenital heart disease is the same as in the normal population.

Subcostal four-chamber view

Two atrioventricular valves are seen which open fully into their respective ventricles. The septal leaflet of the tricuspid valve arises from slightly lower down the septum than the mitral valve, and has some support apparatus arising from the ventricular septum. The right ventricle is further identified by having coarse trabeculations and a muscular band near the apex (known as the 'moderator band'). The left ventricle is smoother walled and has two papillary muscles supporting the mitral valve, and no support apparatus arises from the septum.

Notes Having identified the atria the atrioventricular junction is interrogated – using a combination of subcostal and apical views. The connection may be 'concordant' – right atrium to right ventricle and left atrium to left ventricle (Fig. 8.1a); 'discordant' – right atrium to left ventricle and left atrium to right ventricle; or 'univentricular' – both atria draining to one ventricle, either a double inlet left or right ventricle (Fig. 8.7). There is another form of univentricular connection where either the right or left connection is absent – mitral or tricuspid atresia ('absent left' or 'absent right AV-connection', respectively; see Fig. 8.8). In the presence of atrial isomerism, the atrioventricular connection is of necessity 'ambiguous' as it cannot be either truly concordant or discordant.

The subcostal and apical four-chamber views are best for looking at ventricular morphology, the next step in sequential localization. By convention, we talk about 'anatomical' or 'morphological' right and left ventricles. As already described, the right ventricle has heavy trabeculation, a moderator band across its apex, an infundibulum and a tricuspid valve which attaches directly to the septum and inserts more apically than the mitral valve (Fig. 8.2a,d). An anatomical section is shown in Figure 1.3.9. The left ventricle in contrast has finer trabeculations, no infundibulum and the mitral valve attached to two papillary muscles (usually, not always), but never attached to the septum (Figs 8.2 and 8.3). If there are two ventricles in the heart, then the tricuspid valve is always in the right

☞ *Practical Point*
- **The atrioventricular valve anatomy is the most reliable way to identify the ventricle.**

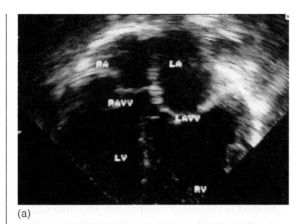

(a)

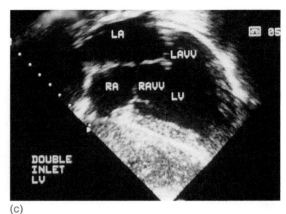

(c)

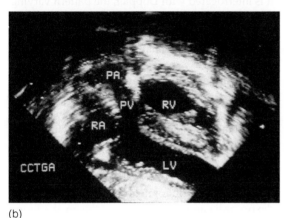

(b)

Fig. 8.7 (a) Atrioventricular discordance. The left ventricle is on the patient's right and the right ventricle on his left. The right atrium connects with the left ventricle and the left atrium with the right ventricle. The atrioventricular valve insertion on to the septum is reversed with the left-sided tricuspid valve lower than the right-sided mitral valves. RAVV, right atrioventricular valve; LAVV, left atrio ventricular valve.
(b) Subcostal cut from a patient with atrioventricular discord. The smooth-walled rather elongated left ventricular cavity is seen inferiorly and to the right and the chunky rough-walled right ventricle is seen superiorly and to the left. CCTGA, congenitally corrected transposition of the great artery.
(c) Echocardiogram from a patient with double inlet left ventricle-univentricular connection. Both atria discharge blood into the left ventricle.

ventricle and the mitral always in the left ventricle. The atrioventricular valve anatomy is therefore the most reliable guide to identifying the ventricle.

Rotated subcostal views to show the right and left ventricular outflow tracts

Rotating the probe anticlockwise generates a subcostal short-axis view. This is particularly good in assessing the RVOT, which is seen to be clear and unobstructed, and 'wrapping around' the central aortic valve with its three leaflets. Rotating in the opposite direction shows the LVOT, clear of obstruction and showing that the anterior leaflet of the mitral valve and the aortic valve are in continuity. Arising from the right ventricle is a large artery which bifurcates early, identifying it as the pulmonary artery. Arising from the left ventricle is a large artery which has no early branches and gently curves to form an arch; small coronary arteries may be seen arising from just above the valve. These features positively identify the aorta.

☞ *Practical Point*
- **The pulmonary artery is identified as a large artery which bifurcates early. The aorta has no early branches, gently curves to form an arch, and small coronary arteries are seen arising just above the valve**

Apical four-chamber view and 'five-chamber' or LV outlet view

The two ventricles are of roughly equal size, both reaching the apex of the heart. The atrioventricular valves are of roughly equal size and both open freely with unobstructed flow through them. The ventricular septum is intact.

Notes One or other of the ventricles may be small or even absent. Patients with double inlet left ventricle usually have a small anterior right ventricle connected to the main chamber by a VSD and leading to a great artery, frequently the aorta

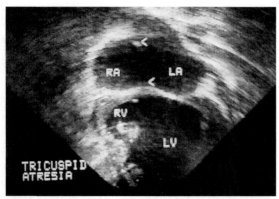

(a)

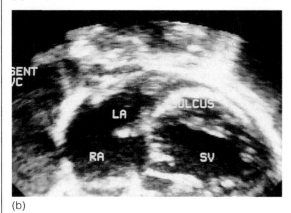

(b)

Fig. 8.8 (a) Echocardiogram from a patient with absent right atrioventricular correction or tricuspid atresia. There is a large interatrial communication (arrowed) between the right atrium and the hypoplastic right ventricle. A wedge of echo dense, fibrous sulcus tissue extends in towards the central fibrous body of the heart.
(b) Echo from a patient with absent left atrioventricular connection – mitral atresia. The dense sulcus tissue this time from the left side of the heart lies between the single ventricle and the left atrium. SV, single ventricle.

(Fig. 8.9). Very occasionally there are truly single ventricle hearts. Double inlet right ventricles with smaller posterior left ventricles are excessively rare.

Once the anatomy of the ventricles and the inflow portions is known, the scan switches to the outlet – the ventricular arterial connections. These can be 'concordant' – right ventricle to the pulmonary artery and left ventricle to the aorta; 'discordant' – right ventricle to aorta and left ventricle to pulmonary artery (also known as complete transposition (Fig. 8.10); or 'double outlet' from either right or left ventricle and 'single outlets' of the heart – pulmonary atresia, aortic atresia and common arterial trunk (Fig. 8.11).

Parasternal-long axis view
This view examines the left heart in more detail, the aortic valve and mitral valves opens fully.

Parasternal short-axis view
This view confirms the normal relationship of the great arteries with the pulmonary artery crossing in front of the aorta; they are not seen in parallel (typical for transposed great arteries). The pulmonary valve opens fully.

High left parasternal and suprasternal views
The duct is visualized and patency and flow within it is interrogated with Doppler, the pattern varying with postnatal age. The aortic arch is left-sided and there is no coarctation, confirmed with careful pulsed Doppler examination.

Identifying associated lesions
Having completed the diagnostic process thus far, it remains to identify the associated lesions such as ventricular septal defects, atrial septal defects and arterial valve stenosis.

At the end of the examination, findings are then described in order. For example, a subject with tricuspid atresia, abdominal situs solitus, dextrocardia and transposition of the great arteries would be described as: 'normal venous connections, normal visceral position, heart in the right chest, absent right AV-connection with atrioventricular concordance and ventriculoarterial discordance'. It can, of course, be long winded and unnecessarily

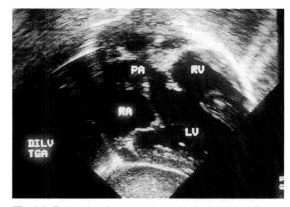

Fig. 8.9 Echo taken from a patient with double inlet left ventricle and transposition of the great arteries. The pulmonary artery arises from the left ventricle. The left ventricle communicates with a small right ventricle on the left shoulder of the ventricular mass. This small ventricle communicates with an aorta which is not seen in this picture.

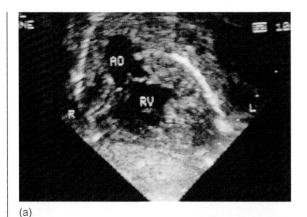

(a)

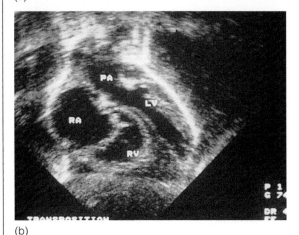

(b)

Fig. 8.10 (a) Subcostal view of the right ventricle in a case of transposition of the great arteries (ventriculoarterial discordance). The rough-walled heavily trabeculated right ventricle gives rise via the aortic valve to the ascending aorta. The right coronary artery can be seen arising from this vessel.
(b) Subcostal view of a patient with transposition of the great arteries – ventriculoarterial discordance. The smooth-walled left ventricle, which lies posteriorly, has an elliptical shape and curves up and forward to meet the pulmonary valve. The pulmonary artery bifurcates thereafter.

cumbersome to enumerate the normal connections in every child with a VSD! In practice such a heart is inferred to have normal connections unless stated and then the associated lesion is described.

Echocardiography is obviously only just part (all be it a vital part) of a diagnostic cascade which includes chest radiography, oximetry, MRI, etc. Catheterization used to be the final stop on this process and is occasionally still necessary. Angiography is still best for making pictures of the most distal structures, the pulmonary arteries,

aortopulmonary collateral connections and the aortic root branches and anomalies.

SUMMARY

Always use the same routine when doing an echocardiogram. Do not assume normality or make short-cuts to focus on one aspect. Positively and sequentially identify structures, their connections and position starting at the inlets and moving to the outlets. Use all of the echocardiographic windows. If in doubt, always seek advice.

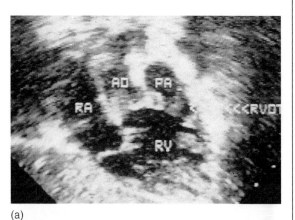

(a)

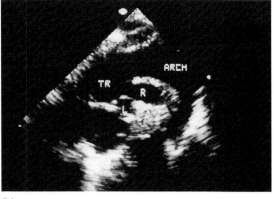

(b)

Fig. 8.11 (a) Subcostal right anterior oblique equivalent view from a patient with double outlet right ventricle and tetralogy of Fallot. The whole of the right heart is seen and between the aorta and the pulmonary artery lies the ventriculoinfundibular fold. There is heavy trabeculation and muscle development in the RVOT.
(b) High parasternal view of a patient with persistent common arterial trunk. The main pulmonary artery is short, comes off the back of the trunk and divides almost immediately into right and left pulmonary arteries. TR, arterial trunk; L, left; R, right.

The cyanosed newborn: excluding structural heart disease

**J Deane Waldman and
Gerard Holmes**

INTRODUCTION

Echocardiography has changed the practice of paediatric cardiology most profoundly in neonates with cyanotic heart disease. Cardiac catheterization is no longer essential for the diagnosis of complex lesions such as tricuspid atresia and an aortogram, often done previously through an umbilical artery, is no longer needed to assess the arterial duct. Instead the heart can be imaged using cross-sectional echocardiography, a colour map of the duct obtained, and the direction of flow through the duct can be assessed with pulsed or continuous wave (CW) Doppler. Whereas it was usual to take a neonate with transposed great arteries to the cardiac catheterization laboratory for balloon septostomy, now many centres do the procedure under echocardiographic guidance in the neonatal unit.

In assessing the cyanotic infant, the newcomer to echocardiography should bear in mind that experience and training are required to exclude congenital cyanotic heart disease reliably. Mistakes are easily made, and potentially fatal conditions (such as total anomalous pulmonary venous connection) can be missed even by experienced echocardiographers. Evaluation of the performance of the structurally normal heart in sick neonates can be learned relatively quickly, and neonatologists may see so much functional heart disease that experience and expertise can be adequately maintained. However, in the cyanotic infant, particularly the infant ventilated for apparent persistent pulmonary hypertension of the newborn (PPHN), experienced echocardiographic assessment is required if the aim of the study is to exclude structural heart disease.

An understanding of the echocardiographic approach to these patients is important for those learning echocardiography. The previous chapter has described a logical, sequential approach to each scan, starting from the subcostal position and identifying situs, vessels and chambers sequentially. This chapter describes characteristic echocardiographic features of some of the common cyanotic congenital heart diseases that might be encountered.

WHEN IS IT NECESSARY TO EXCLUDE CONGENITAL HEART DISEASE WITH ECHOCARDIOGRAPHY IN A CYANOTIC INFANT?

In cyanotic infants a thorough clinical approach to each infant should be carried out; echocardiography cannot and should not replace clinical acumen. The details of clinical, radiological and haematological assessment of the cyanosed infant, very familiar to the neonatologist, are beyond the scope of this book. In brief, cyanosis is most likely to be secondary to a 'cardiac' cause when:

1. the physical examination and chest X-ray suggest the absence of pulmonary disease;
2. haemoglobin level is normal;
3. arterial oxygen saturation is low; and
4. arterial pCO_2 is normal or decreased.

Under these circumstances referral to a paediatric cardiologist or experienced paediatric echocardiographer is mandatory. Infants with obstructed total anomalous pulmonary venous drainage can present with an identical clinical picture to that of PPHN. Without echocardiography, non-invasive differentiation of these two conditions is virtually impossible. For this reason, it is our view that all ventilated infants with hypoxaemia out of proportion to their lung disease should undergo expert echocardiographic review.*

CLASSIFICATION OF CYANOTIC CONGENITAL HEART DISEASE (CHD)

In physiological terms cyanotic CHD has classically been divided into three categories:

1. reduced pulmonary blood flow (due to obstruction, or absence of connection at some point in the right heart, i.e. at the tricuspid valve, pulmonary valve or pulmonary artery);
2. non-serial circulations (due to discordant connections, e.g. transposed great arteries or anomalous pulmonary venous connection);
3. common mixing lesions (e.g. common arterial trunk, single ventricle).

However, the echocardiographer must first think in terms of anatomy, building a mental three-

---

*When expert echocardiography is not available, the hyperoxygenation challenge still remains a useful screening tool to eliminate cyanotic heart disease as the cause of cyanosis, but only in the presence of adequate alveolar ventilation (normal or decreased pCO_2). It is also important to use an arterial pO_2 >200 mmHg as the threshold over which one can eliminate structural cyanotic heart disease. Below 200 mmHg, cyanotic heart disease is possible, especially in conditions with increased pulmonary blood flow.

dimensional picture of the heart starting from venous inflow and ending with arterial outflow, noting abdominal situs and orientation of the heart. The echocardiographic features of eight of the more common cyanotic congenital heart diseases are presented. Important embryological, anatomical or physiological features relevant to the echocardiographer are highlighted in each case.

TOTAL ANOMALOUS PULMONARY VENOUS CONNECTION (TAPVC)

Background

Pulmonary veins normally emerge from the primitive lung buds, grow medially and fuse posterior to the developing heart to form a chamber called the confluence of pulmonary veins (CPV). This CPV later fuses with the left atrium to 'incorporate' the pulmonary veins into the left heart (Fig. 9.1.1a). When the fusion of CPV and LA does not occur, the child has TAPVC. The CPV can connect to *any* systemic venous channel: the portal vein, the coronary sinus or RA directly, or, most commonly, to an ascending vertical vein (Fig. 9.1.1b)

that flows into the innominate vein.

Before echocardiography, TAPVC was the most elusive diagnosis in cyanotic newborns. The electrocardiogram (ECG) is non-specific, the patient often has no murmurs, the chest X-ray shows 'whited-out' lungs and the neonatologist had to guess between obstructed TAPVC, hyaline membrane disease and aspiration syndrome.

Echocardiography

The initial subcostal appearances are similar to those seen in PPHN; the dilated IVC and SVC connect normally to the right atrium and right ventricle, which are also dilated. Abdominal (and thoracic) situs is usually normal. The foramen flap bulges from right to left into an underfilled left atrium. However, the difference is that the pulmonary veins cannot be seen to drain normally into the back of the left atrium.

In the normal heart, a useful way to demonstrate all four pulmonary veins entering the left atrium is to move the transducer up an interspace or two from the parasternal short-axis view and angle inferiorly with some rotation of the transducer so as

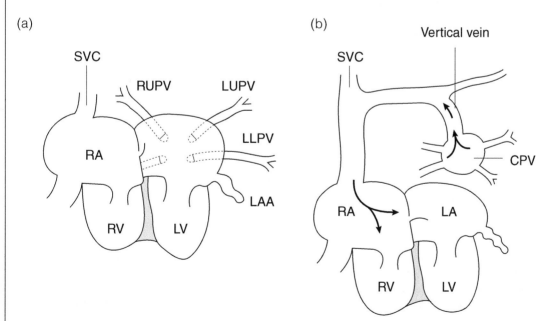

Fig. 9.1.1 Normal and abnormal development of pulmonary venous connections. (a) Normal anatomy is shown including all pulmonary veins connected and draining to the left atrium, a result of complete incorporation of the confluence of pulmonary veins *into* the left atrium. (b) TAPVC. Immediately posterior to the left atrium lies the CPV which receives all pulmonary venous blood and connects to the circulation via an ascending vertical vein, draining to the brachiocephalic anastomosis, which is in turn connected to the right superior vena cava (SVC). There is an obligatory RA to LA shunt.

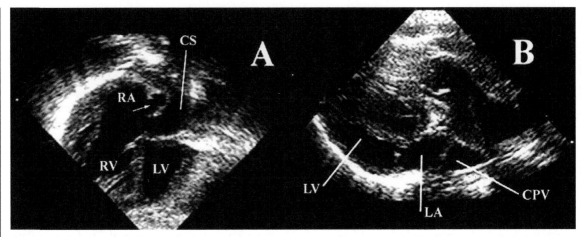

Fig. 9.1.2 Echocardiography in TAPVC. The hallmark of TAPVC is the demonstration of a chamber (usually dilated) behind the left atrium (LA) that receives all pulmonary venous effluent blood. (A) Modified four-chamber view shows a large coronary sinus (CS) which is dilated because it receives the CPV and drains into the right atrium (RA). Arrow shows the atrial septal defect (ASD) through which blood enters the left heart from the RA. (B) Long-axis view (perpendicular to (A)) shows an apparent 'subdivision' within the LA. The chamber which communicates with the mitral valve is the LA and the superior chamber is the CPV which empties into the coronary sinus.

to cut the right pulmonary artery in long axis. Such an echocardiogram is shown in Chapter 2.2 (Figures 2.2.3c and d). When the veins are not demonstrated to connect with the left atrium, however, much skill may be required to demonstrate where they do connect.

There are three basic aspects to the echocardiographic diagnosis of TAPVC:

1. demonstration of a separate chamber – called the confluence of pulmonary veins – behind the left atrium which receives the pulmonary veins and which does not connect with the left atrium (Fig. 9.1.2);
2. demonstration of the connection of the pulmonary venous confluence to systemic veins above, below or behind the heart;
3. evaluation of obstructions within these connections.

When the confluence of pulmonary veins connects superiorly to an anomalous vertical vein, it is described as 'supracardiac TAPVC'. When the CPV connects inferiorly to a descending vertical vein, the term 'infracardiac TAPVC' is used. When the connection is to the coronary sinus lying behind the left atrioventricular (A–V) groove or to the right atrium directly, the child has 'cardiac TAPVC'.

Once TAPVC is suspected, infants must be referred without delay to a cardiac surgical centre. Demonstration of the pulmonary venous confluence

and its connection to the systemic circulation may be a challenge echocardiographically (referral should never be delayed while this is being done!). In this respect colour flow mapping has proved invaluable by demonstrating flow in pulmonary veins, the venous confluence and the systemic venous connection when the structures themselves are not readily apparent by imaging alone. The procedure is to follow back from the pulmonary venous chamber, guided by the colour flow, by angulation and tilt of the probe. In supracardiac TAPVC (Fig. 9.1.1b), the vertical vein is usually large and can be followed upwards to the innominate vein. In infracardiac TAPVC, there is usually a large descending vein lying behind the heart, often best seen in saggital parasternal cuts. Areas of obstruction are seen as mosaic turbulence on colour, and acceleration can be detected using pulsed Doppler study. Infracardiac TAPVC is always obstructed because it connects to the portal vein and therefore the 'obstruction' in the system is the hepatic microcirculation; surgical correction should be done as an emergency in these patients.

The left atrium is usually small in TAPVC and it is routinely enlarged at surgical repair. Prior to repair, the only source of flow into the left atrium is through the atrial septum; therefore, demonstration of a left-to-right atrial shunt rules out TAPVC. The left ventricle is also underfilled and may give the impression of being hypoplastic. However,

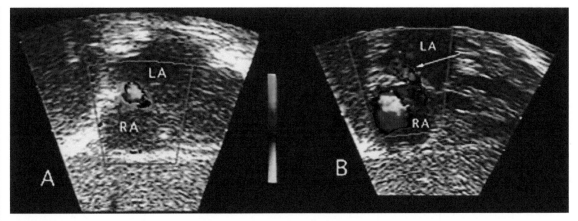

Fig. 9.1.3 Colour maps of atrial shunting. Direction and volume of shunting across the atrial septum is best seen in the subxiphoid view. This is important physiological information in all cyanosed neonates. (A) Red-coded flow is from left atrium to right atrium (see colour code bar) in a normal one-day-old neonate. The colour tends to exaggerate the size of the defect, best determined by 2D imaging rather than on a colour map. (B) Note blue-coded flow from right atrium to left atrium in a child with pulmonary atresia with intact ventricular septum. The flap of the septum primum (arrow) tissue is seen, held open by the flow induced by higher pressure in the right atrium than left atrium.

measurements of left ventricular length usually reveal that the ventricle is adequate to receive the pulmonary venous return after surgical correction. A truly hypoplastic left ventricle does not reach the apex of the heart, which is instead formed by the right ventricular apex.

☞ *Practical Point*
- **Demonstration of a significant left-to-right interatrial shunt on colour or pulsed Doppler interrogation eliminates the diagnosis of TAPVC, since the only source of blood into the LA in this condition is from the right atrium (see Fig. 9.1.3A).**

TRICUSPID ATRESIA

Background
This anomaly, has many anatomical and haemodynamic variations which produce widely different pathophysiological problems.

Systemic venous drainage and abdominal organ arrangement, examined from the subcostal position, are usually normal. There is always an atrial communication; without an ASD, tricuspid atresia is incompatible with survival. However, the ASD may be restrictive, in which case the caval veins will be dilated. The basic feature of tricuspid atresia – lack of a patent right atrium to right ventricle connection – is most easily demonstrated in the apical four-

chamber view, but may also be seen in other views that cut through the right ventricular inlet.

Each of the three key factors in the physiological variations of tricuspid atresia can be evaluated by echocardiography (Fig. 9.1.4):
1. adequacy of the interatrial communication;
2. size of the VSD and resultant size of the right ventricle;
3. ventriculoarterial connections.

Echocardiography
The interatrial shunt, seen best from the subcostal position, is usually large. Flow should be low velocity on pulsed Doppler interrogation, with deep coloured non-turbulent flow on colour mapping.

When the great arteries are normally connected and there is a small VSD (Fig. 9.1.4B), blood flows from RA–LA–LV. Most then goes to the aorta, and the remainder passes into the right ventricle through the small VSD. Restriction to flow to the lungs may be maximal at the VSD or at the right ventricular outflow tract, with reduced pulmonary blood flow and cyanosis as the main clinical features. When the VSD is small ('restrictive') the right ventricle is small as a result of reduced flow through VSD in utero. The degree of restriction to flow is established using a combination of subcostal and apical four-chamber views with superior angulation to take in the great arteries (Fig. 9.1.5); again colour Doppler is very helpful.

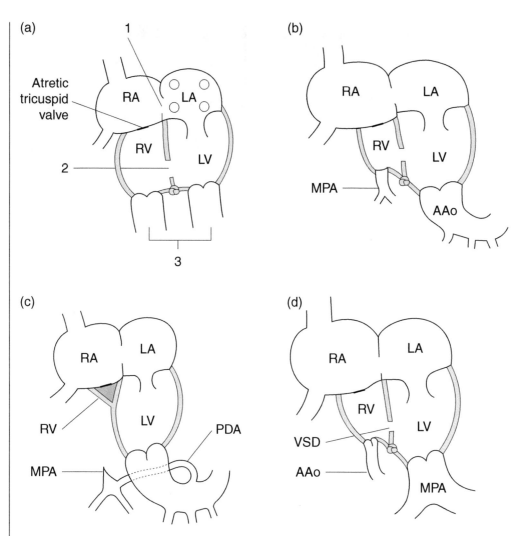

Fig. 9.1.4 Tricuspid atresia: anatomical variations and physiological implications. (a) The basic structural elements are identified with an atretic tricuspid valve and the three key anatomical–pathophysiological factors: (1) status of the ASD, (2) size of the VSD, and (3) great artery connections (normal or transposed). (b) A common form of triscupid atresia with a large ASD, small-to-moderate VSD resulting in a small RV and, with normally related great arteries, a small (stenotic) MPA. This patient is likely to have inadequate pulmonary blood flow and need a neonatal shunt. (c) When there is no VSD and normally related great arteries, the RV is absent and MPA is atretic; pulmonary blood flow is dependent on ductal patency. Such patients always need a systemic-to-pulmonary shunt. (d) A small VSD and transposition results in hypoplasia of the RV and aorta; effectively, this is hypoplastic left heart syndrome.

When the great arteries are transposed (discordant ventriculoarterial connection) in association with tricuspid atresia, the aorta arises from the RV and thus a restrictive VSD will cause subaortic rather than subpulmonary stenosis. As the main pulmonary artery arises from the LV, pulmonary arterial flow and pressure are high. These infants typically present somewhat later than those with restricted pulmonary blood flow, and have features of cardiac failure in association with moderate cyanosis.

When the VSD is large, the RV is large regardless of which great artery arises from the right ventricle.

☞ *Practical Point*
● **Only after one has determined the three anatomical factors separately – ASD, VSD and ventriculoarterial connection – can the physician develop a picture of how blood flows and what physiological adjustments are necessary.**

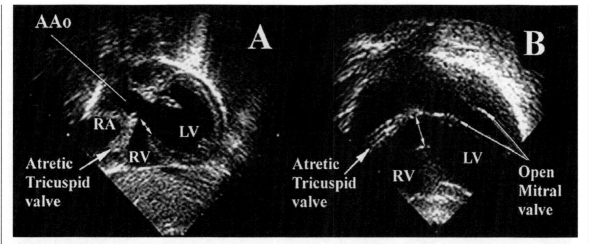

Fig. 9.1.5 Echocardiography in tricuspid atresia. Tricuspid atresia is confirmed echocardiographically by showing the non-patent tricuspid valve 'plate'; this structure can appear to move, but its non-patency must be confirmed by colour map. When there is tricuspid atresia and no VSD, there is no in utero flow to induce development of the right ventricle, which is therefore absent.
(A) When there is a small VSD (double-headed arrow), a small right ventricular cavity is seen.
(B) Although the tricuspid valve is atretic, as in (A), there is a large right ventricular cavity because of a large VSD (double-headed arrow). Note the mitral valve leaflets in open position.

PULMONARY ATRESIA WITH INTACT VENTRICULAR SEPTUM (PAIVS)

Background

This lesion has wide variability, from hearts with good right ventricular size and only an atretic pulmonary valve to those with a tiny round right ventricular cavity and a hypoplastic tricuspid valve. Both present with cyanosis early in the newborn period and depend on ductal flow for pulmonary perfusion. Most need a systemic-to-pulmonary shunt in the neonatal period to assure an adequate source of pulmonary blood flow. Some with a good ventricle are subsequently managed with either surgical or per-catheter pulmonary valve perforation. Those with a diminutive ventricle ('hypoplastic right heart') subsequently are left functionally with a single ventricle and will require a fontan-type operation (atriopulmonary or cavopulmonary connection).

Echocardiography

Abdominal and thoracic situs, systemic and pulmonary venous drainage are usually normal. There is always a right-to-left interatrial shunt because in tricuspid atresia, survival is not possible without an atrial septal defect. The hallmark features, seen on subcostal and apical four-chamber views, include a very thick-walled right ventricle usually with reduced cavity size (Fig. 9.1.6A) and hypoplasia of the tricuspid valve. Tricuspid regurgitation is usually evident from colour and pulsed Doppler study, and the high velocity indicates that right ventricular pressure is at or above systemic pressure (Fig. 9.1.6B). On colour map, there is no direct flow from the right ventricle to the pulmonary artery.

Retrograde flow in the main pulmonary artery is seen from flow through the duct. When the right ventricle and arterial duct are of good size it can be surprisingly difficult to be sure that there is no forward flow through the pulmonary valve; flow from the duct swirls around the pulmonary artery such that on pulsed Doppler interrogation beyond the valve some blood is clearly going forwards. An important difference from the infant with PPHN is that ductal flow is predominantly or entirely left-to-right. In contrast to pulmonary atresia with a VSD, the pulmonary arteries in PAIVS are almost always well formed.

After confirming that the arterial duct is large and unobstructed (and prostaglandin infusion is underway!), the critical features to be noted by echocardiography are:

1. nature of the ASD;
2. tricuspid valve size;
3. right ventricular cavity size;

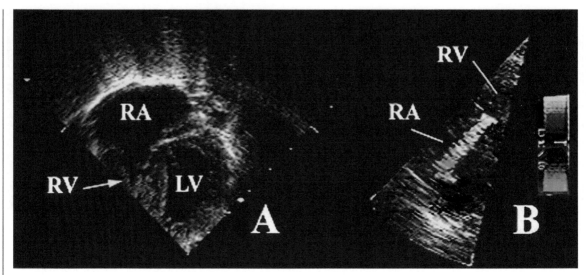

Fig. 9.1.6 Echocardiograph features of pulmonary atresia with intact ventricular septum.
(A) The four-chamber view shows a small right ventricular cavity crowded with muscle, a hypertrophied RV free wall and a small tricuspid valve (open). This view shows only part of the atrial septum.
(B) Colour map of the same image shows a mosaic-colour jet of tricuspid regurgitation in which Doppler interrogation would give a close estimate of RV pressure.

4. length of the atretic segment in the RV; and
5. side of the aortic arch.

All right heart blood volume must traverse the atrial septum; therefore, as with tricuspid atresia, an inadequate ASD causes dilated caval veins and restricts left heart filling, which may lead to low output cardiac failure.

The size of the tricuspid orifice determines right ventricular growth in utero. Judging whether the right ventricle is big enough to support all pulmonary blood flow can be difficult in borderline cases, and it is useful to refer to a table of normal values, indexed to body surface area. Many recent articles link surgical success and survival to size of the tricuspid valve, measured in the four-chamber view. Attempts to quantify right ventricular size directly have met with only limited success; tricuspid valve Z-score value has proved more reliable. Other surgically useful pieces of information are the length of atresia (an easily resectable membrane versus a long segment of fibromuscular obstruction) and the side of the aortic arch, as virtually all of these patients will require a systemic-to-pulmonary shunt. The arterial duct should be reviewed during prostaglandin infusion to assure wide, unrestrictive patency until surgery.

Some hearts with PAIVS have anomalous channels connecting the RV to the coronary artery(ies); this delivers de-oxygenated blood to the coronary circulation in systole and steals oxygenated blood from the coronaries during diastole. RV-to-coronary connections are a critical factor which *cannot* be assessed accurately by present-day echocardiography. When such connections are in the differential diagnosis, cardiac catheterization and selective angiography are required.

☞ *Practical Point*
- **In both tricuspid atresia and PAIVS, restriction to flow across the atrial septal defect may significantly reduce cardiac output; an important echocardiographic sign of this is distension of the right atrium and the caval veins.**

EBSTEIN'S ANOMALY

Background
This is a right heart anomaly characterized by downward displacement of the tricuspid valve leaflets, which may be plastered down to the internal wall of the right ventricle. There is usually an associated atrial septal defect through which there is right-to-left shunting due to several pathophysiological mechanisms.

1. The tricuspid valve itself is regurgitant due to malformation, raising right atrial pressure.
2. There is an 'atrialized' portion of the right ventricle, that is, an area which contracts with the ventricle but is in free communication with the atrium producing a back and forth flow pattern which impedes forward flow through the right heart.
3. The right ventricular cavity itself can be quite small, further restricting forward flow.

There is a broad spectrum of severity from intrauterine death to an almost incidental finding on echocardiography in older children. Infants with Ebstein's anomaly who present with cyanosis in the newborn period usually have severe disease and the prognosis is generally poor.

Echocardiography
The caval veins and right atrium are dilated on subcostal imaging, but pulmonary venous drainage and abdominal situs are normal and the heart is in the left chest. Right-to-left interatrial flow is apparent. Four-chamber views reveal that the tricuspid valve arises from lower down the septum than normally such that the usual small offset of the mitral and tricuspid valves is greatly exaggerated. The area between the true tricuspid anulus (corresponding to the A-V groove), and the coaptation plane of the tricuspid valve leaflets is the 'atrialised right ventricle' (Fig. 9.1.7). There is often

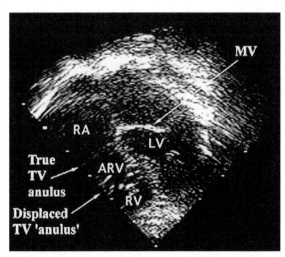

Fig. 9.1.7 Ebstein's anomaly of the tricuspid valve. The tricuspid valve leaflets are displaced downward into the RV cavity. The area between the true anulus and the tricuspid leaflets contracts with the ventricle but communicates with the atrium; this is called the 'atrialised RV'. Note the reduced volume of the remaining 'true' RV.

torrential tricuspid regurgitation, although after the first day or two of life the peak velocity is typically not very high since right ventricular pressure is not elevated unless there is coincident PPHN.

Size of the true right ventricle and status of the pulmonary outflow area, which can be obstructed by the dysplastic valve, must be carefully imaged. Parasternal or subcostal short-axis views are useful in this regard.

TETRALOGY OF FALLOT (ToF)

Background
The four originally described features of ToF were:

1. ventricular septal defect;
2. subpulmonary obstruction;
3. aorta overriding the ventricular septum;
4. right ventricular hypertrophy.

These four components are however the result of a single embryological defect: failure of expansion of the subpulmonary conus. (Compare (a) and (c) in Fig. 9.1.8.) Within ToF there are many variations:

- degree of subpulmonary (conal) obstruction
- size, patency and presence of the pulmonary valve
- size of the pulmonary arteries
- collateral sources of pulmonary blood flow.

There may also be additional VSDs, ASDs and, rarely, mitral stenosis. When ToF presents with cyanosis in the neonatal period, there is severe subpulmonary obstruction or even atresia. This encourages intracardiac right-to-left shunting through the VSD and into the overriding aorta. With severe subpulmonary obstruction or atresia, pulmonary blood flow is dependent on ductal flow.

Echocardiography
Systemic and pulmonary venous drainage are normal; neither atrium is dilated. There may be an ASD. Both A-V valves and their offset at the septum appear normal. The four-chamber views may reveal no abnormalities in ToF because the overriding aorta, the malalignment VSD (Fig. 9.1.9A), and the subpulmonary obstruction are located anteriorly to the plane of examination. Parasternal long-axis imaging demonstrates the large unrestrictive VSD and the aortic override (Fig. 9.1.9B), but will not profile the subpulmonary region or the pulmonary valve. Thus, from this view alone, the distinction

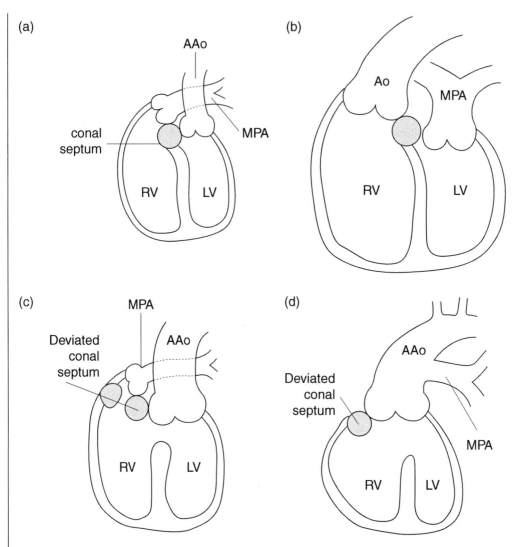

Fig. 9.1.8 Cono-truncal malformations. (a) Normal: lateral view of normal heart showing relationships and location of conal 'infundibular' septum. (b) TGA: great arteries are transposed (aorta from RV and MPA from LV); the conal septum is still in normal position. (c) ToF: deviation of the septum causes the VSD and obstructs the RV outflow tract causing hypoplasia of the MPA. (d) Truncus arteriosus: the VSD is similar to that seen in ToF but there is no MPA; the pulmonary arteries arise from the single arterial trunk.

between ToF, ToF with pulmonary atresia and common arterial trunk cannot be made. The parasternal short-axis view shows the subpulmonary region, pulmonary valve and pulmonary arteries well (Fig. 9.1.9A). Perhaps the best and most inclusive view for demonstration of anatomical features in ToF in the neonate is the subcostal short-axis view through the RVOT (see Fig. 8.11a, p. 179).

Once the diagnosis of ToF is established, the degree of subpulmonary obstruction and pulmonary valvar obstruction should be investigated using

☞ *Practical Point*

● **Four-chamber views are typically normal in ToF because the overriding aorta, the VSD and the subpulmonary obstruction are located anteriorly to the plane of examination.**

colour flow mapping and CW Doppler, as should the contribution of flow through the arterial duct to total pulmonary flow.

Additional anatomical details gleaned from echocardiographic examination in ToF are:

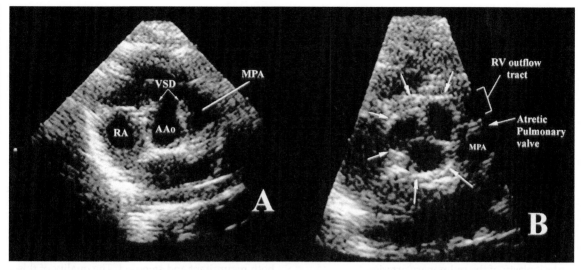

Fig. 9.1.9 Echocardiology in ToF. ToF is characterized by a large, malalignment VSD, and subpulmonary obstruction. In a cyanosed neonate, the obstruction is often complete, i.e. pulmonary atresia. Generally, the more severe the right ventricular outflow obstruction, the more hypoplastic and underdeveloped is the pulmonary artery system and main pulmonary artery. (A) Short-axis view shows the great arteries in normal relationship (crossing) with a large, anterior, 'malalignment' VSD. RA = right atrium, AAo, ascending aorta. (B) ToF with pulmonary atresia: the right ventricular outflow tract is crowded but patent, and there is a very large trileaflet aortic valve, circled by arrows.

- additional defects of the ventricular septum;
- side of the aortic arch; and
- coronary artery origins.

These features are pertinent to shunt surgery or repair.

☞ *Practical Point*
- **Since right and left ventricular pressures are equal in ToF due to the unrestrictive subaortic VSD, other VSDs are less easy to localize with colour Doppler; the ventricular septum must be examined very carefully and thoroughly.**

ToF WITH ABSENT PULMONARY VALVE

Background
Tetralogy with an absent pulmonary valve has the large, unrestrictive VSD and overriding aorta of typical ToF, but there is no subpulmonary obstruction. Instead stenosis is limited to the pulmonary valve anulus where, plastered to the valve ring in place of valve leaflets, there are nubbins of tissue causing stenosis during systole and allowing free pulmonary regurgitation during diastole. In utero, this produces progressive, usually massive, dilatation of the pulmonary arteries (see Fig. 9.1.10) and right ventricle.

After birth, the dilated pulmonary arteries compress and obstruct the bronchi, resulting in respiratory failure and cyanosis. The degree of compression is variable from mild (tachypnoea alone) to severe, where immediate intubation is necessary. The diagnosis can be strongly suspected before echocardiography: the newborn is cyanosed

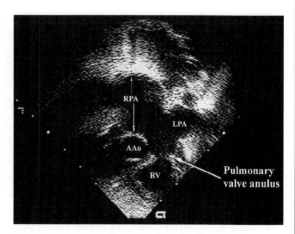

Fig. 9.1.10 Echocardiogram in ToF with absent pulmonary valve syndrome. Subcostal approach angulated superiorly from the four-chamber view demonstrates a stenotic pulmonary anulus with no evident leaflets and massive dilatation of the branch pulmonary arteries (compare with the ascending aorta) which compress the bronchi bilaterally. This patient had cyanosis due to upper airway obstruction.

with respiratory distress, has CO_2 retention and a classic to-and-fro cardiac murmur at the left sternal edge. The chest X-ray shows hyperinflation with greatly enlarged pulmonary arteries.

Echocardiography

On echocardiography the aorta and left ventricle seem underdeveloped compared with the right heart structures, but their size is usually normal in absolute terms. The parasternal and subcostal short-axis views usually demonstrate the anatomy of the pulmonary arteries well.

Operation is deferred if clinically possible because operative risk is inversely proportional to patient size. Repair involves VSD closure, insertion of a bioprosthetic pulmonary valve and reduction arterioplasty of the pulmonary arteries.

COMMON ARTERIAL TRUNK

Background

The common arterial trunk (previously known as truncus arteriosus) is a single central artery arising from the base of the heart giving rise to all *three* circulations – systemic, pulmonary and coronary – and is always associated with a large subarterial VSD. Presentation varies from acyanotic congestive heart failure (with torrential pulmonary blood flow) to severe cyanosis with small branch pulmonary arteries restricting pulmonary blood flow.

Echocardiography

Venous drainage and situs are usually normal, and (as in ToF) the four-chamber views are also typically normal. However, tilting anteriorly from the four-chamber views, a single large artery is seen to leave the heart (Fig. 9.1.11A), overriding a large malalignments VSD. This appearance is similar to ToF with pulmonary atresia. However, the truncal valve in the short-axis view often has more than three leaflets which are usually thickened with rolled edges. Furthermore, the pulmonary artery or arteries are often large and arise from the side of the large common trunk (see Fig. 9.1.8D).

Colour and other Doppler studies carried out from four-chamber, long-axis and suprasternal views often reveal that the truncal valve may be both regurgitant and stenosed. The quality of this valve is crucial in terms of outcome.

Commonly associated lesions which need to be excluded are:

1. interrupted aortic arch
2. truncal valve stenosis or regurgutation
3. mitral stenosis
4. additional VSDs.

The most important anatomical detail is the take-off of the pulmonary artery or arteries from the common trunk. The best views for this are the long-axis parasternal and subcostal four-chamber plus great artery view (Fig. 9.1.11B).

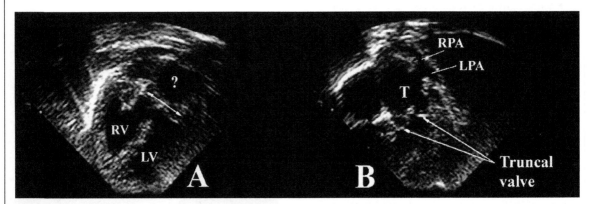

Fig. 9.1.11 Echocardiography in common arterial trunk. It is often difficult to distinguish common arterial trunk (truncus arteriosus) from (ToF) with pulmonary atresia. The diagnostic feature of the former is demonstration of the pulmonary arteries arising from the trunk. It is important to remember, however, that inability to demonstrate the pulmonary arteries does not necessarily mean they are absent. Generally, the arterial duct is absent in common arterial trunk and usually present in tetralogy with pulmonary atresia.
(A) A large dilated artery is seen arising from the base of the heart, shared by both ventricles. From this subcostal view, one cannot differentiate common arterial trunk from ToF.
(B) Gradually angulating the transducer, one sees both pulmonary arteries arising from the common trunk, establishing the diagnosis.

TRANSPOSITION OF THE GREAT ARTERIES

Background

Transposition of the great arteries (TGA) is, by definition, where the aorta arises from the morphological right ventricle and the pulmonary artery arises from the morphological left ventricle. The spatial relationship of the great arteries to each other can vary considerably (compare (A) and (B) in Fig. 9.1.8) but they are never related as in the normal heart where the pulmonary artery crosses in front of the aorta. Transposition can occur in the setting of A-V concordance (right atrium connected to right ventricle, left atrium to left ventricle) or A-V discordance (right atrium connected to left ventricle, left atrium to right ventricle). In the case of concordant A-V connections, transposition is always associated with cyanosis. TGA with discordant A-V connections, also termed 'physiologically or congenitally corrected TGA', is usually not associated with cyanosis, presents later in life, and will not be discussed here further.

Echocardiography

Venous return, situs and the four-chamber views are typically normal, with interatrial flow through a patent oval foramen or ASD. The right atrium leads into the morphological right ventricle (positively identified by the lower septal insertion of the tricuspid valve, with its septal attachments and the moderator band at the apex) and the left atrium leads to the morphological left ventricle, readily identified by the two equal-sized papillary muscles arising from the free wall. However, tilting up from the apical views the vessel arising from the morphological left ventricle bifurcates immediately, defining it as the pulmonary artery (see Fig. 9.2.3). The vessel that arises from the morphological right ventricle gives rise to the head and neck arteries, does not bifurcate, and has the origins of the coronary arteries at its base, identifying it as the aorta.

An important and easily recognizable feature of TGA is the demonstration from the parasternal long- and short-axis views that the great arteries lie parallel to each other, typically with the aorta anteriorly (Fig. 9.1.12). It is never possible to obtain such an image from any projection in a normal heart because of the normal cross-over relationship of these arteries.

After establishing the diagnosis of TGA (A-V concordance with ventriculoarterial discordance), the echocardiographic focus shifts to the assessment

> ☞ Practical Point
> - A characteristic and easily recognizable feature of TGA is the parallel relationship of the great arteries seen from parasternal views.

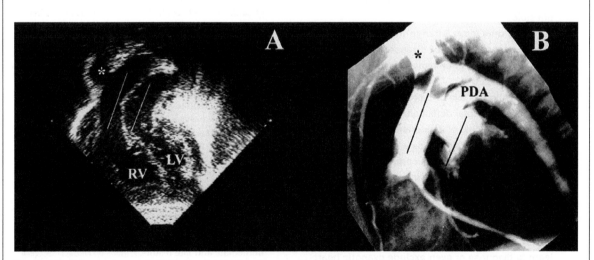

Fig. 9.1.12 Echo-angio correlation in the diagnosis of transposition of the great arteries. The pathognomonic feature of transposition of the great arteries is the presence of parallel, rather than crossing, great arteries arising from the base of the heart. This is best seen in subcostal view. (A) Two parallel, curvilinear vessels arise from the ventricles. One can see a brachiocephalic vessel (*) originating from the anterior great artery, which is thus identified as aorta. (B) Ascending aortography in a neonate with TGA opacifies the main pulmonary artery via a patent ductus arteriosus. Note the parallel relationship of the two proximal great arteries, similar to the image on echocardiogram in (A).

☞ *Practical Point*

- In TGA, adequate mixing at the arterial level is needed regardless of the presence of an arterial duct; if the atrial defect is restrictive, urgent intervention such as atrial balloon septostomy is required.

of associated conditions. Oxygenation is dependent on the mixing of blood between two parallel circuits. This mixing can occur at atrial or ventricular levels and can be assessed by colour flow mapping and conventional Doppler. In the absence of a VSD, adequate mixing at the atrial level is needed regardless of the presence of a patent arterial duct. If the ASD is restrictive, systemic arterial oxygenation is likely to be marginal, and an immediate balloon septostomy is indicated.

☞ *Practical Points*

- Always positively and thoroughly identify structures as you scan from inflow to outflow – failure to see the pulmonary veins or pulmonary arteries, for example, may mean they are genuinely not there (and not just that you are having a bad scanning day!).
- Always check the direction and velocity of flow through the atrial septum and the arterial duct as this gives important information about physiology.
- When the duct looks 'strange' in a baby with cyanotic congenital heart disease, it may be a collateral or other anomalous vessel rather than the arterial duct.
- When a child has two or more anomalies, e.g. complete A-V septal defect plus TAPVC, a complex syndrome of isomerism is more likely (such as 'asplenia' syndrome with right atrial isomerism) than in the less complex cases. In these cases it is especially important to be sure of abdominal situs, and it is worth checking with ultrasound (and blood film) for the presence of a spleen.
- Finally, and most importantly, do not expect to learn to diagnose or even exclude cyanotic heart disease quickly. It takes training, time and continued practice, and in these patients a missed or delayed diagnosis can have serious consequences.

Defects in the ventricular septum – number, size, location and flow – should be assessed. All four valves should also be interrogated by colour flow and conventional Doppler for evidence of obstruction and/or regurgitation. The pulmonary valve will become the neo-aortic valve after the arterial switch operation and thus stenosis in this location will translate to aortic stenosis after repair. Subpulmonary obstruction, which can occur with and without a VSD, should also be identified.

Although many cardiologists assess the coronary arteries by echo (usually best seen with modifications of the parasternal short-axis view cutting through the base of the aorta), only the proximal portions may be well imaged. Virtually all variations of coronary distribution can be surgically relocated to the neo-aorta and, therefore, cine-aortography is usually not necessary.

FURTHER READING

There are literally thousands of articles published on various echocardiographic features of the different cyanotic congenital heart defects; these are of limited interest to neonatologists. To conserve space, they are not included. The articles listed below were chosen either for their conceptual significance or to provide useful clinical or haemodynamic information. In square brackets [ ] are editorial comments citing the significance or utility of each work.

Cetta F, Feldt RH, Facc PW et al. Improved early morbidity and mortality after Fontan operation: the Mayo Clinic experience, 1987 to 1992. *Journal of the American College of Cardiology* 1996;28(2):480–486. [This article is cited to provide neonatologists with long-term follow-up on children with very complex hearts defects (single ventricle, asplenia, etc.) who had Fontan procedures. It is encouraging, especially given that 25 years ago, there was no long-term future for these children.]

DeLisle G, Ando M, Calder AL et al. Total anomalous pulmonary venous connection: Report of 93 autopsied cases with emphasis on diagnostic and surgical considerations. *American Heart Journal* 1976;91:99–122. [This article, first-authored by DeLisle, came from the Praaghs' Registry and is the defining work on TAPVC. It, like the one on ToF by the same team, is a 'must' read. Also make sure it is viewed in an original rather than a xerox copy as the pictures are very important.]

Donahoo JS, Gardner TJ, Zahka K et al. Systemic-pulmonary shunts in neonates and infants using microporous expanded polytetrafluoro-ethylene: immediate and late results. *Annals of Thoracic Surgery* 1980;30(2):146–150. [There are numerous articles on systemic-to-pulmonary shunts each touting the variant practised at that institution. Most centres favour the 'modified Blalock–Taussig' shunt which is a side-to-side connection using a goretex (3.5 or 4 mm) tube graft between the subclavian artery and the ipsilateral branch pulmonary artery. The article cited here has nice drawings of both a central shunt (AAo-MPA using goretex) and the modified B–T shunt; both shunts avoid distortion of the pulmonary artery and are easy to take down.]

Fontan F, Baudet E. Repair of tricuspid atresia. *Thorax* 1971;26:240–248. [This is the original article describing the Fontan procedure. Note that it is only 25 years old; before then, there was no reparative operation for single ventricle. The original concept – using the atrium as a pump – has been modified to use the atrium solely as a conduit and valves are no longer inserted. Nonetheless, this was another seminal work for congenital heart patients. It must also be remembered that low pulmonary artery pressure is the key survival factor; preparations to achieve or maintain low pulmonary resistance start in the newborn nursery.]

Freedom RM. *Pulmonary Atresia with Intact Ventricular Septum*. New York: Futura, 1989. [This book summarizes the body of knowledge on the title material including emphasis on the coronary arterial abnormalities and their implications. The pictures are very well done and quite illustrative.]

Hanley FL, Sade RM, Freedon RM, Blackstone EH, Kirklin JW. Outcomes in critically ill neonates with pulmonary stenosis and intact ventricular septum: a multiinstitutional study. *Journal of the American College of Cardiology* 1993;22:183–192. [The nomogram in this article gives the indexed values for the tricuspid valve anulus which is the critical measurement for determining whether a child is suitable for a three-chamber or four-chamber repair eventually.]

Lakier JB, Stanger P, Heymann M *et al.* Tetralogy of Fallot with absent pulmonary valve. *Circulation* 1974;50:167–174. [This general article nicely explains the haemodynamics and summarizes the clinical problems associated with ToFsPV.]

Mavroudis C, Backer CL. *Cardiac Surgery*, vol 5/1: *The Arterial Switch Operation*. Philadelphia: Hanley & Belfus, 1991. [Children's Memorial Hospital in Chicago has had a compelling interest in TGA – physiology, diagnosis and repair – for over 30 years. Indeed, the original concept for arterial switch was suggested by Dr FS Idriss from that institution in 1961. This book is an excellent summary of the repair of TGA in neonates.]

Rao PS. *Tricuspid Atresia*. New York: Futura, 1992. [A well written and very well illustrated book on tricuspid atresia. Although surgical knowledge has advanced, this still is an excellent summary and 'place-to-start'.]

Van Praagh R, Van Praagh S, Nebesar RA *et al.* Tetralogy of Fallot: underdevelopment of the pulmonary infundibulum and its sequelae. *American Journal of Cardiology* 1970;26:2533. [This is the seminal article on ToF unifying the tetrad into a single understandable construct.]

Yagihara T, Yamamoto F, Nishigaki K *et al.* Unifocalization for pulmonary atresia with ventricular septal defect and major aortopulmonary collateral arteries. *Journal of Thoracic and Cardiovascular Surgery* 1996;112:392–402 [This recent article is representative of the thinking regarding *construction* of pulmonary arteries and recruitment of collaterals in the most severe form of ToF.]

The cyanosed newborn: evaluating the infant with non-structural heart disease

Jon Skinner

INTRODUCTION

After congenital heart disease has been excluded, echocardiography has an important role in haemodynamic assessment during the management of hypoxaemic infants. No two hypoxaemic infants have the same cardiopulmonary haemodynamics, and these change with time.[1] Most infants have a combination of intracardiac and intrapulmonary shunting, and the relative importance of each can change with time.[2] Some profoundly hypoxaemic infants with a normal Pa,CO_2 have evidence of normal or high pulmonary blood flow,[2,3] and all the right-to-left shunting occurs within the lungs. Many of the larger infants with intracardiac shunting have a closed or small arterial duct. The major site of shunting is then the oval foramen. In some infants elevated pulmonary vascular resistance is less of a problem than poor right ventricular function, and these infants clearly need inotropic support. Only echocardiography can assess all these factors. The neonatologist can use echocardiography serially in such patients to determine and evaluate appropriate therapy, obtaining as much information as possible from each echocardiogram rather than measuring one parameter alone.

At present there is no reliable non-invasive way of assessing pulmonary vascular resistance, and the same is true of central venous pressure (CVP).* Echocardiography can roughly assess ventricular filling, ventricular function, and more precisely ventricular output and pulmonary arterial (PA) pressure. Pulmonary blood flow can be assessed by measuring right ventricular output if the arterial duct is closed. If the duct is patent, pulmonary blood flow is assessed by:

1. measuring alterations from normal in left ventricular output (which depends mostly on pulmonary venous return);

---

*A recent study in adults[4] related various echocardiographic measurements to invasive measurements of CVP. They found that the degree of inferior vena cava (IVC) collapse recorded during a phase of positive pressure respiration correlated with mean CVP. A ratio of the smallest to the widest IVC diameter of less than 1:3 signified a low CVP, and greater than 2:3 a high CVP. In the hepatic veins the ratio of forward flow velocity during systole and diastole correlated closely with CVP (r = −0.85); the systolic velocity decreases as CVP increases. A systolic : diastolic flow velocity ratio of 0.25:1 and of 1.5:1 correlated with a CVP of 15–20 mmHg, and 2–10 mmHg, respectively.

2. studying flow velocity in the origin of the branch pulmonary arteries; and
3. assessing left atrial dimension in relation to the aortic root.

A recent study[3] has shown that the haemodynamic feature most linked to outcome in persistent pulmonary hypertension of the newborn (PPHN) is left ventricular output; a value less than 100 ml/kg/min or a stroke volume of less than 1 ml/kg at presentation indicates an infant at very high risk of mortality. No index of PA pressure was closely linked to severity, but persistent pure right-to-left shunting is known to be an ominous sign.[5]

☞ *Practical Point*

- **Pulmonary blood flow is assessed by measuring left ventricular output, flow velocity at the origin of the branch pulmonary arteries and assessing left atrial dimension in relation to the aortic root. If the arterial duct is closed, right ventricular output also reflects pulmonary blood flow.**

WHAT TO LOOK FOR IN THE HYPOXAEMIC INFANT

Each scan begins from the subcostal position as usual.

1. A transverse upper abdominal cut through the IVC is a useful start to the study. With adequate central venous filling, the IVC is distended and does not completely collapse at any stage. Inadequate filling is characterized by periodic collapse of the IVC in relation to inspiration on positive pressure ventilation. Most infants with PPHN need a reasonably high right ventricular filling pressure, and while IVC collapse is a useful sign of hypovolaemia it is a rather late one and most such infants require continuous CVP monitoring anyway.* The site of the pressure line can be assessed echocardiographically. Overdistension of the IVC and hepatic veins is consistent with right ventricular failure.

2. The subcostal and apical four-chamber views classically demonstrate right atrial and right ventricular enlargement, with the atrial septum bulging over to the left (see Figs 9.2.1 and 9.2.2). Note the similarity to the appearance in a baby with transposed great arteries (Fig. 9.2.3). During

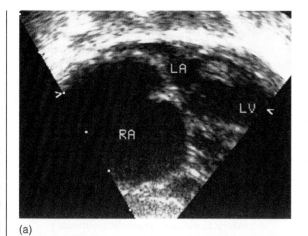

(a)

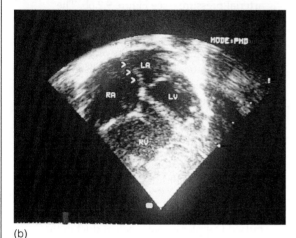

(b)

Fig. 9.2.1 (a) Subcostal view showing a dilated right atrium and atrial septum bulging to the left. The left atrium is underfilled.
(b) This four-chamber view (half-way between an apical and subcostal view) shows that the dilatation also involves the right ventricle. Arrows indicate atrial bulging as in (a).

recovery the septum becomes more central. Colour Doppler demonstrates tricuspid or mitral regurgitation and right-to-left flow across the oval foramen. During recovery, the duration of right-to-left shunting assessed by pulsed Doppler at the oval foramen decreases (see Fig. 3.10). Measurement of peak velocity of tricuspid regurgitation (present in 60–70% of the infants) confirms high pulmonary arterial pressure. If the

☞ *Practical Point*

● **If the heart becomes more difficult to visualize and/or is laterally displaced, consider pneumothorax**

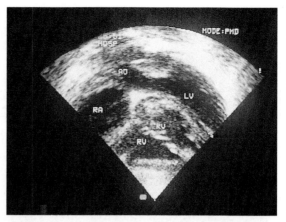

Fig. 9.2.2 Tilting forward from the four-chamber view (Fig. 9.2.1b) shows that the right ventricle is so tense and dilated that it begins to cause narrowing of the left ventricular outflow.

heart is laterally displaced and/or difficult to image, consider recent pneumothorax.[6]
3. The parasternal long-axis view typically shows an enlarged right ventricle anteriorly, and the posterior left ventricle appears underfilled and 'squashed' (Fig. 9.2.4). The left atrium is underfilled and even slit-like. The LA:Ao ratio may be less than 0.5:1, unless there is severe mitral regurgitation, which can occur after severe birth asphyxia or with myocardial ischaemia. The aortic root is measured for later left ventricular output measurement. M-mode assessment typically reveals preserved left ventricular function, although accurate assessment is difficult owing to right ventricular dominance. The septum often moves more with

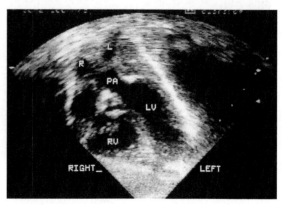

Fig. 9.2.3 A remarkably similar appearance to Figure 9.2.2, but this patient has transposed great arteries. The great artery arising from the left ventricle bifurcates early, and is therefore the pulmonary trunk.

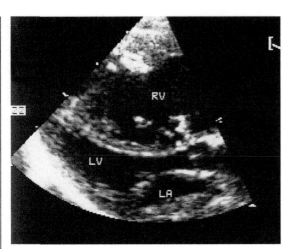

Fig. 9.2.4 In this parasternal long-axis view, the right ventricle is clearly larger than the left ventricle, and both the left atrium and ventricle appear underfilled.

the right ventricle than the left (paradoxical septal motion). Prolonged left ventricular pre-ejection period (LPEP) measured from the Q wave to the opening of the aortic valve may indicate left ventricular dysfunction (LPEP/LVET >0.40).[7,8] Look for marked septal hypertrophy and LVOT obstruction in the macrosomic babies of diabetic mothers; these babies deteriorate with inotropes and cardiac output may improve with β-blockade.

4. Parasternal short-axis views (or long-axis tilted over to the infant's left) reveal the typically

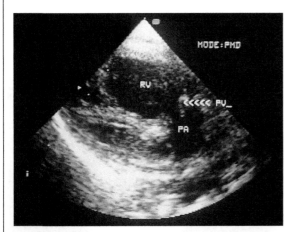

Fig. 9.2.5 Tilting across to the pulmonary artery from the standard long-axis view, the RV outflow is very large, as is the main pulmonary artery. The arrowed pulmonary valve (PV) did not open fully owing to the extremely low RV output. (This appearance is suspicious of pulmonary stenosis, but the movement resolved as the cardiac output improved.)

enlarged main pulmonary artery (Fig. 9.2.5). Pulsed Doppler measurement at the pulmonary valve may reveal a reduced pulmonary stroke distance (less than 6.5 cm) in about half of the patients (Fig. 9.2.6a).[3] The right ventricular pre-ejection period, RPEP, is typically prolonged (RPEP/RVET ratio >0.50 at 0–12 hours, >0.45 at over 12 hours) as a result of combined high pulmonary vascular resistance and/or right ventricular dysfunction.[7,8] (The TPV/RVET ratio is probably of little value in this group of patients.[3]) There may be high-velocity pulmonary valve regurgitation (>2 m/s) secondary to elevated diastolic pulmonary arterial pressure – see Figure 9.2.6b. The pulmonary valve diameter may be measured for the calculation of right ventricular output.

Interrogation of flow at the origin of the branch pulmonary arteries by pulsed Doppler (usually the left pulmonary artery origin) is helpful. This reveals reduced forward flow velocity in the branch pulmonary arteries. The mean velocity throughout the cardiac cycle is typically less than 20 cm/s,[2] and there is little or no forward flow during diastole (diastolic forward flow is profuse with left-to-right ductal shunting).

5. Ductal views and interrogation with colour and pulsed Doppler reveal a patent duct in the majority (80–85%), most of whom (60–70%) have bidirectional ductal flow with a low left-to-right velocity in diastole (<1 m/s) and a prolonged right-to-left shunting phase (typically exceeding the duration of systole (RVET)). A minority have pure right-to-left flow, which persists in severe cases. A few have pure left-to-right flow, but this is always at low velocity. These flow patterns reflect the balance of aortic and PA pressures and are very sensitive to changes; babies may at one minute have pure right-to-left flow, which with minor alteration in ventilation can change to bidirectional flow (see Fig. 9.2.7). During recovery the left-to-right right flow velocity increases, although in term babies the duct typically closes early during recovery. The influence of the ductal shunting depends also on the size of the duct. This is assessed by cross-sectional and colour Doppler as described in Chapter 7, and also by the measurement of differential oxygen saturations from the right arm and a foot.

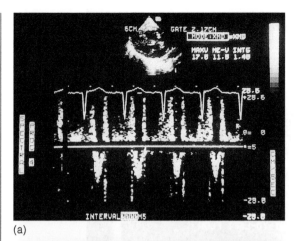

(a)

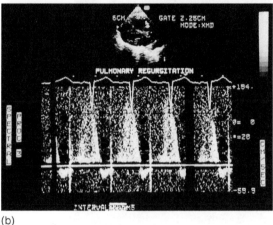

(b)

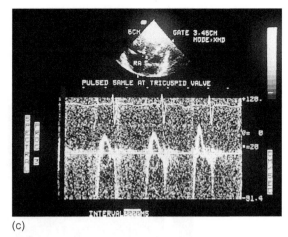

(c)

Fig. 9.2.6 (a) Pulsed Doppler at the pulmonary valve. The RV stroke volume is very low. The second beat has been traced to reveal a stroke distance (flow velocity integral) of 1.48 cm, and a peak velocity of 0.18 cm/s, which are extremely low (pulmonary artery stroke distance is normally over 8 cm in term infants). Regurgitation above the zero line is seen. (b) In the same infant, the scale is now increased to show that the pulmonary valve regurgitation is high velocity. When measured with continuous wave Doppler this was over 2.5 cm/s, suggesting a pressure drop of 25 mmHg between pulmonary artery and RV in diastole (i.e. applying the modified Bernoulli equation, diastolic PA pressure of over 25 mmHg). (c) At the tricuspid valve, peak velocity is also very low, about 0.3 m/s, and flow is brief and not biphasic as normal. The aliasing during systole is from tricuspid regurgitation.

6. From the suprasternal notch continuous or pulsed Doppler reveals reduced ascending aortic flow velocity resulting from low left ventricular output. Aortic stroke distance in term babies with PPHN is usually less than 12 cm, and in preterm babies is less than 8 cm. A stroke volume index after 12 hours of age less than 1 ml/kg or left ventricular output less than 100 ml/kg indicates high risk of mortality.[3]

MONITORING PROGRESS

During a longitudinal study of 30 hypoxaemic newborns, we compared a number of echocardiographic parameters from before and after a sustained 10% rise in SaO_2 in 19 of these infants. Velocity of tricuspid regurgitation and TPV/RVET ratio had no correlation with improvement, whereas there was an increase in left-to-right ductal velocity in 60%, aortic stroke distance in 44% and pulmonary stroke distance in 73%. Thus pulmonary stroke distance was the best indicator of haemodynamic improvement. Large changes in pulmonary and systemic blood flow occurred with little change in systolic pulmonary arterial pressure assessed from TR.

An example of the change in ductal flow following alteration of positive pressure ventilation causing a small reduction in $PaCO_2$ is shown in Figure. 9.2.7.

In another study, increasing velocity of flow at the origin of the left pulmonary artery correlated well with improvement in oxygenation during inhaled nitric oxide therapy in hypoxaemic infants with marked R–L shunting through the oval foramen and arterial duct.[2] Mean velocity in infants before treatment increased significantly from 18 cm/s to 29 cm/s, and the degree of change correlated with the degree of improvement in oxygenation.

The most sensitive echocardiographic indicators of improvement during the minute-to-minute management of such hypoxaemic infants are

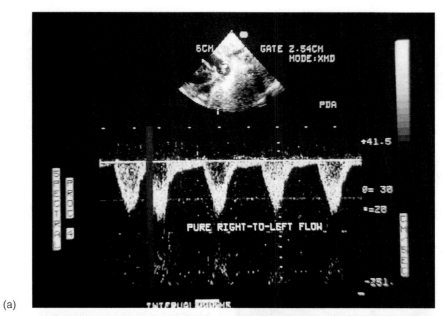

(a)

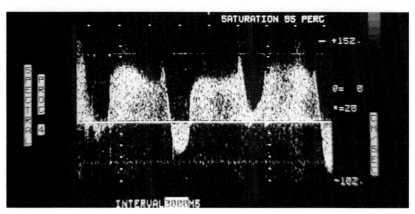

(b)

(c)

Fig. 9.2.7 Serial pulsed Doppler recordings from the arterial duct in an infant with severe meconium aspiration syndrome during an improvement in arterial oxygenation saturation (SaO$_2$) over 30 min due to improved ventilation.

(a) Pure right-to-left ductal flow when SaO$_2$ was less than 80%.

(b) At 83% SaO$_2$ flow in diastole is now partly left-to-right.

(c) At 95% SaO$_2$ flow is mostly left-to-right.

therefore ductal flow velocity and flow pattern, velocity at the origin of the left pulmonary artery, and left and right ventricular outputs. Interatrial flow patterns are also helpful, but repeated subcostal imaging is often less well tolerated by these infants. In the measurement of outputs, the vessel diameter need only be measured once, if at all, because changes in vessel diameter are minimal and are prone to measurement error. Serial change in stroke distance is directly proportional to change in stroke volume and much less prone to measurement error (around 10%). For example, if aortic stroke distance rises from 8 to 12 cm, left ventricualr stroke volume has increased by 50%.

'PPHN', PRESSURE, FLOW AND RESISTANCE

The fact that systolic PA pressure has apparently little correlation to disease severity may be a surprise to the reader. Unfortunately, the term 'PPHN', while a popular name for a well-recognized clinical condition, is not a good name because it suggests that pulmonary hypertension is the main problem. PPHN is complex, multifactorial and varies greatly between subjects. The central haemodynamic problem is low pulmonary blood *flow* secondary to elevated pulmonary vascular resistance. This occurs along with persistence of right-to-left shunting through the fetal channels.

High PA pressure does not necessarily equate with low pulmonary blood flow. Indeed, arterial pressure and flow are *directly* related to each other. If systemic arterial pressure rises we should not assume that systemic cardiac output has fallen. High PA pressure can be associated with high, normal or low pulmonary blood flow, as in an infant with a VSD, a healthy newborn baby and in PPHN, respectively. Almost all babies with hyaline membrane disease have prolonged pulmonary hypertension,[9,10] but most also have normal or high pulmonary blood flow.[11]

Pressure, flow and resistance are related to each other in a manner similar to Ohm's law, $V = IR$, where in this case V = pressure difference across the lungs, I = flow and R = resistance. An increase in pulmonary blood flow associated with a fall in vascular resistance may occur with little or no change in PA pressure. It is thus logical that PA pressure measurements are not reliable indicators of flow or resistance.

Unlike measurement of systolic PA pressure (by TR), the pattern of flow through the duct does tend to reflect improvement because it represents the balance of pressures and resistance across the duct, and the biggest change in pressure as pulmonary vascular resistance falls is during diastole, not in systole. This reflects an increased left-to-right ductal flow velocity (and increased left-to-right *flow*) during diastole. Direct measurement by cardiac catheterization has shown that healthy newborn infants and those with PPHN have systolic PA pressure at systemic levels,[12] but diastolic PA pressure is only at systemic levels in those with PPHN.[13] When the duct is large the balance of systemic and pulmonary vascular resistances is particularly critical because significant amounts of deoxygenated blood can off-load across the duct into the aorta. In these cases in particular, maintaining high systemic vascular resistance (with drugs such as dopamine) may maintain arterial oxygenation better than vasodilators.

It might be better to think of an alternative name to 'PPHN', to avoid focusing on pressure rather than flow. Better names for this condition might be 'pulmonary ischaemia', a name once applied to babies with HMD,[14] or failure or persistence of the transitional circulation (PTC). Persistent fetal circulation (PFC) is reserved by most to describe only babies without associated respiratory disease.

Echocardiography now provides us with the means to assess and treat the individual according to his or her needs at that time such that the 'cookbook' approach to the management of hypoxaemic infants, much criticised by experts in the field, can now be avoided.

REFERENCES

1. Riemenschneider TA, Nielsen HC, Ruttenberg MD, Jaffe RB. Disturbances of the transitional circulation: spectrum of pulmonary hypertension and myocardial dysfunction. *Journal of Pediatrics* 1976;89:622–625.

2. Roze JR, Storme L, Zupan V, Morville P, Dinh-Xua, AT, Mercier JC. Echocardiographic investigation of inhaled nitric oxide in newborn babies with severe hypoxaemia. *Lancet* 1994;344:303–305.

3. Skinner JR, Hunter S, Hey EN. Haemodynamic features at presentation in persistent pulmonary hypertension of the newborn and outcome. *Archives of Disease in Childhood* 1996;74:F26–32.

4. Nagueh SF, Kopelen HA, Zoghbi WA. Relation of mean right atrial pressure to echocardiographic and Doppler parameters of right atrial and right ventricular function. *Circulation* 1996;93:1160–1169.

5. Musewe NN, Poppe D, Smallhorn JF *et al*. Doppler echocardiographic measurement of pulmonary artery pressure from ductal Doppler velocities in the newborn. *Journal of the American College of Cardiology* 1990;15:446–456.

6. Skinner JR, Milligan DWA, Hunter S. Diagnosis of pneumothorax by echocardiography. *Archives of Disease in Childhood* 1991;66:1001–1002 (letter).

7. Johnson GL, Cunningham MD, Desai NS, Cottrill CM, Noonan JA. Echocardiography in hypoxemic neonatal pulmonary disease. *Journal of Pediatrics* 1980;96:716–720.

8. Valdez-Cruz L, Dudell GG, Ferrara A. Utility of m-mode echocardiography for early identification of infants with persistent pulmonary hypertension of the newborn. *Pediatrics* 1981;68:515–525.

9. Skinner JR, Boys RJ, Hunter S, Hey EN. Pulmonary and systemic arterial pressure in hyaline membrane disease. *Archives of Disease in Childhood* 1992;67:366–373.

10. Evans NJ, Archer LNJ. Doppler assessment of pulmonary artery pressure and extrapulmonary shunting in the acute phase of hyaline membrane disease. *Archives of Disease in Childhood* 1991;66:6–11.

11. Mellander M, Larrson LE, Ekstrom-Jodal B, Sabel KG. Prediction of symptomatic patent ductus arteriosus in preterm infants using Doppler and m-mode echocardiography. *Acta Paediatrica Scandinavica* 1987;76:553–559.

12. Emmanouilides GC, Moss AJ, Duffie ER, Adams FH. Pulmonary arterial pressure changes in human newborn infants from birth to 3 days of age. *Journal of Pediatrics* 1964;65:327–333.

13. Drummond WH, Peckham GJ, Fox WW. The clinical profile of the newborn with persistent pulmonary hypertension. Observations of 19 affected neonates. *Clinical Pediatrics* 1977;16:335–341.

14. Chu J, Clements JA, Cotton EK, Klaus MH, Sweet AY, Tooley WH. Neonatal pulmonary ischaemia. Part 1: Clinical and physiological studies. *Pediatrics* 1967;40:709–782.

The cyanosed newborn: echocardiography and ECMO

Dale C Alverson and Mark R Crowley

INTRODUCTION

Extracorporeal membrane oxygenation (ECMO) is a form of partial heart–lung bypass used in term or near-term neonates with potentially reversible respiratory or cardiac failure or pulmonary hypertension, who are likely to die with only conventional therapeutic support.[1] Both venoarterial (V-A) bypass and venovenous (V-V) bypass are available. The method used depends on the underlying pathology and technical limitations in vascular cannulation.

V-A ECMO requires cannulation of both the right common carotid artery and internal jugular vein, which are both usually ligated (Figs 9.3.1 and 9.3.2b). Venous blood is drained out of the right atrium by gravity via a catheter inserted in the right internal jugular vein. Warmed oxygenated blood is returned with the assistance of a roller pump to the aortic arch via a catheter inserted in the right carotid artery. V-A ECMO provides both circulatory and respiratory support since it can do the work of the heart by return of blood flow to the systemic circulation under pressure and can also be used to unload the heart. Thus V-A ECMO allows both cardiac and lung rest while awaiting recovery of these systems.

V-V ECMO usually requires only internal jugular vein cannulation with a double lumen catheter and only venous ligation, thus preserving the carotid artery (Fig. 9.3.2a). Venous blood is drained from the right atrium by gravity via one lumen and the warmed oxygenated blood returns with roller pump assistance via the other lumen. The returning blood is directed towards the tricuspid valve through openings at the cannula's tip. During V-V ECMO, the heart is 'full' and systemic blood flow is dependent upon inherent cardiac function.

Echocardiography is necessary to detect and evaluate structural as well as functional heart disease and to assess pulmonary hypertension, atrial and ductal shunting. It is helpful in guiding the positioning of the cather tips within the heart. During ECMO therapy it is particularly important during episodes of haemodynamic deterioration.

More reliable echocardiographic estimations of cardiac performance are possible on V-V ECMO because the heart is full. Under V-A ECMO the

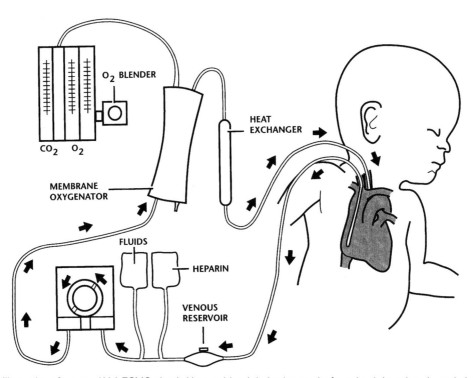

Fig. 9.3.1 Illustration of neonatal V-A ECMO circuit. Venous blood drains by gravity from the right atrium through the venous catheter placed in the internal jugular vein to the venous reservoir. The blood is heparinised and is moved through the circuit via a roller pump and through a membrane oxygenator for gas exchange with the sweep gas mixture passing over the membrane. The oxygenated blood is re-warmed as it passes through a heat exchanger and returns to the infant via the arterial catheter placed in the carotid artery and advanced into the aortic arch (see also Fig. 9.3.2b).

(a)

(b)

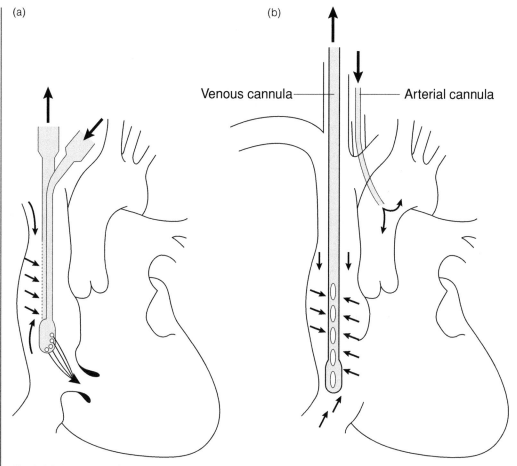

Venous cannula —————————— Arterial cannula

Fig. 9.3.2 Illustration of (a) V-V and (b) V-A ECMO cannulae position. (a) The double lumen venovenous catheter is placed in the jugular vein and advanced into the right atrium. The venous drainage passes through one lumen by gravity to the venous reservoir in the ECMO circuit and the subsequently oxygenated blood returns via the other lumen of the cannula with the distal exit foramina near the tricuspid valve so that flow is directed towards and through the valve into the right ventricle.

heart is unloaded, affecting the load-dependent indices of cardiac function, such as left ventricular fractional shortening and ventricular output. This is particularly important to remember during weaning off ECMO support as the patient recovers.

PRE-ECMO ECHOCARDIOGRAPHIC ASSESSMENT

Even if your department does not offer ECMO, echocardiography may be helpful in predicting the potential need for it and expediting transfer to a nearby unit with ECMO facilities. Major congenital heart defects must be excluded as described in Chapter 9.1. A paediatric echocardiographer with considerable experience in congenital heart disease must perform this part of the assessment. The role of echocardiography in the assessment and

management of PPHN is discussed in Chapter 9.2, and the same principles apply here.

Kinsella *et al.* used echocardiography to assess the role of cardiac dysfunction in determining the need for ECMO in neonates with severe respiratory failure.[2] Their results revealed that patients who went on to require ECMO had significantly lower pulmonary and aortic peak flow velocities, lower pulmonary acceleration, lower left ventricular fractional shortening (FS%) and lower velocity of circumferential fibre shortening (Vcf) ($p < 0.05$). Values for peak pulmonary velocity <0.70 m/s with pulmonary acceleration <14 m/s^2 were associated with the need for ECMO in 7/9 (78%) patients, whereas values above those levels were associated with recovery without ECMO in 11/12 (92%).

However, Karr *et al.* had different results in their neonates with severe lung disease.[3] They found no significant difference in parameters of left ventricular function when comparing those who required ECMO with those who did not. Left ventricular shortening fraction averaged $36.1 \pm 7.6\%$ in the non-ECMO group and $40.5 \pm 8.8\%$ in the ECMO group. As another estimate of contractility, they also calculated 'rate-corrected velocity of circumferential fibre shortening' (Vcfc).* Values were 1.41 ± 0.35 circumferences/s in the non-ECMO group versus 1.58 ± 0.39 in the ECMO group. The authors tried to eliminate the effects of the variation in afterload in their assessments of ventricular function, using 'LV peak systolic wall stress' (LVPWS) as an estimate of afterload.† Relationships between wall stress and ventricular shortening also showed no differences between the two groups. There were also no differences in right or left ventricular pre-ejection period/ejection time ratios. However, systolic pulmonary artery pressure derived from tricuspid regurgitation was somewhat higher in those needing ECMO than in those who did not (63 ± 10 mmHg versus 56 ± 13 mmHg; $p = 0.017$). The authors concluded that cardiac failure was not the primary cause of clinical deterioration in infants with severe lung disease who require ECMO. They also speculated that cardiac performance in the majority of neonates with severe pulmonary hypertension may be adequate to support those infants during V-V ECMO.

Schwartz et al.[4] evaluated LV mass using cross-sectional echocardiography in neonates with left-sided congenital diaphragmatic hernia (CDH) and other causes of pulmonary hypertension.‡ LV mass (indexed to body weight) was significantly *lower* in neonates with CDH as compared with neonates with other causes of pulmonary hypertension; 1.96 ± 0.59 versus 2.84 ± 0.41 g/kg ($p = 0.0001$). The reduced LV mass may reflect poor intrauterine growth of the left ventricle in CDH because of inadequate pulmonary venous return. Infants with CDH who required ECMO before repair had a significantly lower LV mass (1.53 ± 0.50 g/kg) than those who did not (2.20 ± 0.52 gm/kg) ($p = 0.007$). Infants who died also had a significantly lower LV mass compared with survivors; 1.64 ± 0.58 versus 2.09 ± 0.58 g/kg. They concluded that evaluation of LV mass may predict the need for ECMO before surgical repair and that a higher value may indicate good prognosis.

Echocardiography thus plays an important role in predicting the need for ECMO and excluding or diagnosing congenital heart disease in cyanosed infants. Some research also suggests that echocardiographic criteria of ventricular performance or muscle mass may prove to be of prognostic value.

ECHOCARDIOGRAPHIC ASSESSMENT DURING ECMO

Echocardiographic assessment may be useful when an infant fails to make expected progress, during periods of haemodynamic deterioration, and during adjustments in ECMO bypass flow rates, particularly while weaning from ECMO.

The infant not making expected progress

If a patient is responding well to ECMO by other clinical measures, echocardiographic evaluation may not be necessary. However, in patients who are failing to respond or improve as anticipated, a 'second look' can be helpful in ruling out congenital abnormalities that may have been missed initially such as total anomalous pulmonary venous return. This is particularly important with irreversible pulmonary hypertension associated with pulmonary lymphangiectasia, alveolar capillary dysplasia or pulmonary hypoplasia with or without congenital diaphragmatic hernia.

Haemodynamic deterioration

Haemodynamic deterioration can occur for a variety of reasons, most of which are detectable with echocardiography. Myocardial dysfunction

---

*Vcfc is an index of LV function which should theoretically be constant over all ages and heart rates. It is calculated as: Vcfc = SF%/LV ETc, where SF% is LV shortening fraction and LVETc is the left ventricular ejection time measured from the LV outflow tract Doppler signal and corrected to a heart rate of 60 beats per minute (bpm) by dividing by the square root of the R–R interval (the normal value is roughly 0.98 + 0.07 circumferences/s).

†'LV peak systolic wall stress' (LVPWS) was calculated as: LVPWS = BPs × LVESD/LVPWESD, where BPs is the systolic blood pressure (mmHg), M-mode-derived LVESD is LV end-systolic diameter (cm), and LVPWESD is the LV posterior wall thickness at end-systole. Vcfc divided by LVPWS is thought to be a pre- and afterload independent measure of LV function.

‡ The LV mass was calculated using an area–length method: LV mass = 1.055(5/6)(Area-m × [Length + t]), where 1.055 is the density of cardiac muscle, Area-m is the total LV area – LV cavity area, Length is LV length, and t is average LV wall thickness. The average LV wall thickness was calculated as t = (A1/π)1/2 – (A2/π)1/2, where A1 is total LV area and A2 is LV cavity area. All measurements were made at end diastole using the average of three cardiac cycles. The method has not been validated for use in neonates!

may be present for a variety of reasons; it may be one of the prime indications for ECMO, such as post cardiac surgery or with cardiomyopathies, but 'cardiac stun syndrome' has been described upon initiation of ECMO itself.[5]

Several studies have reported a decrease in cardiac output and shortening fraction during ECMO in neonates.[6-11] The changes are most pronounced during the first 24 hours on ECMO and gradually resolve over the course of ECMO support. These studies were primarily performed on patients on V-A ECMO.

Kimball et al. studied 26 newborns with persistent pulmonary hypertension before, during and after V-A ECMO.[8] During ECMO they found that shortening fraction fell from 33% to 25% and cardiac output fell from 205 to 113 ml/kg/min with a fall in heart rate from 158 to 118 bpm. On the

other hand preload increased significantly during ECMO; left ventricular end-diastolic dimension rose from 1.4 to 1.6 cm. All changes resolved when bypass was terminated. They found no significant changes in load-independent indices of contractility (Vcfc/LVPWS) during ECMO.

Berdjis et al. used a load-independent index (Vcfc/LVPWS) to provide a meaningful measure of ventricular performance in critically ill neonates undergoing ECMO.[9] Left ventricular performance was highest before the onset of ECMO and came down towards the normal range during and following ECMO. These changes may reflect exogenous and endogenous catecholamine variation rather than intrinsic variations in myocardial contractility.

Strieper et al. studied cardiac performance in 15

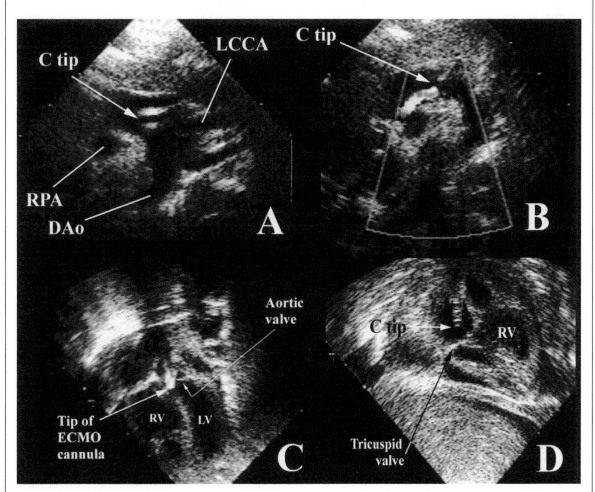

Fig. 9.3.3 Echographic images of cannulae positions. (A) The arterial catheter in the ascending aorta/aortic arch. (B) Colour Doppler flow from the arterial catheter in the ascending aorta/aortic arch. (C) Arterial cannula malpositioned across aortic valve into the LVOT. (D) Venous catheter appropriately positioned in the right atrium (note the small pericardial effusion).

infants before, during, and after *venovenous* ECMO.[10] They reported borderline or normal indices of cardiac function pre ECMO. After initiation of V-V ECMO, cardiac function normalized in all neonates. They concluded that V-V ECMO has no deleterious effects on cardiac performance.

Holley *et al.* studied neonates with meconium aspiration syndrome while on either venoarterial or venovenous ECMO at the end of their course.[11] They showed that load-dependent indices (LV shortening fraction and LV output) were normal at a low bypass flow rate of 25 ml/kg/min and did not change significantly with increasing bypass flow rates up to 125 ml/kg/min. They suggested that previously described decreases in cardiac performance during ECMO are not due to the underlying disease process or the bypass procedure, but are due to changes in loading conditions during partial bypass.

From a practical point of view, in assessing ventricular function on ECMO, straight-forward subjective assessment from cross-sectional images, along with measurement of LV shortening fraction, and possibly LV output, is usually adequate, but large alterations in pre- and afterload need to be borne in mind.

As well as assessing ventricular function, echocardiography can also diagnose pericardial effusion, catheter malposition (e.g. right atrial cannulae can inadvertently cross over into the left atrium (Fig. 9.3.3)), or intravascular thrombus, all of which can result in clinical deterioration.

☞ *Practical Point*

- **When assessing an infant during clinical deterioration on ECMO, the echocardiographer should attempt to exclude worsening myocardial dysfunction, pericardial effusion, catheter malposition and intravascular thrombus.**

Adjusting bypass flow rates

Walther *et al.* used pulsed Doppler techniques to determine right and left ventricular output in newborns on V-A ECMO.[7] They found that during ECMO, left and right ventricular output decreased proportionately to the amount of bypass flow provided. Although this may suggest that weaning from ECMO could be guided by such measurements, the results are rather different from those noted previously by Holley *et al.*,[10] which

suggested that afterload was the major determinant of cardiac performance. Further studies in this area are needed.

CONCLUSIONS

Echocardiography can provide a useful, perhaps even essential, clinical and research tool in the evaluation and management of the neonate on ECMO and during its subsequent transition back to more conventional and less invasive modes of support.

REFERENCES

1. Zwischenberger JB, Bartlett RH (eds). *ECMO Extracorporeal Cardiopulmonary Support in Critical Care.* Ann Arbor, MI: Extracorporeal Life Support Organization, 1995.
2. Kinsella JP, McCurin DC, Clark RH, Lally KP, Null DM. Cardiac performance in ECMO candidates: echocardiographic predictors for ECMO. *Journal of Pediatric Surgery* 1992;27:44–47.
3. Karr SS, Martin GR, Short BL. Cardiac performance in infants referred for extracorporeal membrane oxygenation. *Journal of Pediatrics* 1991;118:437–442.
4. Schwartz SM, Vermillion RP, Hirschl RB. Evaluation of left ventricular mass in children with left-sided congenital diaphragmatic hernia. *Journal of Pediatrics* 1994;125:447–451.
5. Kinsella JP, Gerstmann DR, Rosenberg AA. The effect of extracorporeal membrane oxygenation on coronary perfusion and regional blood flow distribution. *Pediatric Research* 1992;31:80–84.
6. Martin GR, Short BL. Doppler echocardiographic evaluation of cardiac performance in infants on prolonged extracorporeal membrane oxygenation. *American Journal of Cardiology* 1988;62:929–934.
7. Walther FJ, van de Bor M, Gangitano ES, Snyder JR Left and right ventricular output in newborn infants undergoing extracorporeal membrane oxygenation. *Critical Care Medicine* 1990;18(2):148–151.
8. Kimball TR, Daniels SR, Weiss RG *et al.* Changes in cardiac function during extracorporeal membrane oxygenation for persistent pulmonary hypertension in the newborn infant. *Journal of Pediatrics* 1991;118:431–436.
9. Berdjis F, Takahashi M, Lewis AB. Left ventricular performance in neonates on extracorporeal membrane oxygenation. *Pediatric Cardiology* 1992;13:141–145.
10. Strieper MJ, Sharma S, Dooley KJ, Cornish JD, Clark RH. Effects of venovenous extracorporeal membrane oxygenation on cardiac performance as determined by echocardiographic measurements. *Journal of Pediatrics* 1993;122:950–955.
11. Holley DG, Short BL, Karr SS, Martin GR. Mechanisms of change in cardiac performance in infants undergoing extracorporeal membrane oxygenation. *Critical Care Medicine* 1994;22:1865–1870.

The infant with heart failure, hypotension or shock: excluding structural heart disease

Stewart Hunter

INTRODUCTION

The structural heart diseases that cause heart failure in the newborn usually present later than 12–24 hours after birth, and the most common types are obstructive lesions of the left heart. Infants presenting with circulatory failure at or immediately after birth are more likely to have a functional problem such as myocardial insufficiency, typically following perinatal asphyxia. However, there is no clear time distinction, and structural heart disease may coincidentally be present in an infant with perinatal asphyxia. When heart failure is suspected, echocardiography is indicated to find the cause.

Left heart obstructive lesions, including coarctation, aortic stenosis or hypoplastic left heart, need to be considered and excluded. This chapter is concerned with how the echocardiogram can diagnose them, from the left atrium to the arch of the aorta.

The importance of careful clinical examination as part of this process, particularly feeling for the femoral pulses, cannot be overstressed. Nevertheless, the clinical manifestations of heart failure and structural heart disease in the neonate may be very confusing. Many signs elicited and attributed to heart failure can be secondary to lung disease or infection. Tachycardia, tachypnoea, dyspnoea and oedema may all result from respiratory disease or systemic infection as frequently as they do from genuine heart failure with structural or functional heart disease. The only essential criterion for the diagnosis of heart failure is cardiomegaly, which is most reliably diagnosed on the echocardiogram and not on the chest X-ray. The chest X-ray in the neonate is useful for examining the lung fields and the shape of the heart, but is very unreliable as a way of assessing heart size. The echocardiogram is the most important and often the only certain way (short of cardiac catheterization) of identifying the presence of congenital heart disease and differentiating structural from non-structural heart disease and other disease processes.

OBSTRUCTION WITHIN THE LEFT ATRIUM OR AT THE MITRAL VALVE

This is the least common cause of left heart obstruction in the newborn, and can be difficult to diagnose.

Failure to complete the embryological development of the left atrium from its pulmonary venous primordium can lead to a diaphragm across the cavity associated with a small communication. The atrium is divided into two and this rare, but correctable, lesion is known as cortriatriatum (Fig. 10.1.1a). Very rarely a similar lesion can occur on the right side of the heart. Clinical pictures are those of pulmonary venous obstruction and pulmonary hypertension.

A similar haemodynamic abnormality may be seen with a supravalvar mitral membrane (Fig. 10.1.1b). This membrane is often so thin that the ultrasonic diagnosis is very difficult. The embryological origin of this membrane is uncertain.

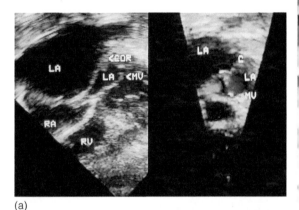

(a)

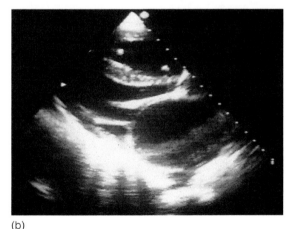

(b)

Fig. 10.1.1 (a) Scan in four-chambered view showing a diaphragm bisecting the left atrium–cor triatriatum of the left side. LA, left atrium; RA, right atrium; MV, mitral valve; RV, right ventricle; C and COR, diaphragm bisecting left atrium. (b) The long-axis view from a child who had clinical evidence of pulmonary hypertension. Just above the opening, leaflets of the mitral valve can be seen the thin curved supravalve membrane which caused obstruction.

Congenital mitral stenosis is a rare neonatal lesion, but is associated with congenital aortic stenosis and coarctation of the aorta. The morphology of the valve is very variable, often with very dysmorphic stenotic leaflets which cannot be repaired surgically, other than by replacement. A common associated problem is the 'parachute mitral valve' malformation, where all the mitral cords insert onto a single papillary muscle group with associated severe obstruction (Fig. 10.1.2a).

Finally, mitral valve hypoplasia and stenosis can be found outside the hypoplastic left heart syndrome in association with univentricular connection abnormality (Fig. 10.1.2b). The haemodynamic effect in this obstruction depends on the patency of the atrial septum, which may have to

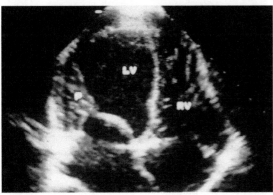

(a)

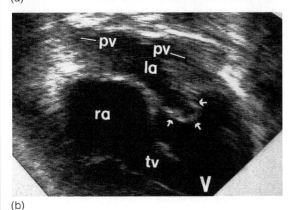

(b)

Fig. 10.1.2 (a) Inverted apical four-chambered view in a child with parachute mitral valve. Both cusps of the mitral valve insert into a single papillary muscle group (P). (b) Echo four-chambered view from a patient with univentricular atrioventricular connection and a hypoplastic stenotic left AV valve (arrowed). pv, pulmonary valve; La, left atrium; ra, right atrium; tv, tricuspid valve.

be removed or ballooned to release the atrial hypertension.

AORTIC VALVE STENOSIS

Critical aortic stenosis is a serious malformation producing morbidity and mortality in the neonatal period. It is now realized that the fetus is also subject to morbidity and mortality as a result of aortic valve stenosis. Dilatation or underdevelopment of the left ventricular cavity in the fetus associated with endocardial fibroelastosis and mitral regurgitation causes gross heart failure and presents with hydrops. Because of the poor outlook for the fetus, attempts have been made to balloon the aortic valve in utero, though with only partial success.[1]

A baby in low output failure with a systolic murmur and poor peripheral pulses should be considered to have aortic stenosis until proved otherwise. The clinical picture may be similar to the coarctation syndrome or interruption of the aortic arch. If in doubt, prostaglandin infusion should be started until specialist cardiology opinion has been obtained. The echocardiogram usually demonstrates a thickened valve (often described as myxomatous) with restricted opening (Fig. 10.1.3a), small aortic root and frequently a dysfunctional left ventricle. Morphology of the aortic valve is often best defined from the parasternal short-axis views (Figs 10.1.3d and e). It may have two cusps, three unequal sized cusps, or even an extremely deformed unicusp.

☞ *Practical Point*
- A baby in low output failure with a systolic murmur and poor peripheral pulses should be considered to have aortic stenosis until proved otherwise.

Critical aortic stenosis in the neonate is associated with a significant mortality whether treatment is attempted by open heart surgery or balloon valvotomy. The critical factor appears to be left ventricular size and function.[2] A small thick-walled cavity indicates poor prognosis (Fig. 10.1.3b). There is probably a critical left ventricular cavity size below which survival with either form of intervention is unlikely. A left ventricular area, measured on a standard long-axis view, of less than 2.2 cm^2 in a term infant usually indicates poor prognosis.

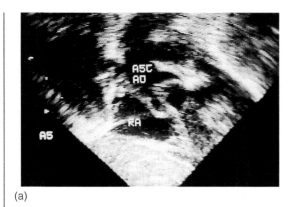

(a)

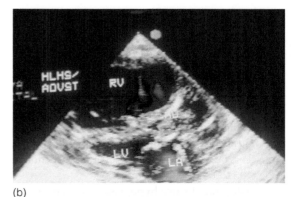

(b)

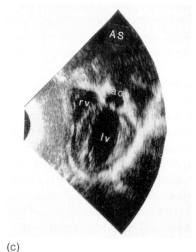

(c)

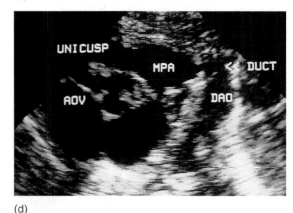

(d)

Fig. 10.1.3 (a) Subcostal four-chambered view, plus aortic root view, in the case of critical aortic stenosis in the newborn. The domed aortic valve with an eccentric orifice is well seen. AS, aortic stenosis; RA, right atrium; ASC AO, ascending aorta.

(b) A long-axis parasternal view from a baby who had a very severe form of neonatal aortic stenosis verging on hypoplasia of the left heart. The right ventricle is enlarged while the left ventricle and left atrium are small. However, there is patency of both the mitral and aortic valves, as shown by the colour flow mapping.

(c) Case of critical aortic stenosis in the neonate, thick-walled, but poorly contracting, somewhat enlarged left ventricle. The aortic valve is shown in the closed position as a thickened structure. rv, right ventricle; lv, left ventricle; ao, aorta; AS, aortic stenosis.

(d) A high parasternal short-axis view in a baby with critical aortic stenosis and a unicusp aortic valve. AOV, aortic valve; MPA main pulmonary artery; DAO, descending aorta.

(e) Parasternal short-axis view of a bicuspid aortic valve with a vertical commissure.

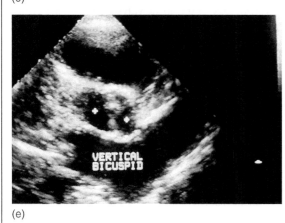

(e)

Nonetheless, balloon dilatation or open heart surgery may buy time and allow growth of the left ventricle. The larger dysfunctional left ventricles which are sometimes seen may show improved systolic function following such intervention.

Doppler studies before intervention usually show turbulent flow in the ascending aorta either from the subcostal views or from the apex (Fig. 10.1.4). Although aortic peak velocity is usually elevated (sometimes as much as 4 m/s), poor left ventricular

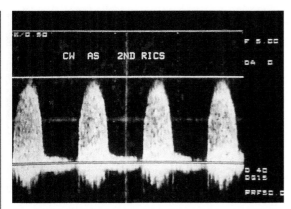

Fig. 10.1.4 Classical second right intercostal space ('2nd Rics') continuous wave (CW) Doppler from a patient with severe aortic stenosis and high-velocity envelope with turbulent flow.

systolic function may lead to lower velocities, even with severe aortic valve stenosis. Not infrequently ballooning or open heart surgery will result in improvement in systolic function and a *rise* in the ascending aortic velocity.

☞ *Practical Point*
- **Severe neonatal aortic stenosis may have surprisingly low ascending aortic velocity on Doppler due to poor left ventricular function and poor cardiac output.**

COARCTATION OF THE AORTA

Without surgery coarctation is a major cause of death in the neonatal period. These babies are often said to suffer from 'coarctation syndrome' because of the typical presentation and the other associated cardiac lesions. Isolated coarctation does present in infancy, but only in about 2% of cases. The associated lesions in descending order of frequency are arterial ducts, bicuspid aortic valves, aortic stenosis and VSD. In the pre-surgical era, more than 80% of children with coarctation died very rapidly, and even today some babies die undiagnosed from coarctation before reaching regional cardiological units.[3]

Clinical presentation and outcome

Of all the neonatal cardiac lesions, coarctation has probably experienced the greatest improvement in outcome. This is largely due to administration of prostaglandin E1 which re-opens the arterial duct,

and also to echocardiography which has replaced invasive catheterization and angiocardiography. Invasive investigation in the past was carried out on sick collapsed oliguric babies, often with lethal results. Coarctation in neonates frequently causes a sudden collapse in a previously well mature infant who had been discharged home with no evidence of congenital heart disease. From failure to feed to full blown circulatory collapse may be only a matter of hours. The cause of this event is a huge increase in afterload from aortic isthmal and arch narrowing and low-flow ischaemic damage to the lower half of the body and its organs – both the result of ductal closure. While the duct remains patent, the fetal circulation is maintained and supply to the lower body is preserved with normal pulses. The classic coarctation in the neonate is at or just before the duct and rarely after it. As soon as the duct closes, renal failure and intestinal ischaemia compound the cardiovascular insult. Before prostaglandin, the best predictor of a poor outlook in neonatal coarctation was a raised blood urea.[4] All neonatologists should be aware of the catastrophic results of ductal closure in babies with coarctation and the almost universally efficacious effect of prostaglandin.

The duct having been reopened, the child's condition is usually allowed to settle with the help of ventilation, inotropic support and correction of the acid–base disturbance. Surgery is no longer a dire emergency, but can be undertaken when the situation settles satisfactorily.

The diagnosis of coarctation is most frequently suspected because of the absence of lower limb pulses. If the circulatory collapse is more extreme, the upper limb pulses may also become difficult to feel. As the child improves on prostaglandin, all the pulses, including the femorals, may return; although the leg blood pressure is usually still less than that in the upper limbs. Careful documentation of blood pressures and pulses in all four limbs is thus essential on admission in the sick neonate. If the clinical signs of coarctation have disappeared following prostaglandin administration, it may be that the only diagnostic findings are present on the echocardiogram.

Echocardiographic diagnosis

Coarctation is best scanned ultrasonically using the suprasternal approach (Figs 10.1.5a–d). Angiography is infrequently used today, even

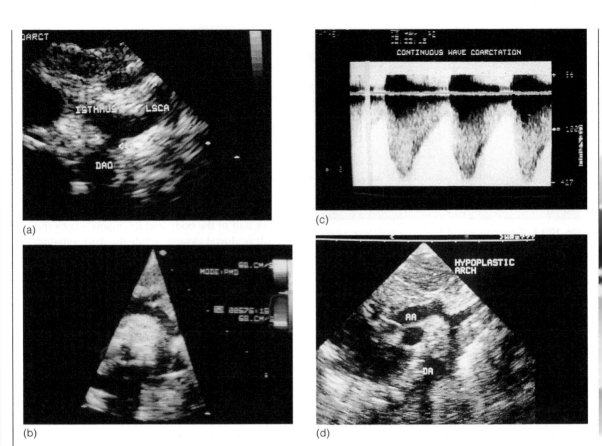

Fig. 10.1.5 (a) High parasternal greatly magnified view of the isthmus of the aorta, the origin of the left subclavian artery (LSCA) and the descending aorta (DAO). Narrowed area of coarctation is arrowed.
(b) Suprasternal view of a baby with coarctation of the aorta. The arch is of reasonable size and the area of coarctation is only clearly identified by the presence of turbulence on the colour flow map.
(c) Continuous wave Doppler from descending aorta via the suprasternal approach. The classical continuous flow which is seen in coarctation is present. The peak velocity is high and the diastolic velocity never returns to the baseline.
(d) Hypoplastic aortic arch in a child who also had coarctation of the aorta. Coarctectomy has been carried out, but there is still isthmal narrowing. AA, ascending aorta; DA, descending aorta.

though it is sometimes difficult to get good ultrasonic pictures of the arch. Doppler has been an advantage to the clinician, but has one or two problems in its use. Often the hypoplastic isthmus is easy to see, but the area of narrowing where the coarctation exists is difficult to identify. Colour flow mapping is invaluable in this situation. The low-velocity primary colours in the flow map are replaced by a mosaic of turbulent flow at the point of coarctation (Fig. 10.1.5b). CW Doppler has a classic flow pattern with an increased systolic velocity and a failure of the signal to return to the baseline in diastole (Fig. 10.1.5c). However, Doppler gradients across the coarctation derived from the continuous wave modality are often misleading, and are probably not as reliable as the upper and lower limb blood pressure differentials,

provided blood pressure measurement is done using Doppler sphygmomanometry and not oscillometry which can seriously overestimate low pressure values. The failure of CW Doppler to assess coarctation severity with reliability is probably related to the long segment isthmal narrowing present in addition to discrete coarctation which seems to invalidate the application of the Bernoulli equation to the Doppler measurements.

☞ *Practical Point*
- **In coarctation, diagnosis is confirmed by a CW Doppler flow pattern in the descending aorta with a long 'tail' during diastole, but the peak velocity correlates poorly with the true gradient.**

Echocardiography demonstrates the associated lesions to perfection. These anomalies are often crucial to the proper management of the cardiovascular situation. Poor left ventricular function and reduced left ventricular cavity are frequently seen with a grossly enlarged right ventricle and right atrium when the ventricular septum is intact. In the presence of a large VSD, on the other hand, left ventricular size is often large and ventricular function is preserved. VSDs are common in coarctation, frequently large, sometimes multiple, and occasionally associated with malalignment of the outlet septum. Such VSDs are probably unlikely to close spontaneously and their demonstration may indicate to the clinician that pulmonary artery banding should be considered at the same time as coarctectomy (Fig. 10.1.6).

INTERRUPTION OF THE AORTIC ARCH

Although the clinical presentation of aortic arch interruption is similar to that of coarctation, there are major differences embryologically and surgically. Interruption of the aortic arch is also associated with VSDs, malalignment of the ventricular septum and arterial ducts, but in addition anomalies of the ventricular outflow tract, such as common arterial trunk, transposition, aortopulmonary window and double outlet right ventricle are frequent. There are three types of interruption of the aortic arch, two of which are very rare. The commonest and easiest to image is when the interruption is after the origin of the left common carotid artery and before the origin of the left subclavian which arises from the distal arch and descending aorta (see Fig. 11.3).

HYPOPLASTIC LEFT HEART SYNDROME

This is the most lethal of the left heart outflow lesions. There is 100% mortality without surgery. The better end of the hypoplastic left heart syndrome merges with the poorer end of critical aortic stenosis. The syndrome includes hypoplasia of the left ventricle, mitral atresia and aortic valve atresia, all of which are present in most cases, making the echocardiographic diagnosis relatively simple (Fig. 10.1.7). The clinical picture has much in common with the coarctation syndrome except that

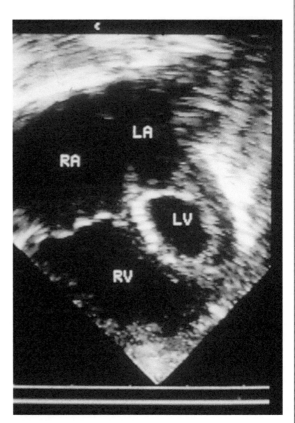

Fig. 10.1.7 A subcostal four-chambered view from a patient with hypoplastic left heart. There is an atrial septal defect. The left ventricle is small and lies above the right ventricular cavity. The colour flow demonstrated preferential (and unrestricted) flow across an atrial septal defect rather than through the mitral valve.

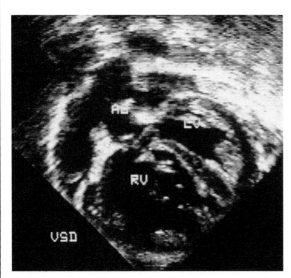

Fig. 10.1.6 A subcostal four-chambered plus aortic route view showing a VSD with malalignment of the ventricular septum of the sort found frequently in association with aortic arch anomalies.

when the duct closes over, pulses diminish or disappear and the post collapse response to prostaglandin, if it occurs, is less good. The surgical options are not particularly encouraging. If a child is diagnosed without full circulatory collapse occurring, then it is possible to carry out the first stage of the Norwood procedure in which the aorta is rebuilt using part of the pulmonary artery and the distal pulmonary artery is detached and supplied by an aortopulmonary shunt. Two further stages of the Norwood procedure follow months or years later. Conversion to a bidirectional Glenn shunt (superior caval vein to right pulmonary artery) is followed eventually by total cavopulmonary connection. Whether this is a viable long-term treatment is as yet unclear. It seems highly likely that transplantation will be required eventually in most cases. Echocardiography is the best way to make this diagnosis and hopefully this can be done early enough in fetal life to allow the opportunity for termination, or immediately after birth to facilitate the first part of the Norwood procedure.

REFERENCES

1. Maxwell D, Allan L, Tynan MJ. Balloon dilatation of the aortic valve in the fetus: a report of two cases. *British Heart Journal* 1991;65(5):256–258.
2. Zeevi B, Keane JF, Castaneda AR, Perry SB, Locke JE. Neonatal critical valvar aortic stenosis. *Circulation* 1989;80:831–839.
3. Abu-Harb M, Hey E, Wren C. Death in infancy from unrecognised congenital heart disease. *Archives of Disease in Childhood* 1994;71:3–8.
4. Macartney FJ, Taylor JFN, Graham GR, De Leval M, Stark J. The fate of survivors of cardiac surgery in infancy. *Circulation* 1980;62:80–91.

The infant with heart failure, hypotension or shock: evaluating the infant with non-structural heart disease

Jonathan P Wyllie
Jon Skinner

INTRODUCTION

This chapter gives examples demonstrating the importance of echocardiography in the assessment of the hypotensive or shocked newborn infant. All of the methods that can be used have previously been outlined in earlier chapters, particularly Chapters 4 and 5.

Although structural heart disease rarely presents immediately at birth, the logical and detailed approach outlined in Chapter 8 should always be used when assessing the shocked infant. Watch out carefully for left heart obstructive lesions as stressed in Chapter 10.1. Always combine your usual clinical skills with echocardiography. Clinical suspicion of congenital heart disease requires immediate expert referral.

CAUSES OF CIRCULATORY FAILURE IN THE NEWBORN

Circulatory failure and/or hypotension

Circulatory failure and/or hypotension commonly occurs for four reasons in the newborn.

1. Poor myocardial contractility, e.g. in perinatal asphyxia, particularly in extreme prematurity, or in association with sepsis.
2. Hypovolaemia, e.g. in early clamping of the umbilical cord.
3. Large left-to-right ductal shunt, particularly in extreme prematurity, even in the first day of life.
4. Secondary to sepsis, often with a high cardiac output, but sometimes with added myocardial failure.

Less common causes

Two less common causes which are very important because treatment is fundamentally different are:

1. Hypertrophic cardiomyopathy in association with maternal diabetes.
2. Pericardial effusion, e.g. secondary to fetal anaemia or haemorrhagic tamponade following vascular instrumentation (e.g. jugular line insertion). These are both detected easily, efficiently and reliably with echocardiography.

Circulatory failure with hypertension

Circulatory failure can also occur with hypertension, typically due to renal dysfunction and treatment is with vasodilators (not inotropes).

EXAMPLES

Myocardial failure

Cross-sectional views typically show a large 'baggy' looking heart, and Doppler examination shows low cardiac output and often atrioventricular valve regurgitation. It can be difficult to detect improvement. Often the infants look better before the echocardiogram does! Serial assessment of aortic or pulmonary stroke distance is especially helpful, but improvement in contractility can be assessed with M-mode and fractional shortening (FS). An example is shown in Figure 10.2.1; FS is 15%.

Hypovolaemia

With only a little practice, the underfilled heart is easy to recognize. The inferior vena cava (IVC) periodically collapses and is difficult to see on the subcostal cuts. All of the chambers appear small, and there is usually a profound tachycardia. In severe hypovolaemia, the ventricles appear hypertrophic since the muscle bulk collapses down onto the small ventricular cavities and is thicker. Aortic and pulmonary stroke distances are low, and ejection times often very brief. An example is shown in Figure 10.2.2.

Large left-to-right ductal shunt

It is important to recognize that good ventricular function does not always mean good or adequate cardiac output. The example in Figure 10.2.3 is typical of the hyperdynamic appearance of a left

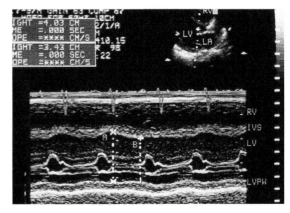

Fig. 10.2.1 Pump failure. This M-mode interrogation through the left ventricle of a four-month-old infant shows gross LV dilatation and very poor movement of both the interventricular septum and the LV posterior wall. LVEDD is 4.03 cm, LVESD is 3.43 cm. Fractional shortening is therefore (4.03–3.43)/4.03 × 100, i.e. 15%.

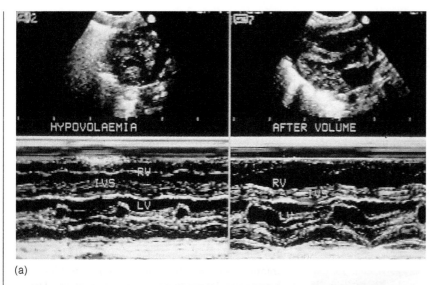

(a)

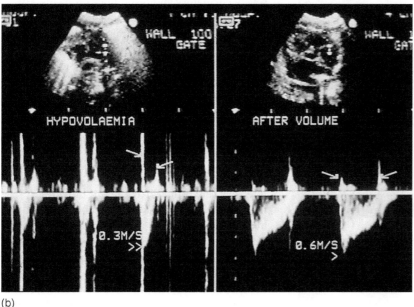

(b)

Fig. 10.2.2 Hypovolaemia. This 28-week preterm infant became extremely hypovolaemic during a severe candidal skin sepsis. Echocardiograms are shown before and after volume replacement, using the same scale. (a) M-mode of the left ventricle. The LV cavity is not much thicker than the septum and the mitral valve leaflets do not separate widely before closing again. After volume replacement, the heart rate is lower, both the RV and LV are better filled, and the mitral valve excursion is greater. (b) Pulsed Doppler at the pulmonary valve. The arrows indicate the opening and closing clicks of the valve. During hypovolaemia the time between the clicks (ejection time) is very brief, and with the second beat on the screen, no forward flow registers. After volume replacement, the ejection time is greatly prolonged, the peak velocity has increased. The stroke distance (not measured on these images) rose from less than 1 cm to about 7 cm.

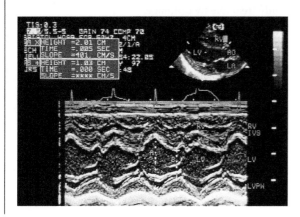

Fig. 10.2.3 Large left-to-right ductal shunt. This LV M-mode shows a typically hyperdynamic ventricle in this setting of high preload and low afterload. LVEDD is 2.01 cm, LVESD is 1.03 cm; LV FS is 49%.

ventricle in a well infant with a large ductal shunt; the FS is 49%. If there is a large shunt, and the ventricle appears even a little subnormal, inotropic support (such as dobutamine) is to be recommended early.

Pericardial tamponade

Once seen, never forgotten, so take a good look at Figure 10.2.4. The dark area around the heart can only be fluid. Fluid which has accumulated slowly can be well tolerated, but rapid accumulation is not. Diastolic atrial collapse is shown in this figure and is a sign of imminent tamponade. Another useful sign is marked swing in the inflow or outflow Doppler signals. Tricuspid and pulmonary valve

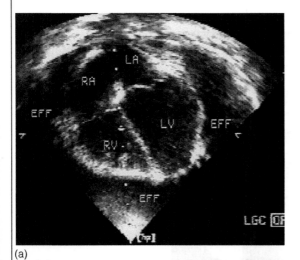

(a)

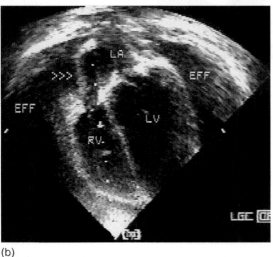

(b)

Fig. 10.2.4 Pericardial tamponade. The dark area around the heart (EFF, effusion) can only be fluid. The arrows in (b) show diastolic right atrial collapse.

Doppler velocities increase by 60–100% with inspiration.

Myocardial hypertrophy

Cardiac hypertrophy is common following intrauterine stress, and is a feature of hypertension. Of itself it is not usually a problem since it is reactive and, once the cause is resolved, it goes away (see Fig. 10.2.5). However, steroid therapy and maternal diabetes can cause profound hypertrophy and even cause LVOT obstruction. Even if the cause is transient, it seems reasonable to call these hypertrophic cardiomyopathies.

Hypertrophic cardiomyopathy

An example is shown in Figure 10.2.6. This preterm infant was born with hyperinsulinism and had severe circulatory and respiratory problems. His cardiac output was helped by using β-blockers (positive inotropes are contraindicated; they make the dynamic subaortic obstruction worse). The dynamic obstruction involves systolic anterior motion of the mitral valve during systole – an example is shown from an older patient (though it does occur in neonates with HCM).

CONCLUSION

Echocardiography is crucial in modern neonatal intensive care primarily because it provides information on the underlying problem not available by any other means. 'Blind' therapy of the shocked or hypotensive infant is outdated and unwise. Volume resuscitation is inappropriate when the myocardium needs support, while inotropes are dangerous in hypertrophic cardiomyopathy; neither is the treatment for a large ductal shunt which may need to be closed, and pericardial tamponade is only treatable by drainage.

Aside from diagnosing the problem, echocardiography provides a means to monitor treatment effectively. The mainstay of this is FS of the left ventricle, and serial assessment of aortic and/or pulmonary artery stroke distance. Valuable adjuncts are central venous pressure monitoring (probably measured too little in neonatology), core–peripheral temperature difference, capillary refill time and acid–base status.

Echocardiography is a part of the haemodynamic diagnostic armamentarium that no neonatal intensivist should be without.

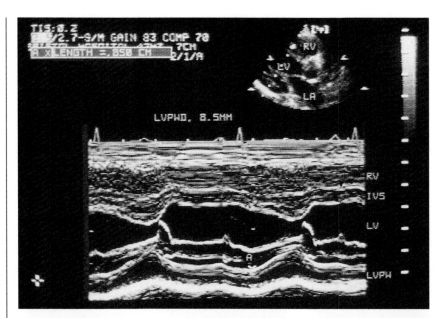

Fig. 10.2.5 Myocardial hypertrophy. This infant had aortic stenosis with preserved ventricular function. The left ventricular posterior wall thickness in diastole (LVPWD) is roughly twice the upper normal range at 8.5 mm.

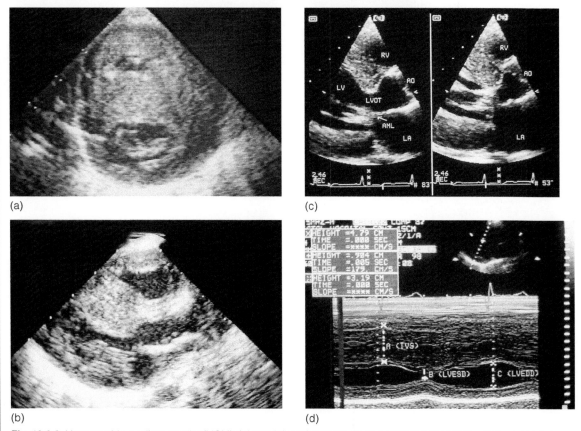

(a)

(b)

(c)

(d)

Fig. 10.2.6 Hypertrophic cardiomyopathy (HCM). (a) and (b) are from a 28-week gestational age infant with hyperinsulinism. (a) Parasternal short-axis view shows the hypertrophy affecting mostly the septum and right ventricular free wall. (b) The enormity of the septum is even more apparent in the long-axis view. (c) and (d) are from adolescents with familial hypertrophic cardiomyopathy. (c) 'SAM' systolic anterior motion of the mitral valve. The anterior mitral valve leaflet (AML, arrowed) moves forwards during systole into the left ventricular outflow tract (LVOT) to obstruct it, causing subaortic stenosis. (d) M-mode through the left ventricle shows virtual cavity obliteration during systole (LVESD 0.9 cm, LVEDD 3.2 cm, septum (IVS) 4.8 cm).

CHAPTER 11

The dysmorphic baby and congenital heart defects

J Deane Waldman
John Plowden
Carol Clericuzio

INTRODUCTION

This chapter highlights some of the more common syndromes and systemic conditions presenting in the neonate that can be associated with congenital heart disease. It also covers some structural heart diseases not presented elsewhere in the book.

The clinical approach to the dysmorphic neonate should be a *team* effort. The neonatologist should confer with the cardiologist and other relevant consultants (clinical geneticist, endocrinologist, neurologist, etc.) *prior to* detailed discussions with the family.

All of the conditions discussed are familiar to the neonatologist so only a brief background to each condition is presented before concentrating on the cardiac abnormalities and highlighting important echocardiographic features not covered elsewhere in the book.

DOWN SYNDROME

Features of Down syndrome are illustrated in Figure 11.1.

Background

Down syndrome is the most common chromosome disorder in newborns with an incidence of 1 in 800 live births. Trisomy 21 due to non-disjunction accounts for 95%; the remaining 5% are due to mosaic trisomy 21 or translocation. Rapid karyotype of peripheral blood lymphocytes is usually available within 72 hours. Newly available fluoresence in situ hybridization (FISH) probes can be used to demonstrate trisomy 21 within 24 hours, although this technology will not distinguish non-disjunction from translocation.

Associated abnormalities

In addition to congenital heart disease, there is an increased risk of congenital gastrointestinal atresias or malformations such as malrotation and annular pancreas.

Congenital heart disease

Approximately 40–50% of neonates with Down syndrome have congenital heart disease. The most common abnormality (60%) is a defect of the A-V

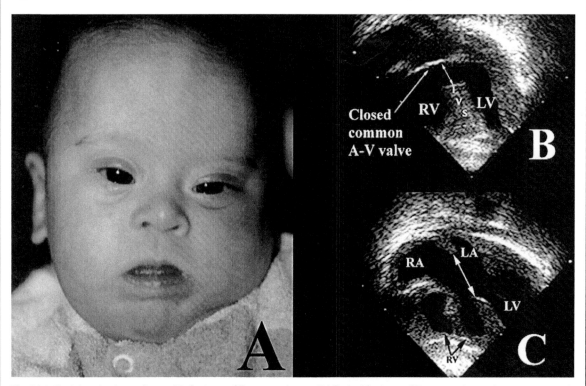

Fig. 11.1 Facial and echocardiographic features of Down syndrome. (A) Typical features of Down syndrome: large tongue and upslanted palpebral fissures. (B) Closed common atrioventricular (A-V) valve inserting medially at the same point, with the VSD between the coaptation plane and the crest of the interventricular septum (IVS). The atrial septal defect (ASD) is 'above' the A-V valve. (C) The A-V valve is open. The large single septal defect (double arrow) is no longer subdivided by the A-V valve.

septum, which may be 'partial' (primum ASD) or complete (both ASD and VSD as well as valvar abnormalities). Perimembranous ventricular septal defects, secundum atrial septal defects, and patent ductus arteriosus (PDA) make up 30% of the heart disease seen; tetralogy of Fallot (ToF) and other complex conditions comprise about 10%. The combination of A-V septal defect with ToF is almost exclusively seen in Down syndrome. Conversely, over 60% of infants with A-V septal defect have Down syndrome.

Echocardiographic features of complete A-V septal defect include:

1. A-V valves insert at same level on the septum;
2. the septal defect 'under' (caudad to) the closed valve is the VSD;
3. the septal defect 'above' (cephalad to) the closed valve is the ASD;
4. when the valves are open, there is a single, central hole;
5. A-V valve regurgitation is common;
6. the A-V canal may be malapportioned such that there is preferential flow into one ventricle and hypoplasia of the other.

These features are seen well in standard four-chambered views. The absence of normal offsetting of the right and left A-V valves is especially important. The large common A-V valve orifice can be profiled from a subcostal short-axis view, demonstrating one large orifice instead of two separate ones.

☞ *Practical Point*
- **Complete A-V septal defect (CAVSD) can occur along with other cardiac abnormalities, such as ToF or patent arterial duct, particularly in Down syndrome.**

NOONAN SYNDROME

The features of Noonan syndrome are illustrated in Figure 11.2.

Background
Noonan syndrome is a multiple malformation syndrome characterized by low posterior hairline with short or webbed neck, pectus excavatum, cryptorchidism in males and dysplastic pulmonary valve. Figure 11.2 illustrates the typical facies of a baby with Noonan syndrome. The disorder has been called the 'male Turner syndrome', but as it can affect both males and females, this terminology is inappropriate. Facial features include downslanting palpebral fissures, ocular hypertelorism, ptosis and low-set and/or abnormal pinnae. The other signs such as shield chest, pectus deformities, scoliosis and mental retardation are usually more apparent as the child matures. It should be suspected in any newborn with dysplastic pulmonary valve. Most cases represent sporadic occurrences although autosomal dominant inheritance has been documented in many families. There is currently no genetic testing available for Noonan syndrome and the diagnosis is made on clinical grounds.

Associated defects
A variety of bleeding diatheses have been documented, including deficiencies of factors 8, 11 and 12, and platelet disorders.

Congenital heart disease
Approximately 50–65% of these patients have congenital heart disease. The most frequent is valvar pulmonary stenosis with a thickened, nodular, dysplastic valve and poorly formed commissures. Although balloon dilatation is often attempted in these children, the success rate is lower than in more common valve stenosis. There is also an association with hypertrophic cardiomyopathy (HCM), which may be obstructive. ASDs, VSDs, and rarely anomalous pulmonary venous return can occur. Interestingly, about 1% of all patients with ToF have Noonan syndrome.

The most striking echocardiographic finding is thickened, poorly mobile pulmonary valve leaflets often without doming, best demonstrated in the parasternal short-axis view. Doppler study may show a significant increase in the velocity across the pulmonary valve. Prominent post-stenotic dilatation such as is seen in the usual form of pulmonary stenosis is unusual in patients with Noonan syndrome. The ventricular walls and interventricular septum should be evaluated for evidence of HCM and the velocity through the LVOT should be determined for evidence of obstruction.

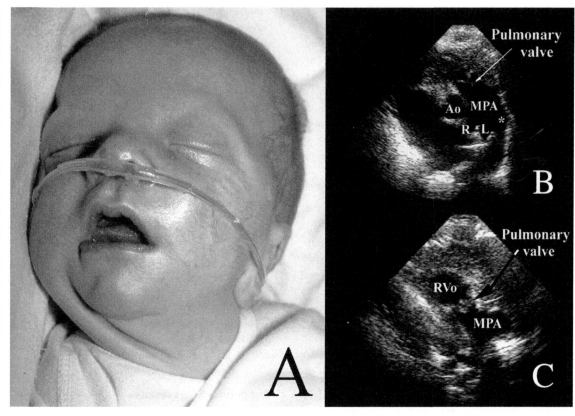

Fig. 11.2 Typical Noonan's facies and representative echocardiograms. (A) Note the downward sloping palpebral fissures, excess nuchal skin and mild congenital lymphoedema. A nasal cannula is in place to provide oxygen because of RV outflow (RVO) tract obstruction and reduced pulmonary blood flow. (B) Type of pulmonary valve seen in *non-dysmorphic* children. There is doming and some thickening as well as post-stenotic dilatation (*) in the main pulmonary artery (MPA). R, right pulmonary artery; L, left pulmonary artery. (C) Typical dysplastic valve seen in children with Noonan syndrome. Compare this with the valve in (B).

22q11 DELETION SYNDROMES

Features of 22q11 deletion syndromes are illustrated in Figure 11.3.

Background

The DiGeorge, Velo-Cardio-Facial (VCF) and CATCH-22 syndromes are part of a family of conditions associated with chromosome 22q11 deletion. Because of the phenotypic overlap between these syndromes, particularly in the neonatal period, they will be discussed together as the '22q11 deletion syndrome'. The disorder should be suspected in neonates with the classic DiGeorge syndrome, findings of hypocalcaemia, absent thymus and conotruncal cardiac defect (e.g. common arterial trunk, ToF, interrupted aortic arch), as well as those with more typical VCF features of cleft palate, with or without the Pierre–Robin malformation sequence, long flexible digits and congenital heart disease (most commonly a VSD). Subtle facial findings in some DiGeorge syndrome patients include lateral placement of inner canthi and small ears. The majority of DiGeorge/VCF/ CATCH-22 patients will have a deletion 22q11 demonstrated by FISH studies, usually performed on peripheral blood lymphocyte chromosomes.

Associated abnormalities

The identification of this chromosomal deletion should prompt a search for the other associated DiGeorge problems such as T cell deficiency and hypocalcaemia. There are recent reports of 22q11 deletion in individuals with apparently isolated congenital heart disease, particularly ToF. A number of phenotypically normal parents of affected children have been found to have 22q11 deletion and therefore FISH probe testing of parents is suggested for recurrence risk counselling.

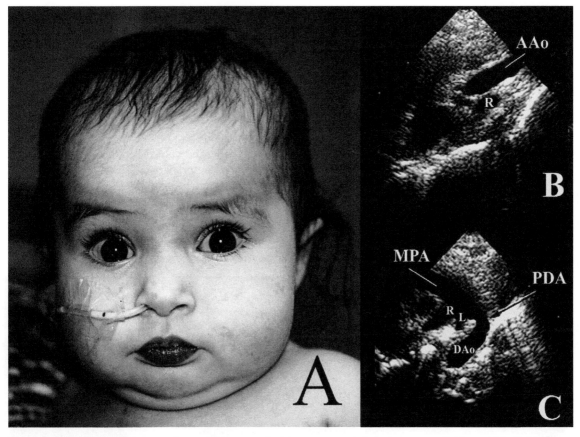

Fig. 11.3 Features of DiGeorge syndrome. (A) Common facial appearance (relatively non-specific) for a child with 22q11 deletion. Note the gavage feeding tube; these children often have feeding difficulties. (B) The ascending aorta is completely straight with no (normal) curvature towards the descending portion of the arch. The branch right pulmonary artery (RPA) is in normal position (R). (C) The main pulmonary artery (MPA) has three 'branches': the right (R) and left (L) branch pulmonary arteries and the PDA, from which the descending aorta (DAo) extends.

Congenital heart disease

Interrupted aortic arch (see Fig. 11.3B and C) and/or common arterial trunk (see Chapter 9.1) are the most common cardiac abnormalities. Other anomalies found include right aortic arch, aberrant right subclavian artery, VSD and ToF. Surgery is often required within the first few days of life, especially with interrupted aortic arch. Genetic consultation is recommended, as approximately 68% of all patients with an interruption between the left common carotid and left subclavian arteries (type B) and about one-third of those with common arterial trunk have 22q11 deletion. Until the presence of a functioning T cell system is *confirmed*, the administration of ***irradiated blood products*** is vital in order to prevent graft-versus-host reaction in all neonates with interrupted aortic arch, truncus arteriosus or ToF.

> ☞ *Practical Point*
> - Until the presence of a functioning T cell system is confirmed, the administration of *irradiated blood products* is vital in order to prevent graft-versus-host reaction in all neonates with interrupted aortic arch, truncus arteriosus or ToF.

On echocardiography, interrupted aortic arch is best seen from the suprasternal long-axis view. The descending aorta is supplied by the arterial duct, which is essential to survival. The size and flow characteristics of the duct must be determined. When the diagnosis is made, even prior to completion of the echocardiographic study, prostaglandins should be started in order to maintain or improve ductal patency. The relationship of the aortic arch and the trachea should be established since a right aortic arch is common and will have surgical implications. In the parasternal long-axis view, common arterial trunk and ToF may look identical with an overriding artery and a large malalignment VSD. In ToF the patent but stenotic main pulmonary artery arises from the right ventricle; in those with ToF and pulmonary atresia, the main pulmonary artery is either absent or markedly hypoplastic and fills solely by retrograde flow from the PDA. In common arterial trunk, the pulmonary artery system arises from the ascending aorta. In most cases of ToF there is evidence of reduced pulmonary blood flow and marked cyanosis, while patients with common arterial trunk often have minimal cyanosis and

evidence of increased pulmonary blood flow both by physical examination and chest X-ray.

HETEROTAXY SYNDROMES

Images of the heterotaxy syndromes are illustrated in Figure 11.4.

Background

The asplenia and polysplenia (heterotaxy) syndromes are primary defects of visceral laterality. They represent 'bilateral right-sidedness' and 'bilateral left-sidedness' respectively, and are associated with a characteristic pattern of complex congenital heart defects, as well as abnormalities of the lungs, liver and stomach. Asplenia syndrome

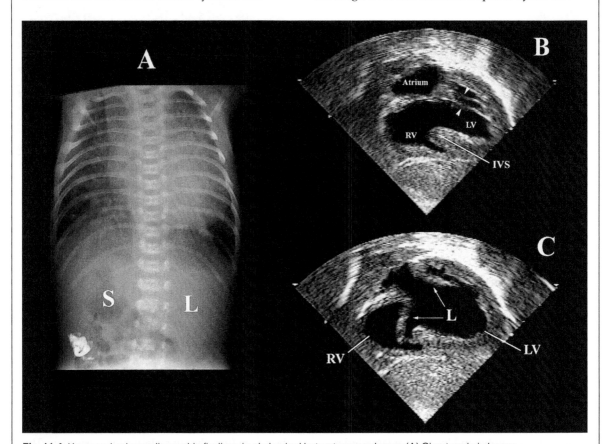

Fig. 11.4 X-ray and echocardiographic findings in abdominal heterotaxy syndrome. (A) Chest and abdomen roentgenogram in a patient with asplenia showing cardiomegaly, pulmonary overcirculation and abdominal situs inversus (stomach on right (S) and liver (L) on left). Note that the cardiac apex and liver are on the same side; this is almost always associated with congenital heart disease. A small residuum of barium is noted in the right lower quadrant. (B) there are two unequal ventricles separated by an incomplete IVS. A single, closed A-V valve guards the atrium with attachments only to the lateral free wall. This appearance suggests a single A-V valve that preferentially flows into one ventricle. (C) in the same patient, the valve leaflets (L) are in open position. Note that the anterior leaflet extends only to and slightly across the IVS; this restricts inflow to the RV which is secondarily hypoplastic. In addition to an A-V canal defect, this child with asplenia syndrome had single ventricle physiology, transposition and total anomalous pulmonary venous connections.

was described by Ivemark in 1955 and features bilateral trilobed lungs, asplenia, bilateral liver (isomerism) and right-sided stomach in addition to cardiac defects. It is more common in males, and should be suspected in neonates with cyanotic heart disease and visceral heterotaxy. The identification of associated anomalies (e.g. absent spleen and secondary immune compromise, intestinal and renal malformations) is important for medical management.

The less common polysplenia syndrome is usually accompanied by milder congenital heart defects. While both disorders usually occur sporadically, there are a number of familial cases. The genetics of the familial cases is complex and undoubtedly more than one gene locus is involved.

Congenital heart disease

Patients with asplenia always have multiple cardiac abnormalities such as CAVSD, transposition of the great arteries, pulmonary stenosis or atresia, total anomalous pulmonary venous connection (TAPVC) and right isomerism. The overall prognosis is poor since they not only have severe cardiac defects, but often die from sepsis as they have problems combatting infection with encapsulated organisms. Continuous coverage against both Gram-positive and Gram-negative organisms is important; administration of pneumococcal and *Haemophilus influenzae* vaccines is also recommended.

Polysplenic patients may have common atrium, absent inferior or bilateral superior vena cave, partial anomalous pulmonary venous connection, and left pulmonary isomerism. Dextrocardia is found in roughly 40% of asplenic or polysplenic patients.

On echocardiographic study one begins with a subxiphoid short-axis view to show the positions and relationships of the IVC and aorta (see Fig. 8.5, p. 175). Absence of the suprarenal IVC may suggest a heterotaxy syndrome. The apex of the heart is often noted in the midline or to the right. In many instances, one large ventricle is noted with a large, single central A-V valve and little or no atrial septum. Marked enlargement of the SVC or coronary sinus may be a clue to TAPVC draining to those locations. The size and spatial relationships of the great arteries must be determined as both transposition and malposition are common. A small pulmonary annulus with a thickened pulmonary valve is often noted and in some cases there may be

pulmonary atresia. As in all newborns with heart disease, the presence of an arterial duct must be noted as well as its size and flow characteristics. In patients with significant pulmonary stenosis or atresia, ductal patency must be maintained with a continuous infusion of prostaglandins.

> ☞ *Practical Point*
> ● **The presence of two or more major congenital cardiac anomalies, especially A-V canal defect and anomalous pulmonary venous drainage, should strongly suggest the presence of asplenia syndrome.**

TURNER SYNDROME

Features of Turner syndrome are illustrated in Figure 11.5.

Background

Turner syndrome occurs in 1:2000 females. In half there is deficiency of one entire X chromosome; the other half show a wide variety of X chromosomal abnormalities, including mosaicism and partial deletions of X. The diagnosis of Turner syndrome should be considered not only in those with the typical dysmorphic features, but also in those with lymphoedema of the hands and feet and in any female neonate with left heart obstruction (coarctation, hypoplastic left heart syndrome). Recurrence risk is not thought to be increased for parents, and parental chromosome studies are not indicated.

Associated abnormalities

Neonates with Turner syndrome should undergo renal ultrasound because of the high incidence (60%) of associated renal anomalies.

Congenital heart defects

Congenital cardiac abnormalities are present in 20–35%; over half of these are coarctation of the aorta. The echocardiographic findings of coarctation (described in Chapter 10) are best noted from the suprasternal position. Other forms of congenital heart disease include hypoplastic left heart syndrome, bicuspid aortic valve (with or without stenosis) and mitral valve abnormalities. Aortic root dilatation, dissection and rupture have been reported in older children or adults.

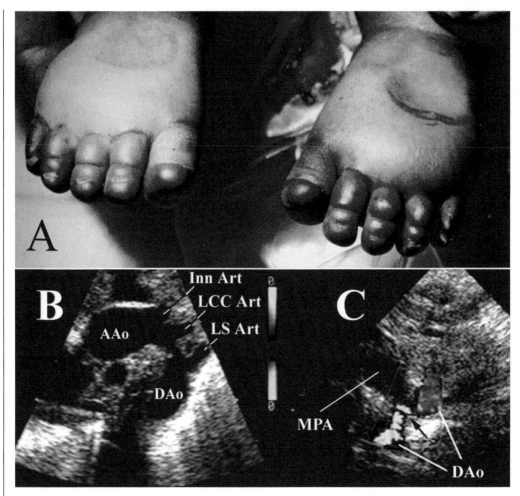

Fig. 11.5 Features of Turner syndrome. (A) Note the general suffusion and severe pedal oedema in this neonate, with pitting seen on the left foot. (B) Note the general hypoplasia of the aorta between the left common carotid artery (LCC Art) and the left subclavian artery (LS Art) as well as the shelf of tissue within the lumen. The poststenotic dilatation of the ascending aorta suggests valvar aortic stenosis as well. (C) Colour flow map in a different patient shows the normal velocity (deep blue) in the proximal descending aorta until the obstruction is reached, where angulation and stenosis are noted as well as multi-hue (turbulent) high-velocity flow through the obstructed segment (black arrow).

WILLIAMS SYNDROME

Features of Williams syndrome are illustrated in Figure 11.6.

Background

Williams syndrome is usually first suspected in late infancy and is not easily diagnosed in the neonate. The characteristic phenotype includes prenatal and postnatal growth deficiency, mild microcephaly, characteristic facies with prominent lips, long philtrum, short nose with anteverted nares, and periorbital fullness of subcutaneous tissues. There may be fifth finger clinodactyly and hoarse cry.

Idiopathic hypercalcaemia occurs in about 15% of infants and is usually managed with a low-calcium diet. These infants are fussy eaters, often with failure-to-thrive. The diagnosis should be suspected in infants with any of these features, particularly in conjunction with characteristic congenital heart disease.

Williams syndrome is caused by a microdeletion of chromosome 7q11.23, a region which includes a gene for elastin. In normal individuals, two copies of the elastin gene are present, one on each of their #7 chromosomes. In Williams syndrome (either with or without heart disease), one of the copies has been deleted as a sporadic event. Routine

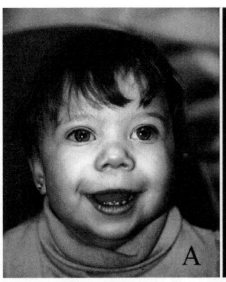
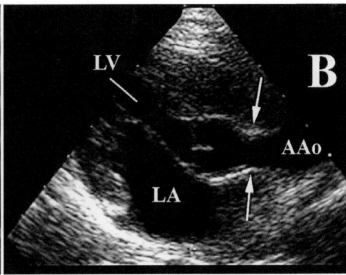

Fig. 11.6 Features of Williams syndrome in an older child. (A) An older child with the typical facies of Williams syndrome: long philtrum, upturned nose and large mouth. (B) Note the symmetrical indentation (arrows) at the sinotubular junction of the ascending aorta. This is a mild form of supravalvar stenosis; the disparity between the sinus of Valsalva and the ascending aorta can be severe.

chromosome studies are normal, but the microdeletion can be detected by commercially available FISH probes for 7q11.23. It is hypothesized that the elastin gene deletion causes a progressive arteriopathy, leading to arterial stenosis, especially above the aortic valve. Most cases represent sporadic new deletions but parent-to-child transmission has been documented.

Associated abnormalities
A variety of associated renal abnormalities have been reported such that renal ultrasound is indicated at the time of diagnosis.

Congenital heart disease
The primary cardiac abnormalities in Williams syndrome are supravalvar aortic stenosis (60%) and peripheral pulmonary artery stenosis (PPAS). The former can progress rapidly and should be followed closely, especially during infancy. On the other hand, PPAS can improve over time. Less commonly, stenoses of other vessels can occur, including renal, mesenteric and coronary arteries.

Supravalvar aortic stenosis is well seen in the parasternal long-axis view, but evaluation of the gradient by Doppler is best determined from the suprasternal approach. Gradient obtained by Doppler in this condition often markedly exceeds that obtained at cardiac catheter. The gradient

usually becomes more severe as the patient gets older. PPAS is noted in a high parasternal short-axis view which demonstrates the main and branch pulmonary arteries. Cross-sectional imaging may show significant narrowing at the origin of the right and/or left pulmonary arteries, while colour flow Doppler shows turbulence into the branch pulmonary arteries. An increase in velocity of over 2.5 m/s by Doppler through this area suggests the diagnosis of PPAS.

INFANT OF A DIABETIC MOTHER

Features of the infant of a diabetic mother (IDM) are illustrated in Figure 11.7.

Background
In insulin-dependent diabetic women the incidence of major malformations in the fetus is 200–300% greater than in the general population. Fetal complications of both pre-conceptional diabetes and gestational diabetes are common and well known to the neonatologist.

Congenital heart disease
Cardiac abnormalities occur in approximately 2.5–4% of babies born to mothers with insulin-dependent diabetes. All types of congenital heart disease are seen in increased numbers but the most

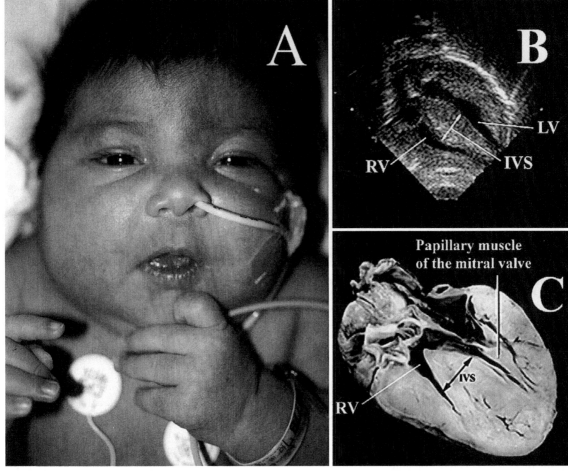

Fig. 11.7 Typical facial and cardiac findings in an infant of a diabetic mother. (A) The classic plethoric, 'swollen' facies of an IDM. (B) Echocardiogram in subxiphoid view shows massive hypertrophy of the free walls and septum, encroaching on the cavities of the LV and RV. (C) Pathology specimen in the same projection shows the extremely thick walls and even papillary muscles limiting the volume of the ventricles.

common cardiac abnormality is HCM. This is thought to be related to high insulin levels in the fetus, an increased number of insulin receptors in the fetal heart, and increased protein and fat synthesis resulting in myocardial cell hyperplasia and hypertrophy as well as glycogen deposition. The hypertrophy occurs primarily in the interventricular septum but can affect any portion of the ventricular walls. This may result in dynamic and clinically significant LVOT obstruction. Fortunately, spontaneous resolution typically occurs, although this may take months. Since the LVOT obstruction is dynamic, inotropic agents are generally contraindicated. β-blockers can be of dramatic benefit since they reduce heart rate and

contractility and thus decrease the degree of obstruction.

The echocardiographic appearance of HCM in IDM patients can be striking. The parasternal long-axis shows prominent hypertrophy of the interventricular septum, often out of proportion to the RV and LV free walls, which are also frequently thickened. In addition, the anterior leaflet of the mitral valve may move in an anterior direction during systole, resulting in increased LVOT obstruction. The LV cavity may be small. Left ventricular shortening fraction may be normal or increased. Doppler may show high velocity from the left ventricle into the aorta and colour flow Doppler often reveals turbulence. Over time, the echocardiographic appearance improves and typically normalizes by 12 months of age.

TUBEROUS SCLEROSIS

Features of tuberous sclerosis (TS) are illustrated in Figure 11.8.

Background

TS is usually diagnosed in the neonatal period only when a search is made for features of the condition because of an affected parent, or because a cardiac tumour (rhabdomyoma) is identified. Typical hypopigmented skin macules are more commonly seen in older children. The diagnosis is made on clinical grounds. At present, it is not known how many infants with apparently isolated cardiac rhabdomyoma, who do not meet current diagnostic criteria for TS, actually harbour a gene mutation for TS. Two genetic loci for TS have been identified to date (9q34 and 16p13) and in the future, DNA testing for TS mutations may be possible. Family history may be helpful since TS is transmitted as an

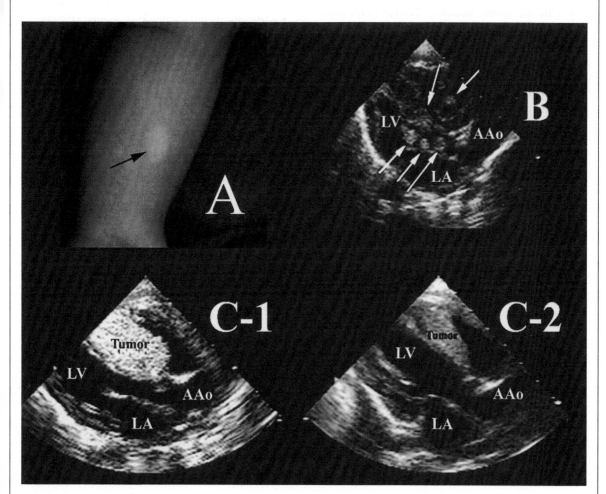

Fig. 11.8 Features of tuberous sclerosis. (A) Hypopigmented skin macule seen in a four month old with tuberous sclerosis. In tuberous sclerosis the cardiac abnormality is usually rhabdomyoma, which may be multiple (arrows in (B)) or solitary (C-1). Both forms tend to regress spontaneously. The image in (C-1) was taken when the patient was 6 weeks old. (C-2) was taken from the same patient two years later; note the reduction in tumour size both absolutely and in relation to the size of the ascending aorta.

autosomal dominant trait with variable penetrance. However, greater than 50% of cases appear to be the result of spontaneous mutation.

Congenital heart disease

Rhabdomyomas of the heart are noted in a third to a half of patients with TS. Conversely, TS is diagnosed in a third to a half of patients with cardiac rhabdomyomas. In many instances, more than one tumour is present. The natural history of the tumours is resolution, and therefore management is primarily observation. Endomyocardial biopsy is not necessary for diagnosis and surgical excision is indicated only in those (rare) patients with life-threatening ventricular outflow tract obstruction or arrhythmias. Rarely, lesions at the crux of the heart may affect the conduction system causing heart block.

Echocardiographically, the cardiac rhabdomyomas are often striking (see Fig. 11.8). They are usually bright and echo-dense in their appearance and ventricular (especially left) in location. In some cases, there is outflow tract obstruction underneath the aortic and/or pulmonary valves. Occasionally, tumours may also be noted in the atria or atrial septum. In contrast to the other hamartomatous lesions in TS, the cardiac rhabdomyomas usually resolve over time, even very large ones, and can be followed with sequential echocardiographic studies. These tumours are generally not pedunculated and the risk of embolization is low.

OTHER SYNDROMES

Trisomy 18

Background

Trisomy 18 syndrome is the second most common autosomal trisomy in newborns, with an incidence of 1 in 3000. The classical dysmorphic features can usually lead to a clinical diagnosis. As with trisomy 21, there is rapid FISH chromosome study available, but routine karyotyping is recommended to identify translocation cases.

Congenital heart disease

Structural cardiac defects are seen in virtually every case: malalignment ventricular septal defects, ToF and double-outlet right ventricle are common; 20%

have A-V septal defects. Although over 90% have congenital nodular polyvalvar dysplasia with redundant or myxomatous leaflets, this is rarely a clinically important condition. Most of these infants also have a patent arterial duct. Cardiac surgery is generally not considered for these infants because of the grave prognosis of the syndrome, and most die by three months of age.

Trisomy 13

Background

Trisomy 13 syndrome is the third most common autosomal trisomy in newborns, with an incidence of 1 in 5000. The diagnosis can usually be firmly made on clinical grounds. As with trisomies 18 and 21, there is rapid FISH chromosome study available for trisomy 18, but routine karyotyping is recommended to identify translocation cases. The outlook for these infants is poor, but long-term survivors have been noted.

Congenital heart defects

Congenital heart defects are present in 50–80%. Most commonly, ventricular and atrial septal defects are seen as well as PDA. Other cardiac anomalies include bicuspid aortic and pulmonary valves, malalignment VSD, double-outlet right ventricle and ToF. Cardiac surgical repair is not indicated because of the poor prognosis associated with this chromosomal abnormality.

VACTERL association

Background

The VACTERL acronym refers to Vertebral anomalies, Anal atresia, Cardiac defects, Tracheo-Esophageal fistula, Renal/Radial defects and other Limb defects. Other anomalies include hemifacial microsomia/microtia and genital anomalies. A subgroup have aqueductal stenosis and secondary hydrocephalus but other CNS involvement is uncommon and intellect is typically normal. About 50% of newborns with VACTERL are <2500 gs at birth and one-third are premature. Failure-to-thrive is common. Most cases are sporadic, and occur at increased frequency in infants of diabetic mothers.

Congenital heart disease

Congenital heart disease occurs in 50–80%. The most common defects are VSD and ASD, patent arterial duct and ToF. Other defects include other conotruncal defects such as common arterial trunk and transposition of the great arteries as well as coarctation of the aorta. A single umbilical artery is noted in about 15% of patients.

CHARGE association

Background

The acronym CHARGE association refers to the non-random association of ocular Coloboma, Heart defects, Atresia choanae, Retarded growth and development, Genital hypoplasia and Ear anomalies, including deafness. Like VACTERL, this condition is of unknown aetiology and is sporadic. Unlike VACTERL, CHARGE is relatively uncommon. It is essentially a diagnosis of exclusion after syndromic and chromosomal disorders have been ruled out since it shares phenotypic features with a number of other chromosomal abnormalities and syndromes, including trisomies 13, 18 and 8q-, VACTERL, DiGeorge (22q11 deletion), Treacher–Collins and Crouzon syndromes.

Congenital heart disease

Cardiac defects are common. In one large study, 16 of 50 patients had ToF, either alone or in association with other heart defects such as A-V septal defect, pulmonary atresia, or Ebstein's anomaly. Other forms of CHD noted include VSD, ASD, double-outlet right ventricle, single ventricle, and transposition of the great arteries. Over three quarters required cardiac surgical intervention.

Holt–Oram syndrome

Background

The Holt–Oram syndrome should be suspected in neonates with bilateral upper limb (particularly radial/thumb) defects and congenital heart disease (usually septal defects). The shoulder girdle is frequently hypoplastic as well. It has an autosomal dominant inheritance pattern with marked clinical variability of expression; parents of a newly diagnosed child should be carefully evaluated for subtle features of the syndrome. A candidate genetic locus has been identified on chromosome 12q2, but as other families have not shown linkage to this locus, there may be multiple genes responsible.

Congenital heart disease

Up to 95% of children with Holt–Oram have an ASD. These can be difficult to distinguish from a widely patent oval foramen in the newborn and the subcostal views are the most helpful (see Chapter 3). Surgery is not urgently required so review can be done later when the oval foramen should have closed. Rhythm abnormalities, first-degree A-V block or a junctional rhythm are also common. Less common associations include VSDs, hypoplastic peripheral blood vessels and other forms of congenital heart disease.

FURTHER READING

Journal articles

Giddins NS, Finley JP, Nanton MA, Roy DL. The natural course of supravalvar aortic stenosis and peripheral pulmonary artery stenosis in Williams syndrome. *British Heart Journal* 1989;62:315–319.

Goldberg R, Motzkin B, Marion R, Scambler PJ, Shprintzen RJ. Velo-cardio-facial syndrome: a review of 120 patients. *American Journal of Medical Genetics* 1993;45:313–319.

Ivemark B. Implications of agenesis of the spleen on the pathogenesis of conotruncus anomalies in childhood. *Acta Paediatrica Scandinavica* 1955;441(Suppl 104):590–592.

Morris CA, Demsey SA, Leonard CO, Dilts C, Blackburn BL. Natural history of Williams syndrome: physical characteristics. *Journal of Pediatrics* 1988;113:318–326.

Smith AT, Sack GH, Taylor GJ. Holt–Oram syndrome. *Journal of Pediatrics* 1979;95:538–543.

Van Praagh S, Truman T, Firpo A, Bano-Rodrigo A, Fried R, McManus B, Engle MA, Van Praagh R. Cardiac malformations in Trisomy-18: a study of 41 postmortem cases. *Journal of the American College of Cardiology* 1989;13:1586–1597.

Waldman JD, Rosenthal A, Smith AL, Shurin S, Nadas AS. Sepsis and congenital asplenia. *Journal of Pediatrics* 1977;90:555–559.

Webb DW, Thomas RD, Osborne JP. Cardiac rhabdomyomas and their association with tuberous sclerosis. *Archives of Diseases in Childhood* 1993;68:367–370.

Wyse RKH, Al-Mahdawi S, Burn J, Blake K. Congenital heart disease in CHARGE association. *Pediatric Cardiology* 1993;14:75–81.

Books

Greenberg F, Rudolph AJ. *The science and practice of pediatric cardiology*, ch 144, pp 2397–2413. Philadelphia: Lea & Febiger, 1990.

Jones KL. *Smith's recognizable patterns of human malformation*, 4th edn, pp 10–25, 106–109, 272, 450–451, 543–544, 556–557, 602–603, 606–607. Philadelphia: WB Saunders, 1988.

Noonan JA. *Fetal and neonatal cardiology*, ch 48, pp 578–594; IDM, pp 137–138, 502–503. Philadelphia: WB Saunders, 1990.

Zahka K. *Moss and Adams heart disease in infants, children and adolescents including the fetus and young adult*, 5th edn, ch 41, pp 614–625. Baltimore: Williams & Wilkins, 1995.

Index

Note: Page references in *italics* refer to Figures

Printed and bound by CPI Group (UK) Ltd, Croydon, CR0 4YY

03/10/2024

01040349-0015